Learning
Radiology

SECOND EDITION

Learning Radiology

RECOGNIZING THE BASICS

William Herring, MD, FACR
Vice Chairman and Residency Program Director
Department of Radiology
Albert Einstein Medical Center
Philadelphia, Pennsylvania

ELSEVIER
SAUNDERS

ELSEVIER
MOSBY

1600 John F. Kennedy Blvd.
Ste 1800
Philadelphia, PA 19103-2899

LEARNING RADIOLOGY   978-0-323-07444-5
Copyright © 2012, 2007 by Mosby, Inc., an affiliate of Elsevier Inc.

Notices

Knowledge and best practice in this field are constantly changing. As new research and experience broaden our understanding, changes in research methods, professional practices, or medical treatment may become necessary.

Practitioners and researchers must always rely on their own experience and knowledge in evaluating and using any information, methods, compounds, or experiments described herein. In using such information or methods they should be mindful of their own safety and the safety of others, including parties for whom they have a professional responsibility.

With respect to any drug or pharmaceutical products identified, readers are advised to check the most current information provided (i) on procedures featured or (ii) by the manufacturer of each product to be administered, to verify the recommended dose or formula, the method and duration of administration, and contraindications. It is the responsibility of practitioners, relying on their own experience and knowledge of their patients, to make diagnoses, to determine dosages and the best treatment for each individual patient, and to take all appropriate safety precautions.

To the fullest extent of the law, neither the Publisher nor the authors, contributors, or editors, assume any liability for any injury and/or damage to persons or property as a matter of products liability, negligence or otherwise, or from any use or operation of any methods, products, instructions, or ideas contained in the material herein.

Library of Congress Cataloging-in-Publication Data
Herring, William.
   Learning radiology : recognizing the basics / William Herring. — 2nd ed.
       p. ; cm.
   Includes bibliographical references and index.
   ISBN 978-0-323-07444-5 (pbk. : alk. paper)
   1. Radiology, Medical—Study and teaching.   I. Title.
   [DNLM: 1. Radiography—methods.   2. Diagnosis, Differential. WN 200]
   R899.H472 2012
   616.07′572—dc22
                         2011006507

Acquisitions Editor: James Merritt
Developmental Editor: Andrea Vosburgh
Publishing Services Manager: Deborah Vogel
Project Manager: Brandilyn Tidwell
Designer: Ellen Zanolle
Illustrations Manager: Michael Carcel
Marketing Manager: Jason Oberacker

Printed in the United States of America

Last digit is the print number: 9   8   7   6   5   4

To my wife, Patricia,

and our family

Contributor

Daniel J. Kowal, MD
Computed Tomography Division Director
Radiology Elective Director
Department of Radiology
Saint Vincent Hospital
Worcester, Massachusetts
Chapter 20, Magnetic Resonance Imaging

Preface to the First Edition

If you're the kind of person, like I am, who reads the preface after you've read the book, I hope you enjoyed it. If you're the kind of person who reads the preface before reading the book, then you're in for a real treat.

Suppose for a moment that you wanted to know what kind of bird with a red beak just landed on your windowsill (don't ask why). You could get a book on birds that listed all of them alphabetically from albatross to woodpecker and spend time looking at hundreds of bird pictures. Or you could get a book that lists birds by the colors of their beaks and thumb through a much shorter list to find that it was a cardinal.

This is a red-beak book. Where possible, groups of diseases are first described by the way they *look* rather than by what they're *called*. Imaging diagnoses frequently, but not always, rest on a recognition of a reproducible visual picture of that abnormality. That is called the *pattern recognition approach* to identifying abnormalities, and the more experience you have and more proficient you become at looking at imaging studies, the more comfortable and confident you'll be with that approach.

Before diagnostic images can help you decide what disease the patient may have, you must first be able to differentiate between what is normal and what is not. That isn't as easy as it may sound. Recognizing the difference between normal and abnormal probably takes as much, if not more, practice than deciding what disease the person has.

In fact, it takes so much practice, some people—I believe they are called *radiologists*—have actually been known to spend their entire life doing it. You won't be a radiologist after you've completed this book, but you should be able to recognize abnormalities and interpret images better. By so doing, perhaps you can participate in the care of patients with more assurance and confidence.

In this text, you'll spend time in each section learning how to recognize what is normal so that you can differentiate between such things as a skin fold and a pneumothorax or so that you can recognize whether that fuzzy white stuff at the lung bases is pneumonia or the patient simply hasn't taken a deep breath.

Where pattern recognition doesn't work, we'll try whenever possible to give you a logical *approach* to reaching a diagnosis based on simple yet effective decision trees. These will be little decision trees—saplings with only a few branches—so that they are relatively easy to remember.

By learning an approach, you'll have a method you can apply to similar problems again and again. Have you ever heard the saying "Give a man a fish; you have fed him for today. Teach a man to fish, and you have fed him for a lifetime"? Learning an imaging approach is like learning how to fish, except a lot less smelly. An approach will enable you to apply a rational solution to diagnostic imaging problems.

This text was written, in part, to make complementary use of the medium for which radiologic images are ideally suited: the computer screen. The web is ideal for accessing and displaying images, but many people do not want to read large volumes of text from their computer screens. So we've joined the text in the printed book with photos, quizzes, and tutorials available online at StudentConsult.com in a series of *web enhancements* that accompany every chapter.

This text is not intended to be encyclopedic. There are many wonderful radiology reference texts available, some of which contain thousands of pages and weigh slightly less than a Volkswagen. This text is oriented more towards students, interns, and residents or residents-to-be.

Not every imaging modality is covered equally in this book, and some are not covered at all. This book emphasizes conventional radiography because that is the type of study most patients have first and because the same imaging principles that apply to recognizing the diagnosis on conventional radiographs can be applied to making the diagnosis on more complex modalities.

With a better appreciation and understanding of why images look the way they do, you'll soon be recognizing abnormalities and making diagnoses that will impress your mentors and peers and astound your friends and relatives.

Let's get started.

William Herring, MD

Preface to the Second Edition

This second edition of *Learning Radiology: Recognizing the Basics* includes numerous changes and additions. There are additional chapters, over a hundred new photos, reorganization of key material throughout the text, and an increased emphasis on the cross-sectional imaging modalities of computed tomography (CT), magnetic resonance imaging (MRI), and ultrasound.

Two entirely new chapters have been added to help you understand the basic principles and fundamental observations of ultrasound and MRI. Trauma has moved to its own chapter, bringing together related material to provide cohesive coverage of this important subject. A new and helpful appendix has been added, which lists the most appropriate imaging study to order for each of a myriad of clinical scenarios. This information should prove indispensable on clinical rounds.

Many chapters have been reorganized. The chapter on Recognizing Adult Heart Disease has been restructured to include relevant material featuring CT and MRI. The chapters on Diseases of the Chest and Diseases of the GI and Urinary Tracts have been updated with increased emphasis on CT,

ultrasound, and MRI. The chapters on Recognizing Arthritis and Common Causes of Neck and Back Pain incorporate more MRI imaging. The chapter on Recognizing Bowel Obstruction and Ileus now includes additional CT imaging.

There are enhancements to the printed text again available to registered users on the StudentConsult.com website, including access to the full text and all of its photos. Also available on the website are 24 interactive modules to help you learn radiologic anatomy. An algorithm for diagnosing adult heart disease using conventional radiography is available online. A new section on nuclear medicine has also been added to StudentConsult.com.

The first edition suggested that you'd soon be recognizing abnormalities and making diagnoses that would impress your mentors and peers and astonish your friends and relatives. With this edition, you hold the potential to be even more astounding.

Prepare to amaze.

William Herring, MD

Acknowledgments

First, I am grateful to the many thousands of you whom I have never met but who found a website called Learning Radiology helpful, and made it so popular it played a role leading to the first edition of this book, which was so popular that it led to this second edition.

For their help and suggestions, I would like to thank my colleague Mindy Horrow, MD, who read and critiqued several chapters with her usual expert eye and fine mind, and Thomas Reilly, MD, one of our radiology residents, who made invaluable suggestions about how the first edition could be changed. Daniel Kowal, MD, a radiologist who graduated from our program, did an absolutely wonderful job in simplifying the complexities of MRI for a great new chapter he wrote for this edition.

I want to thank Shuchi Rodgers, MD, Jenifer Slone, MD, Susan Summerton, MD, Mindy Horrow, MD, Morrie Kricun, MD, Huyen Tran, MD, Joanne Lee, MD, Jeffrey Weinstein, MD, and Michael Chen, MD for supplying additional photos for this edition. Thanks to Ryan Smith, MD for reviewing the StudentConsult chapter on nuclear medicine.

I certainly want to recognize and again thank Jim Merritt and Andrea Vosburgh from Elsevier for their continued support and assistance.

I also want to acknowledge the hundreds of radiology residents and medical students who, over the years, have provided me with an audience of motivated learners without whom no teacher could teach.

Finally, I want to thank my wonderful wife, Pat, who has encouraged me throughout the project, and my family.

Contents

Chapter 13
Recognizing the Normal Abdomen: Conventional Radiographs 127

Chapter 14
Recognizing Bowel Obstruction and Ileus 138

Chapter 15
Recognizing Extraluminal Air in the Abdomen 148

Chapter 16
Recognizing Abnormal Calcifications and Their Causes 156

Chapter 17
Recognizing the Imaging Findings of Trauma 164

Chapter 18
Recognizing Gastrointestinal, Hepatic, and Urinary Tract Abnormalities 172

Chapter 19
Ultrasonography: Understanding the Principles and Recognizing Normal and Abnormal Findings 193

Chapter 20
Magnetic Resonance Imaging: Understanding the Principles and Recognizing the Basics 209
DANIEL J. KOWAL

Chapter 21
Recognizing Abnormalities of Bone Density 218

Chapter 22
Recognizing Fractures and Dislocations 232

Chapter 23
Recognizing Joint Disease: An Approach to Arthritis 249

Chapter 24
Recognizing Some Common Causes of Neck and Back Pain 261

Chapter 1

Recognizing Anything: An Introduction to Imaging Modalities

Up for a challenge? Look at these four images (Fig. 1-1). Each is diagnostic. How many can you recognize? "None" would be a good start. The answers are at the end of this book, both literally and figuratively. Literally, because the answers **really** are at the end of this book—on the last printed page, to be exact. Figuratively, because you will learn about each of these modalities, about these four diseases and many others, about how to approach imaging studies, and much more as you complete this text.

LET THERE BE LIGHT ... AND DARK, AND SHADES OF GRAY

- Once upon a time, not too long ago, radiographic images lived on the medium of film. In some places, film is still used, but it is becoming much less common.
- Images were produced by a combination of x-rays and light striking a piece of photographic film, which in turn produced a latent image that was subsequently processed in a darkroom filled with chemicals and then, literally, hung up to dry.
  - When an immediate reading was requested, the films were interpreted while still dripping with chemicals, and the term **wet reading** for a "stat" interpretation was born.
  - Films were viewed on lighted view boxes (almost always backward or upside-down if the film placement was being done as part of a movie or TV show).
- This workflow lasted for decades, but it had two major drawbacks:
  - It required lots of physical storage space for the growing number of films.
  - The radiographic film itself could only be in one place at one time, which was not necessarily where it might be needed to help in the care of the patient.
- And so **digital radiography** came to be, in which the photographic film was replaced by a **photosensitive cassette or plate** that could be processed by an electronic reader so that the image could be stored digitally.
  - Countless images could be stored in the space of one spinning hard disk on a computer server.
  - Even more importantly, the images could be viewed by anyone with the right to do so, anywhere in the world, at any time.
- The studies were maintained on computer servers on which the images could be archived, communicated, and stored. This was and is called **PACS**, a **Picture Archiving, Communications, and Storage** system.
- Using PACS systems, all sorts of images can be stored and retrieved, including **conventional radiographs (CR)**, computed tomographic scans (CT), ultrasound images (US), and magnetic resonance imaging studies (MRI).
- Let's look briefly at each of these modalities.

CONVENTIONAL RADIOGRAPHY (PLAIN FILMS)

- Images produced through the use of ionizing radiation, i.e., x-rays, but without added contrast material like barium or iodine, are called *conventional radiographs* or, more often, "plain films."
- These images are relatively inexpensive to produce, can be obtained almost anywhere using portable or mobile machines, and are still the most widely obtained imaging studies.
- They require a source to produce the x-rays (the "x-ray machine"), a method to record the image (a film, cassette, or plate) and a way to process the recorded image (either using chemicals or a digital reader).
- Common uses for conventional radiography include the ubiquitous chest x-ray, plain films of the abdomen, and virtually every initial image of the skeletal system to exclude fractures or arthritis.
- Ionizing radiation in large doses, substantially higher than any medical radiographic procedure, is known to produce cell mutations that can lead to many forms of cancer or anomalies. Public health data on lower levels of radiation vary as to their assessment of risk, but it is generally held that only medically necessary diagnostic examinations should be performed and that studies using x-rays should be avoided during potentially teratogenic times, such as pregnancy.

COMPUTED TOMOGRAPHY (CT OR CAT SCANS)

- CT scanners, first introduced in the 1970s, brought a quantum leap to medical imaging.
- Using a gantry with a rotating x-ray beam and multiple detectors in various arrays (which themselves are rotating continuously around the patient) along with sophisticated computer algorithms to process the data, a large number of two-dimensional, slicelike images could be formatted in multiple imaging planes.
- CT scans can also be "windowed" (see Chapter 11) in a way that optimizes the visibility of different types of pathology after they are obtained, a benefit called **postprocessing** that digital imaging, in general, markedly advanced.

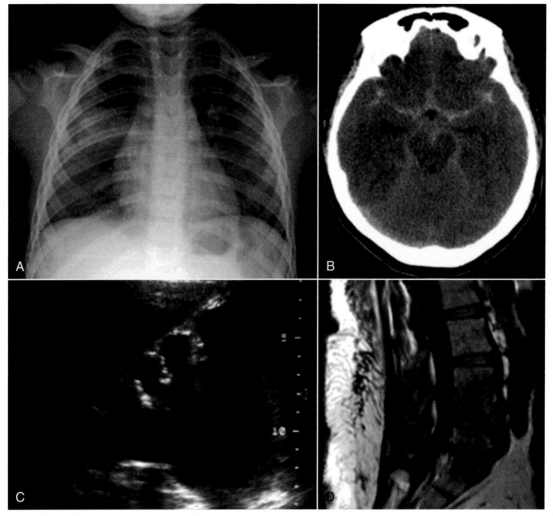

Figure 1-1 Images of four different patients with four different diseases, each in a different imaging modality. How many do you know? The answers are on the last printed page of this text.

Postprocessing allows for additional manipulation of the raw data to best demonstrate the abnormality without repeating a study and reexposing the patient.

- Producing CT images requires an expensive scanner, a space dedicated to its installation, and sophisticated computer processing power.
- CT scans, though, are the cornerstone of cross-sectional imaging and are widely available, although not as yet truly portable. CT scanners are more expensive to acquire and operate than conventional radiographic units and, like them, still utilize ionizing radiation (x-rays) to produce their images.

ULTRASOUND (US)

- Ultrasound utilizes acoustical energy above the audible frequency of human hearing to produce images, instead of using x-rays as both conventional radiography and CT scans do.
- It employs a **transducer,** which both produces the ultrasonic signal and records it. The signal is processed for its characteristics by an onboard computer. Ultrasound images

are recorded digitally and are easily stored in a PACS system.

- Ultrasound scanners are relatively inexpensive compared to CT and MRI scanners. They are widely available and can be made portable to the point of being handheld.
- Because ultrasound utilizes no ionizing radiation, it is particularly useful in imaging women of child-bearing age, pregnant women, and children.
- Ultrasound is especially useful in imaging soft tissues and for delineating solid from cystic structures. It is also widely used for image-guided biopsies and is a noninvasive means of studying blood flow.
- Ultrasound is generally considered to be a very safe imaging modality without any known major side effects when used at medically diagnostic levels.

MAGNETIC RESONANCE IMAGING (MRI)

- Magnetic resonance imaging utilizes the potential energy stored in the body's **hydrogen atoms**. The atoms are manipulated by very strong magnetic fields and radio-frequency pulses to produce enough localizing and tissue-specific energy to allow highly sophisticated computer programs to generate 2- or 3-dimensional images (see Chapter 20).

- MRI scanners are not as widely available as CT scanners; they are expensive to acquire and require careful site construction to operate properly. In general, they also have a relatively high, ongoing operating cost.
- However, they utilize no ionizing radiation and produce much higher contrast between different types of soft tissues than can CT.
- MRI is widely used in neurologic imaging and is particularly sensitive in imaging soft tissues like muscles, tendons, and ligaments.
- Safety issues are associated with the extremely strong magnetic fields of an MRI scanner, both for objects within the body (e.g., pacemakers) and for ferromagnetic projectiles in the MRI scanner environment (e.g., metal oxygen tanks). There are also known side effects from the radiofrequency waves such scanners produce, and possible adverse effects from some MRI contrast agents.

TERMINOLOGY

- "Oh no," you say, "must we have this section? Let me skip to the good parts." You can do that: just remember where this section is because you may have to refer to it later.
- Like politics, all terminology is local. Follow the terminology conventions used in your hospital or, alternatively, the person rendering your course grade, even if those conventions are different from what is described here.

Terminology Conventions Used in This Book

- **Image**: a good, all-around term that can be used to describe any type of rendering of a radiologic examination.
  - It works for all modalities; you may use it freely.
  - You could say you were looking at an "*image* of the abdomen on a conventional radiograph," or a "CT *image* of the abdomen," or an "ultrasound *image* of the abdomen," and so on. (Don't use the term *picture* to refer to a radiologic image; *image* will make you sound much smarter.)
  - When you view your images, **remember you and the patient are always looking at each other face-to-face.** This is the convention by which most images are viewed **no matter what the position of the patient when the image was exposed.**
    - The patient's right side, whether it is on conventional radiographs or a CT scan, is on your left side, and the patient's left side should be on your right side.
- **Cassette:** a cassette is the flat device that looks like a huge iPad that **holds either a piece of film** or a **special digital plate** on which the latent image resides until it is *processed* in one of two ways, depending on whether the cassette contains **film** or a **digital phosphor plate** without film.
  - **If the cassette contains film,** the film will be removed from the cassette in a **darkroom** (or by something called a *daylight loader* that simulates a darkroom) and **sent through an automatic processor** that contains a series of chemicals **that will develop the image,** make it visible to the human eye, and fix it permanently on the film. A new, unexposed piece of film will then be loaded into the cassette, and the cassette will be ready for the next exposure.
  - **If it is a digital cassette and contains no film,** it will be **processed through an electronic reader** that will decipher the electronic image stored on the phosphor plate in the cassette and transmit that digital image to another system to store it. The electronic image in the cassette is then "erased" and the cassette is used again and again.
  - Another, similar method of recording the image is on a digital plate connected directly to the processing computers without the need to ferry digital cassettes back and forth to an electronic reader. This is sometimes called **direct digital radiography.**
- **Study** or **examination:** used interchangeably, they refer to a **collection of images that examine a particular part of the body or system,** as in "double contrast *study* of the colon" (a series of images of the colon using air and barium and produced through the use of x-rays); or an "MRI *examination* of the brain" (a collection of images of the brain using MRI to produce the images).
- **Contrast material (contrast agent):** usually a substance that is administered to a patient in order to make certain structures more easily visible (frequently referred to simply as **contrast**).
  - The **most widely used examples of radiologic contrast materials** include liquid **barium,** which is administered orally for upper gastrointestinal (UGI) examinations and rectally for barium enema (BE) examinations, and **iodine,** which is administered intravenously for contrast-enhanced CT scans of the body.
  - Contrast agents also are used for MRI (most often, some solutions of gadolinium injected intravenously for its paramagnetic properties) and for ultrasound (gas-filled microbubbles).
- **Dye:** the lay term for contrast. Although *contrast* is the better term, many patients, and some radiologists in explaining tests to patients, use the term *dye.* Don't use the word dye unless you are talking to a patient explaining a test; use the term *contrast* or *contrast agent.* In fact, if you can use the words **contrast** and **image** in the same sentence, people will think you are a genius.
- **Flat plate:** an archaic, but still used, term meaning a conventional radiograph or plain film of the abdomen, almost always obtained with the patient lying supine. This term is left over from the pioneer days of radiology before film was used as the recording medium and the image was produced on a flat, glass plate.
- **White and black:** these are not radiologic terms, but almost every modality displays its images in white, black, and various shades of gray.
  - With conventional radiography, an object's inherent density will determine whether it appears white, black, or one of those shades of gray.
- **"En face" and "in profile":** used primarily in conventional radiography and barium studies.
  - When you look at a lesion directly "head-on," you are seeing it *en face.* A lesion seen tangentially (from the side) is seen *in profile.*
  - Only a sphere, which, by definition, is perfectly round in every dimension, will appear exactly the same shape

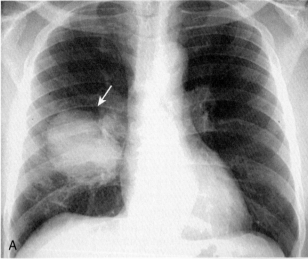

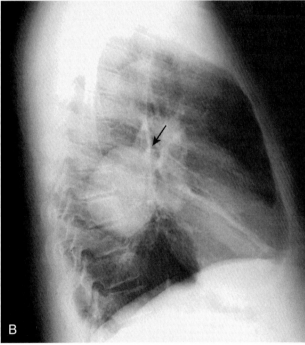

Figure 1-2 Right lower lobe bronchogenic carcinoma. A nearly spherical mass is in the right lower lobe of the lung seen on the frontal **(A)** (*solid white arrow*) and lateral **(B)** (*solid black arrow*) radiographs of this patient. Because the mass is nearly spherical, it has relatively the same shape when viewed *en face* and **in profile.**

no matter in which plane it is viewed (e.g., a nodule in the lung) (Fig. 1-2).
- Naturally occurring structures, whether normal or abnormal, of any shape other than a sphere will appear slightly different in shape if viewed *en face* or *in profile.*
- This is not an easy concept to grasp because it **involves making a mental reconstruction of a three-dimensional object from the two-dimensional projections** conventional radiographs provide.
- For example, a disk-shaped object (one that looks like a playing piece used in the game of checkers), such as an ingested coin, will appear circular when viewed *en face* but rectangular when viewed in *perfect profile* (Fig. 1-3).

- **Horizontal versus vertical x-ray beams:** terms that describe the orientation of x-ray beams.
  - Horizontal and vertical beam orientation is an important concept to understand because it will help you in interpreting all kinds of conventional radiographic studies and in understanding their limitations. This may, in turn, prevent you from falling for a diagnostic pitfall.
  - An x-ray beam is usually directed either *horizontally* between the tube and the cassette (as in an upright chest examination) or *vertically* between the tube and the cassette (as in a supine radiograph of the abdomen with the patient lying on the examining table).
  - **Horizontal x-ray beams are usually parallel to the floor** of the examining room (unless the room was built by do-it-yourselfers on weekends).
  - In conventional radiography, **an air-fluid or fat-fluid level will be visible only if the x-ray beam is horizontal,** *regardless of the position of the patient* (Fig. 1-4).
  - An **air-fluid** or **fat-fluid** level is an interface between two substances of different densities in which the lighter substance rises above and forms a straight-edge interface with the heavier substance below.
  - **You** usually **don't have to specify whether you want the x-ray beam to be horizontal or vertical when ordering a study;** by convention, certain studies are always done using one method or the other (Table 1-1). In general, any study with the terms *erect, upright, cross-table,* or *decubitus* is always **done with a horizontal beam. You can see fluid levels (if present) with any of these types of studies.**

The Five Basic Densities

- **Conventional radiography is limited to demonstrating five basic densities,** arranged here from least to most dense (Table 1-2):
  - **Air,** which appears the blackest on a radiograph.
  - **Fat,** which is a lighter shade of gray than air.
  - **Soft tissue or fluid** (because both soft tissue and fluid appear the same on conventional radiographs, you can't differentiate between heart muscle and the blood inside of the heart on a chest radiograph).
  - **Calcium** (usually contained within bones).
  - **Metal,** which appears the whitest on a radiograph.
    - Objects of metal density are not normally present in the body. Radiologic **contrast media** and **prosthetic knees or hips** are **examples of metal densities** artificially placed in the body (Fig. 1-5).
- One of the major benefits of CT scanning is its ability to **expand the gray scale,** which enables us to differentiate many more than these five basic densities.
- Remember, the denser an object is, the more x-rays it absorbs, and the whiter it appears on radiographic images.
- The less dense an object is, the fewer x-rays it absorbs, and the blacker it will appear on radiographs.
- Unfortunately, the specific terms used to describe what appears as *white* on an image and what appears as *black* on an image change from one modality to another. Table 1-3 is a handy chart that describes the terms used for black and white using various modalities.

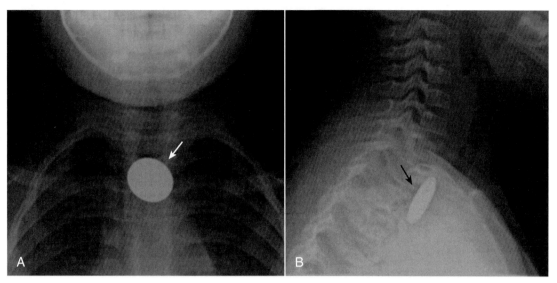

Figure 1-3 Coin in the esophagus. Both the frontal **(A)** and the lateral **(B)** images of this child's upper thorax demonstrate a radiopaque (white) metallic density in the region of the upper esophagus. The child swallowed a quarter, which is temporarily lodged in the esophagus just above the aortic arch. Notice how different the coin looks when viewed ***en face*** in **(A)** (*solid white arrow*) where it is seen as a circle and **in profile (B)** where it is seen on end (*solid black arrow*).

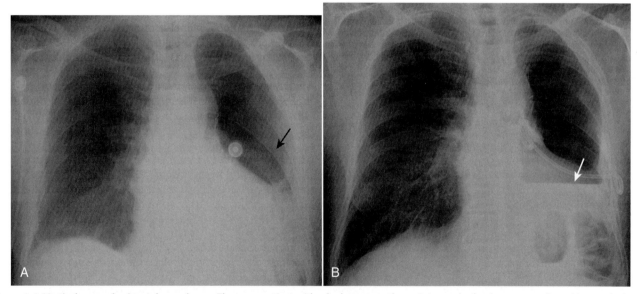

Figure 1-4 Vertical versus horizontal x-ray beam. The same patient with a hydropneumothorax is imaged a few hours apart, first with a vertical x-ray beam (**A,** supine chest) (*solid black arrow*) and then with a horizontal x-beam (**B,** upright chest) (*solid white arrow*). In both images, the patient has both air and fluid in the left hemithorax, but only in image **B** with the horizontal beam is the distinctive flat, air-fluid interface seen. An air-fluid interface will only be visible with an x-ray beam that is parallel to the floor (horizontal) no matter what position the patient is in.

THE BEST SYSTEM IS THE ONE THAT WORKS

- Some folks systematically look at imaging studies, such as chest radiographs, from the outside of the image to the inside of the image; others look at them from the inside out or from top to bottom. Some systems for reminding you to examine every part of an image have catchy acronyms and mnemonics.

- The fact is: **it doesn't matter what system you use as long as you look at everything** on the image.
  - So use whatever system works for you but be sure to look at everything. "Looking at everything," by the way, includes looking at all of the views available in a given study, not just everything on one view. (Don't forget the lateral chest radiograph in a two-view study of the chest).
- Experienced radiologists usually have no system at all.
  - "Burned-in" images are bad for computer monitors but they're great for radiologists. "Burned" into the neurons of a radiologist's brain are mental images of what a normal frontal chest radiograph looks like, what thoracic sarcoidosis looks like, and so on.
  - They frequently use a "**gestalt**" impression of a study, which they see in their mind's eye within seconds of looking at an image. If the image does or does not correspond to the mental image that resides in their brains, **then** they systematically study the images.
    - This is not magic; this ability comes only with experience so, at least for now, you are probably not quite ready to use the "gestalt" approach.

TABLE 1-1 HORIZONTAL VERSUS VERTICAL X-RAY BEAM

Examples of Types of Studies	Orientation of Beam	Implications
Upright view of the abdomen	Horizontal	Air-fluid levels will be visible; free air will rise to undersurface of diaphragm
Left lateral decubitus view of the abdomen	Horizontal	Air-fluid levels will be visible; free air will rise over liver
Supine abdomen	Vertical	Air-fluid levels will not be visible: free air will rise to undersurface of anterior abdominal wall and may not be visible until large amounts are present
Upright chest	Horizontal	Pneumothorax, if present, will usually be visible at apex of lung; air-fluid levels (e.g., in cavities) will be visible
Supine chest	Vertical	Pneumothorax may not be visible unless large; air-fluid levels will not be visible
Cross-table lateral examination of the knee	Horizontal	Fat-fluid levels (*lipohemarthrosis*), if present, will be visible
Supine examination of the knee	Vertical	Fat-fluid levels will not be visible

TABLE 1-2 FIVE BASIC DENSITIES SEEN ON CONVENTIONAL RADIOGRAPHY

Density	Appearance
Air	Absorbs the least x-ray and appears "blackest" on conventional radiographs
Fat	Gray, somewhat darker (blacker) than soft tissue
Fluid or soft tissue	Both fluid (e.g., blood) and soft tissue (e.g., muscle) have the same densities on conventional radiographs
Calcium	The most dense, naturally occurring material (e.g., bones) absorbs most x-rays
Metal	Usually absorbs all x-rays and appears the "whitest" (e.g., bullets, barium)

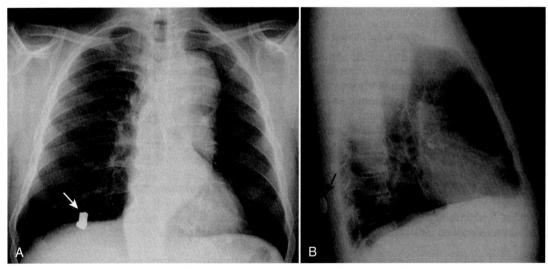

Figure 1-5 Bullet in the chest. The dense (white) metallic foreign body overlying the right lower lung field (*arrows*) is a bullet. It is much denser (whiter) than the bones (calcium density), represented by the ribs, clavicles, and spine. Fluid (like the blood in the heart) and soft tissue density (like the muscle of the heart) have the same density, which is why we can't differentiate the two using conventional radiography. The air in the lungs is the least dense (blackest). Two views at 90° angles to each other, such as these frontal **(A)** and lateral **(B)** chest radiographs, are called **orthogonal** views. With only one view, it would be impossible to know the location of the bullet. Orthogonal views are used throughout conventional radiography to localize structures in all parts of the body.

TABLE 1-3 WHITE AND BLACK: TERMS FOR EACH MODALITY

Modality	Terms Used for "White"	Terms Used for "Black"
Conventional radiographs	Increased density Opaque	Decreased density Lucent
CT	Increased (high) attenuation Hyperintense or hyperdense	Decreased (low) attenuation Hypodense
MRI	Increased (high) signal intensity Bright	Decreased (low) signal intensity Dark
US	Increased echogenicity Sonodense	Decreased echogenicity Sonolucent
Nuclear medicine	Increased tracer uptake	Decreased tracer uptake
Barium studies	Radiopaque	Nonopaque Radiolucent

■ The most valuable system to use in interpreting images is the **system in which you routinely increase your knowledge.**
  • If you don't know what you are looking for, you can stare at an image for hours or days or, in the case of the lateral chest radiograph, you can ignore an image entirely, and the end result will be the same: you won't see the findings.
    • There is an axiom in radiology: **You only see what you look for and you only look for what you know.** So, if you don't know what to look for, you will never recognize the finding no matter what system you use or how long you stare at the image.
■ So, by reading this book, you will gain the knowledge that will allow you to recognize what it is you're looking at—the best system of all.

CONVENTIONS USED IN THIS BOOK

■ **Bold type** is used liberally throughout this text to **highlight important points, and** because this is a book filled with a large number of extraordinarily important points, **you will see much bold type.**
■ **Diagnostic pitfalls,** potential false-positive or false-negative traps on the way to the correct interpretation of an image, are signaled by this icon:

■ **Important points** that are so important that not even **boldface** type does them justice are signaled by this icon:

■ The **Weblink** symbol means additional instructional material is available on the StudentConsult.com website for registered users:

■ **"Take-home" points** at the end of chapters are signaled by this icon:

• You may use these points anywhere, not only your home.

WEBLINK

Registered users may obtain more information on Recognizing Anything: An Introduction to Imaging Modalities on StudentConsult.com.

 TAKE-HOME POINTS

Recognizing Anything: An Introduction to Imaging Modalities

Conventional radiographs are produced using ionizing radiation generated by x-ray machines and viewed on a monitor or light box.

Such x-ray machines are relatively inexpensive, widely available and can be made portable. The images are limited as to the sensitivity of findings they are capable of displaying.

Computed tomography utilizes rapidly spinning arrays of x-ray sources and detectors and sophisticated computer processing to increase the sensitivity of findings visible and display them in any geometric plane.

CT scanners have become the foundation of cross-sectional imaging. They are moderately expensive and also use ionizing radiation to produce their images.

Ultrasound produces its images using the acoustical properties of tissue and does not employ ionizing radiation. It is thus safe for use in pregnant women, children, and women of child-bearing age. It is particularly useful in analyzing soft tissues and blood flow.

Ultrasound units are less expensive, in widespread use, and have been produced as small as handheld devices.

Magnetic resonance imaging produces its images based on the energy derived from hydrogen atoms placed in a very strong magnetic field and subjected to radio-frequency pulsing. Powerful computer algorithms analyze the data to produce images in any plane.

MRI units are relatively expensive, require site construction for their placement, and are usually higher in cost to operate. They have become the cornerstone of neuro-imaging and are of particular use in studying muscles, ligaments, and tendons.

Five basic radiographic densities, arranged in order from that which appears the whitest to that which appears the blackest are metal, calcium (bone), fluid (soft tissue), fat, and air.

You only see what you look for and you only look for what you know, so the best way to interpret radiologic images correctly is to know as much about them as you can.

Chapter 2

Recognizing Normal Chest Anatomy and a Technically Adequate Chest Radiograph

- In order to become more comfortable interpreting chest radiographs, you **first** need to be able to recognize **fundamental, normal anatomy** so you can differentiate it from what is abnormal.
- **Second**, you have to be able to quickly determine if a study is **technically adequate** so that you don't mistake technical deficiencies for abnormalities.
- **Third**, if you decide a finding is abnormal, **you need to have some strategy for deciding what the abnormality is**.
- **First (and second) things first**: This chapter will familiarize you with normal chest radiographic anatomy and enable you to evaluate the technical adequacy of a radiograph by helping you become more familiar with the diagnostic pitfalls certain technical artifacts can introduce.

THE NORMAL FRONTAL CHEST RADIOGRAPH

- Figure 2-1 displays some of the normal anatomic features visible on the frontal chest radiograph.
- **Vessels and bronchi: normal lung markings**
  - **Virtually all of the "white lines" you see in the lungs on a chest radiograph are blood vessels.** Blood vessels characteristically branch and taper gradually from the hila centrally to the peripheral margins of the lung. You cannot accurately differentiate between pulmonary arteries and pulmonary veins on a conventional radiograph.
  - **Bronchi are mostly invisible** on a normal chest radiograph because they are normally very **thin-walled**, they **contain air,** and they are **surrounded by air.**
- Pleura: normal anatomy
  - The **pleura is composed of two layers, the outer parietal and inner visceral, with the pleural space between them.** The visceral pleura is adherent to the lung and enfolds to form the major and minor fissures.
  - Normally **several milliliters of fluid, but no air, are in the pleural space.**
  - Neither the parietal pleura nor the visceral pleura is **normally visible** on a conventional chest radiograph, except on occasion where the two layers of visceral pleura enfold to form the fissures. Even then, they **are usually no thicker than a line drawn with the point of a sharpened pencil.**

THE LATERAL CHEST RADIOGRAPH

- As part of the standard two-view chest examination, patients usually have an **upright, frontal** chest radiograph and an **upright, left lateral** view of the chest.

- A **left lateral chest x-ray** (the patient's left side is against the film) is of **great diagnostic value** but is **sometimes ignored by beginners** because of their lack of familiarity with the findings visible in that projection.
- Figure 2-2 displays some of the normal anatomic features visible on the lateral chest radiograph.
- **Why look at the lateral chest?**
  - It can help you **determine the location** of disease you already identified as being present on the frontal image.
  - It can **confirm the presence of disease** you may be unsure of on the basis of the frontal image alone, such as a mass or pneumonia.
  - It can **demonstrate disease not visible on the frontal image** (Fig. 2-3).

FIVE KEY AREAS ON THE LATERAL CHEST X-RAY (FIG. 2-2 AND TABLE 2-1)

- **The retrosternal clear space**
- **The hilar region**
- **The fissures**
- **The thoracic spine**
- **The diaphragm and posterior costophrenic sulci**

The Retrosternal Clear Space

- Normally, a relatively lucent crescent is present just behind the sternum and anterior to the shadow of the ascending aorta.
  - Look for this clear space to "fill-in" with soft tissue density when an anterior mediastinal mass is present (Fig. 2-4).

⚠ **Pitfall:** Be careful not to mistake the soft tissue of the patient's superimposed arms for "filling-in" of the clear space. Although patients are asked to hold their arms over their head for a lateral chest exposure, many are too weak to raise their arms.

  - **Solution:** You should be able to identify the patient's arm by spotting the humerus (Fig. 2-5).

The Hilar Region

- The hila may be difficult to assess on the frontal view, especially if both hila are slightly enlarged, since comparison with the opposite normal side is impossible.
- The lateral view may help. Most of the hilar densities are made up of the pulmonary arteries. Normally, no discrete mass is visible in the hila on the lateral view.

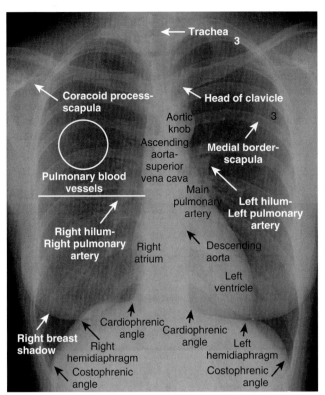

Figure 2-1 Well-exposed frontal view of a normal chest. Notice how the spine is just visible through the heart shadow. Both the right and left lateral costophrenic angles are sharply and acutely angled. The *white line* demarcates the approximate level of the minor or horizontal fissure, which is usually visible on the frontal view because it is seen **en face**. There is no minor fissure on the left side. The *white circle* contains lung markings that are blood vessels. Note that the left hilum is normally slightly higher than the right. The *white "3"* lies on the posterior 3rd rib while the *black "3"* lies on the anterior 3rd rib.

■ When there is a hilar mass, such as might occur with enlargement of hilar lymph nodes, the hilum (or hila) will cast a distinct, lobulated masslike shadow on the lateral radiograph (Fig. 2-6).

The Fissures

■ On the **lateral film**, both the **major (oblique) and minor (horizontal) fissures may be visible** as a fine, white line (about as thick as a line made with the point of a sharpened pencil).
  - The **major fissures** course obliquely, roughly **from the level of the 5th thoracic vertebra to** a point on the diaphragmatic surface of the pleura **a few centimeters behind the sternum**.
  - The **minor fissure lies at the level of the 4th anterior rib** (on the right side only) and is **horizontally** oriented (see Figs. 2-1 and 2-2).
  - Both the major and minor fissures may be visible on the lateral view, but because of the oblique plane of the major fissure, **only the minor fissure is usually visible on the frontal view**.
■ The fissures demarcate the upper and lower lobes on the left and the upper, middle, and lower lobes on the right.
■ When a fissure contains fluid or develops fibrosis from a chronic process, it will become thickened (Fig. 2-7).

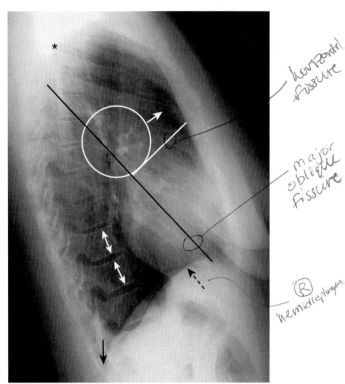

Figure 2-2 Normal left lateral chest radiograph. A clear space is present behind the sternum (*solid white arrow*). The hila produce no discrete shadow (*white circle*). The vertebral bodies are approximately of equal height and their endplates are parallel to each other (*double white arrows*). The posterior costophrenic angles (*solid black arrow*) are sharp. Notice how the thoracic spine appears to become blacker (darker) from the shoulder girdle (*black star*) to the diaphragm because there is less dense tissue for the x-ray beam to traverse at the level of the diaphragm. The heart normally touches the anterior aspect of the left hemidiaphragm and usually obscures (silhouettes) it. The superior surface of the right hemidiaphragm is frequently seen continuously from back to front (*dotted black arrow*) because it is not obscured by the heart. Notice the normal space posterior to the heart and anterior to the spine; this will be important in assessing cardiomegaly (Chapter 9). The *black line* represents the approximate location of the major or oblique fissure; the *white line* is the approximate location of the minor or horizontal fissure. Both are visible because they are seen *en face* on the lateral view.

  - **Thickening of the fissure by fluid is almost always associated with other signs of fluid in the chest** such as Kerley B lines and pleural effusions (see Chapter 6).
  - **Thickening of the fissure by fibrosis** is the more likely cause if there are **no other signs of fluid in the chest**.

The Thoracic Spine

■ Normally, the **thoracic vertebral bodies** are roughly **rectangular in shape**, and **each** vertebral body's **endplate parallels the endplate of the vertebral body above and below it**.
■ **Each intervertebral disk space becomes slightly taller than or remains the same as the one above it** throughout the thoracic spine.
■ Degeneration of the disk can lead to narrowing of the disk space and the development of small, bony spurs (*osteophytes*) at the margins of the vertebral bodies.
■ When there is a compression fracture, most often from osteoporosis, the vertebral body loses height. Compression

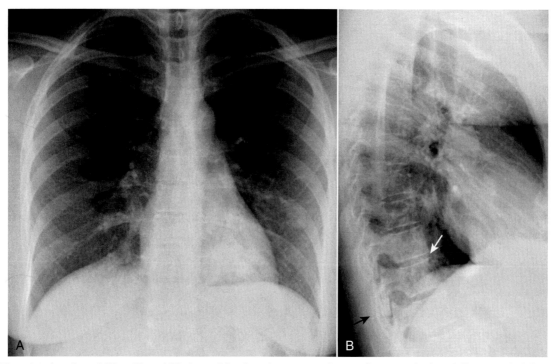

Figure 2-3 **The spine sign.** Frontal **(A)** and lateral **(B)** views of the chest demonstrate airspace disease on the lateral film **(B)** in the left lower lobe that may not be immediately apparent on the frontal film (look closely at **A** and you may see the pneumonia in the left lower lobe behind the heart). Normally, the thoracic spine appears to get "blacker" as you view it from the neck to the diaphragm because there is less dense tissue for the x-ray beam to traverse just above the diaphragm than in the region of the shoulder girdle (see also Fig. 2-2). In this case, a left lower lobe pneumonia superimposed on the lower spine in the lateral view (*solid white arrow*) makes the spine appear "whiter" (more dense) just above the diaphragm. This is called the **spine sign**. Note that on a well-positioned lateral projection, the right and left posterior ribs almost superimpose on each other (*solid black arrow*), a sign of a true lateral.

TABLE 2-1 THE LATERAL CHEST: A QUICK GUIDE OF WHAT TO LOOK FOR

Region	What You Should See
Retrosternal clear space	Lucent crescent between sternum and ascending aorta
Hilar region	No discrete mass present
Fissures	Major and minor fissures should be pencil-point thin, if visible at all
Thoracic spine	Rectangular vertebral bodies with parallel end plates; disk spaces maintain height from top to bottom of thoracic spine
Diaphragm and posterior costophrenic sulci	Right hemidiaphragm slightly higher than left; sharp posterior costophrenic sulci

fractures very commonly first involve depression of the superior endplate of the vertebral body (Fig. 2-8).

- **Don't forget to look at the thoracic spine when studying the lateral chest radiograph** for valuable clues about systemic disorders (see Chapter 24).

The Diaphragm and Posterior Costophrenic Sulci

- Because the diaphragm is composed of soft tissue (muscle) and the abdomen below it contains soft tissue structures like the liver and spleen, only the upper border of the diaphragm, abutting the air-filled lung, is usually visible on conventional radiographs.
- Even though we have one diaphragm that separates the thorax from the abdomen, we usually do not see the entire diaphragm from side-to-side on conventional radiographs because of the position of the heart in the center of the chest.
  - Therefore, we refer to the right half of the diaphragm as the *right hemidiaphragm* and the left half of the diaphragm as the *left hemidiaphragm*.
- **How to tell the right from the left hemidiaphragm on the lateral radiograph:**
  - The **right hemidiaphragm is usually visible for its entire length from front to back**. Normally, **the right hemidiaphragm is slightly higher than the left**, a relationship that tends to hold true on the lateral radiograph as well as on the frontal.
  - The **left hemidiaphragm** is seen sharply posteriorly but **is silhouetted by the muscle of the heart anteriorly** (i.e., its edge disappears anteriorly) (see Fig. 2-2).
  - **Air in the stomach** or splenic flexure of the colon appears immediately **below the left hemidiaphragm**. The liver lies below the right hemidiaphragm, and bowel gas is usually not seen between the liver and the right hemidiaphragm.
- **The posterior costophrenic angles (posterior costophrenic sulci)**
  - Each hemidiaphragm produces a rounded dome that indents the central portion of the base of each lung, like the bottom of a wine bottle.
    - This produces a depression, or *sulcus,* that surrounds the periphery of each lung and represents the lowest point of the pleural space when the patient is upright.

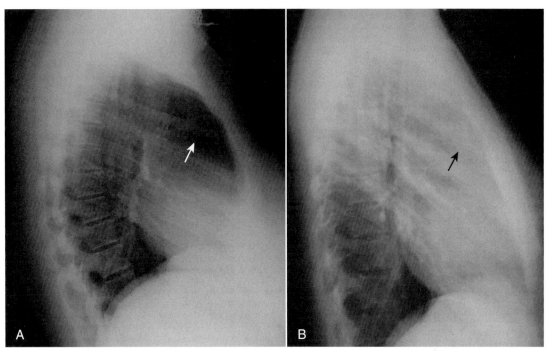

Figure 2-4 Anterior mediastinal adenopathy. A normal lateral **(A)** shows a clear space behind the sternum (*solid white arrow*). Left lateral view of the chest **(B)** demonstrates soft tissue that is filling in the normal clear space behind the sternum (*solid black arrow*). This represents anterior mediastinal lymphadenopathy in a patient with lymphoma. Adenopathy is probably the most frequent reason the retrosternal clear space is obscured. Thymoma, teratoma, and substernal thyroid enlargement also can produce anterior mediastinal masses but do not usually produce exactly this appearance.

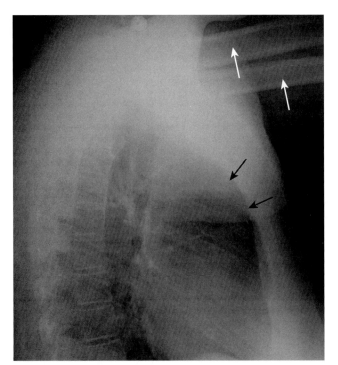

Figure 2-5 Arms obscure retrosternal clear space. In this example, the patient was not able to hold her arms over her head for the lateral chest examination, as patients are instructed to do in order to eliminate the shadows of the arms from overlapping the lateral chest. The humeri are clearly visible (*solid white arrows*) so even though the soft tissue of the patient's arms appears to fill in the retrosternal clear space (*solid black arrows*), this should not be mistaken for an abnormality such as anterior mediastinal adenopathy (see Fig. 2-4).

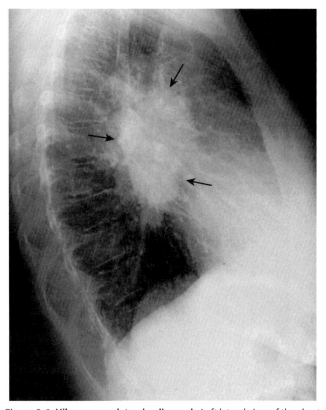

Figure 2-6 Hilar mass on lateral radiograph. Left lateral view of the chest shows a discrete lobulated mass in the region of the hila (*solid black arrows*). Normally, the hila do not cast a shadow that is easily detectable on the lateral projection. This patient had bilateral hilar adenopathy from sarcoidosis but any cause of hilar adenopathy or a primary tumor in the hilum would have a similar appearance.

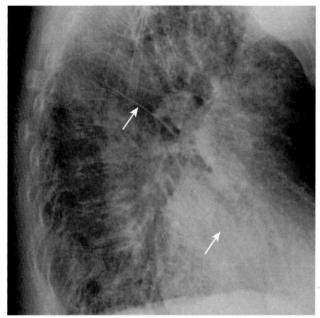

Figure 2-7 Fluid in the major fissures. Left lateral view of the chest shows thickening of both the right and left major fissures (*solid white arrows*). This patient was in congestive heart failure and this thickening represents fluid in the fissures. Normally, the fissures are either invisible or, if visible, they are fine, white lines of uniform thickness no larger than a line made with the point of a sharpened pencil. The major or oblique fissure runs from the level of the 5th thoracic vertebral body to a point on the anterior diaphragm about 2 cm behind the sternum. Notice the increased interstitial markings that are visible throughout the lungs and are due to fluid in the interstitium of the lung.

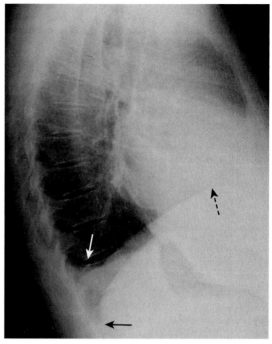

Figure 2-9 Blunting of the posterior costophrenic sulcus by a small pleural effusion. Left lateral view of the chest shows fluid blunting the posterior costophrenic sulcus (*solid white arrow*). The other posterior costophrenic angle (*solid black arrow*) is sharp. The pleural effusion is on the right side because the hemidiaphragm involved can be traced anteriorly farther forward (*dotted black arrow*) than the other hemidiaphragm (the left), which is normally silhouetted by the heart and not visible anteriorly.

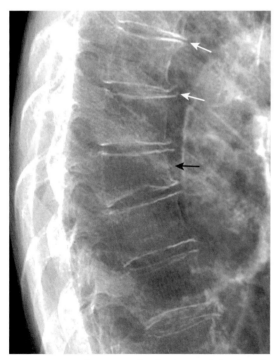

Figure 2-8 Osteoporotic compression fracture and degenerative disk disease. Don't forget to look at the thoracic spine when studying the lateral chest radiograph for valuable information about a host of systemic diseases (see Chapter 24). In this study, loss of stature of the 8th thoracic vertebral body is due to osteoporosis (*solid black arrow*). Compression fractures frequently involve the superior endplate first. Small osteophytes are present at multiple levels from degenerative disk disease (*solid white arrows*).

- On a frontal chest radiograph, this sulcus is most easily viewed in profile at the outer edge of the lung as the *lateral costophrenic sulcus* (also called the *lateral costophrenic angle*) and on the lateral radiograph as the *posterior costophrenic sulcus* (also known as the *posterior costophrenic angle*) (see Figs. 2-1 and 2-2).
- **Normally, all of the costophrenic sulci are sharply outlined and acutely angled.**
- Pleural effusions accumulate in the deep recesses of the costophrenic sulci, filling in their acute angles with the patient upright. This is called **blunting of the costophrenic angles** (see Chapter 6).
- It takes only about **75 cc** of fluid (or less) to **blunt the posterior costophrenic** *angle on the lateral film, while* it takes about **250-300 cc** to **blunt the lateral costophrenic angles** on the frontal film (Fig. 2-9).

EVALUATING THE CHEST RADIOGRAPH FOR TECHNICAL ADEQUACY

- Evaluating **five technical factors** will help you determine if a chest radiograph is **adequate** for interpretation or whether certain artifacts may have been introduced that can lead you astray (Table 2-2):
  - **Penetration**
  - **Inspiration**
  - **Rotation**
  - **Magnification**
  - **Angulation**

TABLE 2-2 WHAT DEFINES A TECHNICALLY ADEQUATE CHEST RADIOGRAPH?

Factor	What You Should See
Penetration	The spine should be visible through the heart
Inspiration	At least eight to nine posterior ribs should be visible
Rotation	Spinous process should fall equidistant between the medial ends of the clavicles
Magnification	AP films (mostly portable chest x-rays) will magnify the heart slightly
Angulation	Clavicle normally has an "S" shape and superimposes on the 3rd or 4th rib

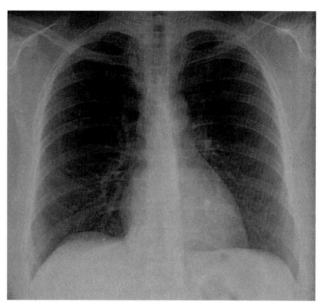

Figure 2-11 Overpenetrated frontal chest radiograph. Overpenetration makes lung markings difficult to see, mimicking some of the findings in emphysema or possibly suggesting a pneumothorax. How lucent (dark) the lungs appear on a radiograph is a poor way of evaluating for the presence of emphysema because of artifacts introduced by technique. In emphysema, the lungs are frequently hyperinflated and the diaphragm flattened (see Chapter 12). In order to diagnose a pneumothorax, you should see the pleural white line (see Chapter 8).

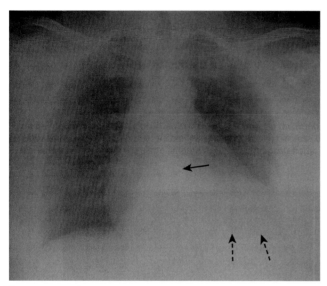

Figure 2-10 Underpenetrated frontal chest radiograph. The spine (*solid black arrow*) is not visible through the cardiac shadow. The left hemidiaphragm is also not visible (*dotted black arrows*) and the degree of underpenetration makes it impossible to differentiate between actual disease at the left base versus nonvisualization of the left hemidiaphragm from underpenetration. A lateral radiograph of the chest would help to differentiate between artifact of technique and true disease.

Penetration

- Unless x-rays adequately pass through the body part being studied, you may not visualize everything necessary on the image produced.
  - To determine if a frontal chest radiograph is adequately penetrated, you should be able to see the thoracic spine through the heart shadow (see Fig. 2-1).

 Pitfalls of underpenetration (inadequate penetration): You can tell a frontal chest radiograph is underpenetrated (too light) if you are not able to see the spine through the heart (Fig. 2-10). Underpenetration can introduce at least **two errors** into your interpretation.

- First, the left hemidiaphragm may not be visible on the frontal film because the left lung base may appear opaque. This technical artifact could either mimic or hide true disease in the left lower lung field (e.g., left lower lobe pneumonia or left pleural effusion) (see Fig. 2-10).
  - **Solution:** Look at the lateral chest radiograph to confirm the presence of disease at the left base (see "The Lateral Chest Radiograph" in this chapter).

- Second, the pulmonary markings, which are mostly the blood vessels in the lung, may appear more prominent than they really are. You may mistakenly think the patient is in congestive heart failure or has pulmonary fibrosis.
  - **Solutions:** Look for other radiologic signs of congestive heart failure (see Chapter 9). Look at the lateral chest film to confirm the presence of increased markings, airspace disease, or effusion at the left base that you suspected from the frontal radiograph.

Pitfall of overpenetration

- If the study is overpenetrated (too dark), the lung markings may seem decreased or absent (Fig. 2-11). You could mistakenly think the patient has emphysema or a pneumothorax or, if the degree of overpenetration is marked, it could render findings like a pulmonary nodule almost invisible.
  - **Solutions:** Look for other radiographic signs of emphysema (see Chapter 12) or pneumothorax (see Chapter 8). Ask the radiologist if the film should be repeated.

Inspiration

- A full inspiration ensures a reproducible radiograph from one time to the next and eliminates artifacts that may be confused for or obscure disease.
  - The **degree of inspiration can be assessed by counting the number of posterior ribs visible** above the diaphragm on the frontal chest radiograph.

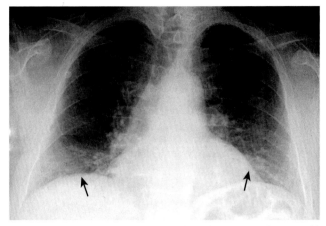

Figure 2-13 Sub-optimal inspiration. Only eight posterior ribs are visible on this frontal chest radiograph. A poor inspiration may "crowd" and therefore accentuate the lung markings at the bases (*solid black arrows*) and may make the heart seem larger than it actually is. The crowded lung markings may mimic the appearance of aspiration or pneumonia. A lateral chest radiograph should help in eliminating the possibility, or confirming the presence, of basilar airspace disease suspected from the frontal radiograph.

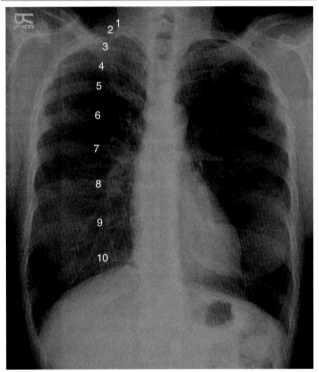

Figure 2-12 Counting ribs. The posterior ribs are numbered in this photograph. Ten posterior ribs are visible above the right hemidiaphragm, an excellent inspiration. In most hospitalized patients, eight to nine visible posterior ribs in the frontal projection is an inspiration that is adequate for accurate interpretation of the image. When counting ribs, make sure you don't miss counting the 2nd posterior rib, which frequently overlaps the 1st rib.

- To help in differentiating the **anterior** from the **posterior ribs**, consult Box 2-1.
- **If 10 posterior ribs are visible, it is an excellent inspiration** (Fig. 2-12).
- In many **hospitalized patients, visualization of eight to nine posterior ribs** is a degree of inspiration usually **adequate** for accurate interpretation of the image.

 Pitfall: Poor inspiration

- A **poor inspiratory effort will compress and crowd the lung markings**, especially at the bases of the lungs near the diaphragm (Fig. 2-13). This may lead you to mistakenly think the study shows lower lobe pneumonia.
  - **Solution:** Look at the lateral chest radiograph to confirm the presence of pneumonia (see "The Lateral Chest Radiograph" in this chapter and Chapter 7).

Rotation

- **Significant rotation** (the patient turns the body to one side or the other) **may alter the expected contours of the heart and great vessels, the hila, and hemidiaphragms**.
- The easiest way to assess whether the patient is rotated toward the left or right is by studying **the position of the medial ends of each clavicle relative to the spinous process** of the thoracic vertebral body between the clavicles (Fig. 2-14).
  - The **medial ends of the clavicles are anterior structures**.
  - The **spinous process is a posterior structure**.
  - **If the spinous process appears to lie equidistant from the medial ends of each clavicle** on the frontal chest radiograph, **there is no rotation** (Fig. 2-15A).
  - If the spinous process appears **closer to the medial end of the left clavicle, the patient is rotated toward his own right side** (Fig. 2-15B).
  - If the spinous process appears **closer to the medial end of the right clavicle, the patient is rotated toward his own left side** (Fig. 2-15C).
  - These relationships hold true regardless of whether the patient was facing the x-ray tube or the cassette at the time of exposure.

 Pitfalls of excessive rotation

- Even minor degrees of rotation can distort the normal anatomic appearance of the heart and great vessels, the hila, and hemidiaphragms.
- **Marked rotation can introduce errors in interpretation: The hilum may appear larger** on the side rotated farther away from the imaging cassette because objects farther from the imaging cassette tend to be more magnified than objects closer to the cassette.
- **Solutions: Look at the hilum on the lateral chest view** to see if that view confirms hilar enlargement (see "The Hilar Region" in this chapter). Compare the current

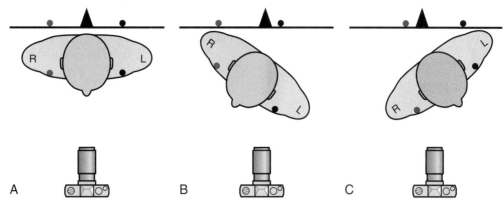

Figure 2-14 How to determine if the patient is rotated. In **A,** the patient is not rotated and the medial ends of the right (*orange dot*) and left (*black dot*) clavicles are projected on the radiograph (*black line*) equidistant from the spinous process (*black triangle*). In **B,** the patient is rotated toward his own right. Notice how the medial end of the left clavicle (*black dot*) is projected closer to the spinous process than is the medial end of the right clavicle (*orange dot*). In **C,** the patient is rotated toward his own left. The medial end of the right clavicle (*orange dot*) is projected closer to the spinous process than is the medial end of the left clavicle (*black dot*). The camera icon depicts this as an AP projection, but the same relationships would be true for a PA projection as well. Figure 2-15 shows how this applies to radiographs.

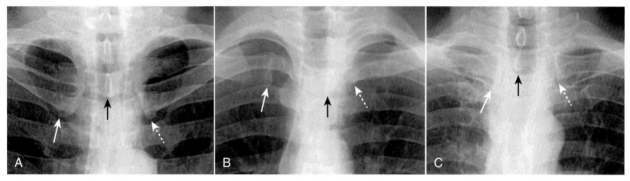

Figure 2-15 How to evaluate for rotation. A, Close-up view of the heads of the clavicles demonstrates that each (*white arrows*) is about equidistant from the spinous process of the vertebral body between them (*black arrow*). This indicates the patient is not rotated. **B,** Close-up view of the heads of the clavicles in a patient rotated toward his own right (remember that you are viewing the study as if the patient were facing you). The spinous process (*black arrow*) is much closer to the left clavicular head (*dotted white arrow*) than it is to the right clavicular head (*solid white arrow*). **C,** Close-up view of the heads of the clavicles in a patient rotated toward his own left. The spinous process (*black arrow*) is much closer to the right clavicular head (*solid white arrow*) than it is to the left (*dotted white arrow*).

study to a previous study of the same patient to assess for change.

- Rotation may also distort the appearance of the normal contours of the heart and hila.
- The **hemidiaphragm may appear higher** on the side rotated away from the imaging cassette (Fig. 2-16).
  - **Solution:** Compare the current study to a previous study of the same patient.

Magnification

- Depending on the position of the patient relative to the imaging cassette, magnification can play a role in assessing the size of the heart.

The closer any object is to the surface on which it is being imaged, the more true to its actual size the resultant image will be. As a corollary, the farther any object is from the surface on which it is being imaged, the more magnified that object will appear.

- In the standard **PA** chest radiograph, i.e., one obtained in the **posteroanterior projection, the heart**, being an anterior structure, **is closer** to the imaging surface and

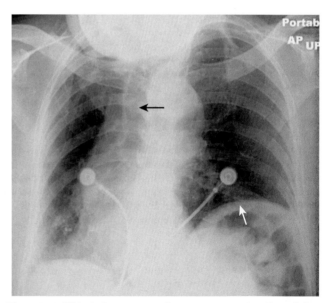

Figure 2-16 Distorted appearance due to severe rotation. Frontal chest radiograph of a patient markedly rotated toward her own right. Notice how the left hemidiaphragm, being farther from the cassette than the right hemidiaphragm because of the rotation, appears higher than it normally would (*solid white arrow*). The heart and the trachea (*solid black arrow*) appear displaced into the right hemithorax because of the rotation.

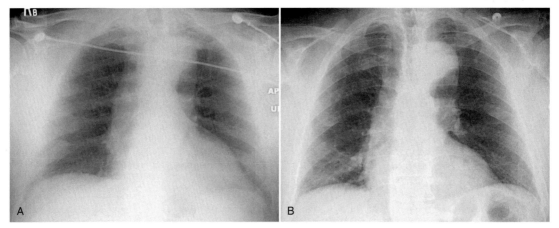

Figure 2-17 Effect of positioning on magnification of the heart. Frontal chest radiograph done in the AP projection **(A)** shows the heart to be slightly larger than in **B,** which is the same patient's chest exposed minutes later in the PA projection. Because the heart lies anteriorly in the chest, it is farther from the imaging surface in **A** and is therefore magnified more than in **B,** in which the heart is closer to the imaging surface. In actual practice, there is very little difference in the heart size between an AP and PA exposure so long as the patient has taken an equal inspiration on both.

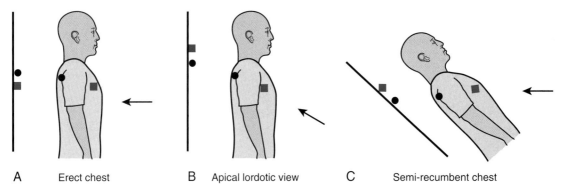

| | A | Erect chest | B | Apical lordotic view | C | Semi-recumbent chest |

Figure 2-18 Diagram of apical lordotic effect. In **A,** the x-ray beam (*black arrow*) is correctly oriented perpendicular to the plane of the cassette (*black line*). The *orange square* symbolizes an anterior structure (like the clavicles) and the *black circle* a posterior structure (like the spine). In **B,** the x-ray beam is angled upward, which is the manner in which an apical lordotic view of the chest is obtained. The x-ray beam is no longer perpendicular to the cassette, which has the effect of projecting anterior structures higher on the radiograph than posterior structures. The position of the x-ray beam and patient in **C** leads to the exact same end result as **B** and is how semirecumbent, bedside studies are frequently obtained on patients who are not able to sit or stand upright. Anterior structures in **C** are projected higher than posterior structures.

thus **truer to its actual size**. In a PA study, the x-ray beam enters at "P" (posterior) and exits at "A" (anterior). The standard frontal chest radiograph is usually a PA exposure.

- In an **AP** image, i.e., one obtained in the **anteroposterior projection, the heart** is **farther** from the imaging cassette and is therefore **slightly magnified**. In an AP study, the x-ray beam enters at "A" (anterior) and exits at "P" (posterior). Portable, bedside chest radiographs are almost always AP.
- Therefore, **the heart will appear slightly larger on an AP image than will the same heart on a PA image** (Fig. 2-17).
- There's another reason the heart looks larger on a portable AP chest image than a standard PA chest radiograph:
  - The distance between the x-ray tube and the patient is shorter when a portable AP image is obtained (about 40 inches) than when a standard PA chest radiograph is exposed (taken by convention at 72 inches). The greater the distance the x-ray source is from the patient, the less the degree of magnification.

- To learn how to determine if the heart is really enlarged on an AP chest radiograph, see Chapter 9.

Angulation

- Normally, the x-ray beam passes **horizontally** (parallel to the floor) **for an upright chest** study, and in that position, the **plane of the thorax** is **perpendicular** to the x-ray beam.
- **Hospitalized patients**, in particular, may not be able to sit completely upright in bed so that **the x-ray beam may enter the thorax with the patient's head and thorax tilted backwards**.
  - This **has the same effect as angling the x-ray beam towards the patient's head** and the image so obtained is called an *apical lordotic view* of the chest.
  - On apical lordotic views, **anterior structures in the chest** (like the clavicles) are projected **higher** on the resultant radiographic image **than posterior structures** in the chest, which are projected lower (Fig. 2-18).

 Pitfall of excessive angulation

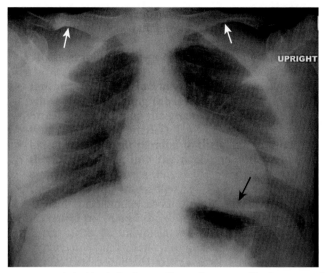

Figure 2-19 **Apical lordotic chest radiograph.** An apical lordotic view of the chest is now most frequently obtained inadvertently in patients who are semirecumbent at the time of the study. Notice how the clavicles are projected above the first ribs and their usual "S" shape is now straight (*solid white arrows*). The lordotic view also distorts the shape of the heart and produces spurious obscuration of the left hemidiaphragm (*solid black arrow*). Unless the artifacts of technique are understood, these findings could be mistaken for disease that doesn't exist.

- You can recognize an apical lordotic chest study when you see the clavicles project at or above the posterior first ribs on the frontal image. An apical lordotic view distorts the appearance of the clavicles, straightening their normal "S" shape appearance (Fig. 2-19).
- Apical lordotic views may also distort the appearance of other structures in the thorax. The **heart may have an unusual shape**, which sometimes mimics cardiomegaly and distorts the normal appearance of the cardiac borders. The **sharp border of the left hemidiaphragm may be lost**, which could be mistaken as a sign of a left pleural effusion or left lower lobe pneumonia.
  - **Solutions:** Know how to recognize technical artifacts and understand how they can distort normal anatomy. Consult with a radiologist about confusing images.

WEBLINK

Registered users may obtain more information on Recognizing Normal Chest Anatomy and a Technically Adequate Chest Radiograph on StudentConsult.com.

TAKE-HOME POINTS

Recognizing Normal Chest Anatomy and a Technically Adequate Chest Radiograph

Virtually all of the lung markings are composed of pulmonary blood vessels; the minor fissure may be visible on both the frontal and lateral views, the major fissure only on the lateral.

The lateral chest radiograph can provide invaluable information and should always be studied when available.

Five key areas to inspect on the lateral projection include the retrosternal clear space, the hilar region, the fissures, the thoracic spine, and the diaphragm/posterior costophrenic sulci.

Five parameters define an adequate chest examination, and recognition of them is important to accurately differentiate abnormalities from technically produced artifacts.

They are **penetration, inspiration, rotation, magnification, and angulation.**

If the chest is **adequately penetrated**, you should be able to see spine through the heart; underpenetrated (too light) studies obscure the left lung base and tend to spuriously accentuate the lung markings, while overpenetrated studies (too dark) may mimic emphysema or pneumothorax.

If the patient has taken an **adequate inspiration**, you should see at least eight to nine posterior ribs above the diaphragm; poor inspiratory efforts may mimic basilar lung disease and may make the heart appear larger.

The spinous process should fall equidistant between the medial ends of the clavicles to indicate the patient is not rotated; rotation can introduce numerous artifactual anomalies affecting the contour of the heart and the appearance of the hila and diaphragm.

Anteroposterior (AP) films (mostly portable chest x-rays) will magnify the heart slightly compared to the standard posteroanterior (PA) chest radiograph (usually done in the radiology department).

Frontal views of the chest obtained with the patient semiupright in bed (tilted backwards) may produce apical lordotic images that distort normal anatomy.

Chapter 3

Recognizing Airspace Versus Interstitial Lung Disease

CLASSIFYING PARENCHYMAL LUNG DISEASE

- **Diseases** that affect the lung **can be arbitrarily divided into two main categories** based in part on their pathology and in part on the pattern they typically produce on a chest imaging study.
  - Airspace (alveolar) disease
  - Interstitial (infiltrative) disease
- Why learn the difference?
  - While many diseases produce abnormalities that display both patterns, recognition of these patterns frequently helps narrow the disease possibilities so that you can form a reasonable differential diagnosis (Box 3-1).

CHARACTERISTICS OF AIRSPACE DISEASE

Airspace disease characteristically produces opacities in the lung that can be described as **fluffy, cloudlike, or hazy**.

- These fluffy opacities tend to be **confluent**, meaning they blend into one another with imperceptible margins.
- The **margins of airspace disease are indistinct**, meaning it is frequently difficult to identify a clear demarcation point between the disease and the adjacent normal lung.
- Airspace disease may be **distributed throughout the lungs**, as in pulmonary edema (Fig. 3-1), **or** it may **appear to be more localized** as in a segmental or lobar pneumonia (Fig. 3-2).
- Airspace disease may contain **air bronchograms**.
  - The visibility of air in the bronchus because of surrounding airspace disease is called an *air bronchogram*.
  - An air bronchogram is a **sign of airspace disease**.
- Bronchi are normally not visible because their walls are very thin, they contain air, and they are surrounded by air. When something like fluid or soft tissue replaces the air normally surrounding the bronchus, then the air inside of the bronchus becomes visible as **a series of black, branching tubular structures**—this is the *air bronchogram* (Fig. 3-3).
- What can fill the airspaces besides air?
  - **Fluid**, such as occurs in pulmonary edema
  - **Blood**, e.g., pulmonary hemorrhage
  - **Gastric juices**, e.g., aspiration
  - **Inflammatory exudate**, e.g., pneumonia
  - **Water**, e.g., near-drowning

Airspace disease may demonstrate the *silhouette sign* (Fig. 3-4).

- The silhouette sign occurs when two objects **of the same radiographic density** (fat, water, etc.) **touch each other so that the edge or margin between them disappears.** It will be impossible to tell where one object begins and the other ends. **The *silhouette sign* is valuable not only in the chest but as an aid in the analysis of imaging studies throughout the body.**
- The characteristics of airspace disease are summarized in Box 3-2.

SOME CAUSES OF AIRSPACE DISEASE

- Three of the many causes of airspace disease are highlighted here and will be described in greater detail later in the text.
- **Pneumonia** (see also Chapter 7)
  - About 90% of the time, community-acquired lobar or segmental pneumonia is caused by *Streptococcus pneumoniae* (formerly known as *Diplococcus pneumoniae*) (Fig. 3-5).
  - Pneumonia usually manifests as patchy, segmental, or lobar airspace disease.
  - Pneumonias may contain air bronchograms.
  - Clearing usually occurs in less than 10 days (pneumococcal pneumonia may clear within 48 hours).
- **Pulmonary alveolar edema** (see also Chapter 9)
  - Acute alveolar pulmonary edema classically produces bilateral, perihilar airspace disease sometimes described as having a *bat-wing* or *angel-wing configuration* (Fig. 3-6).
  - It may be asymmetrical but is usually not unilateral.
  - Pulmonary edema, which is cardiac in origin, is frequently associated with pleural effusions and fluid that thickens the major and minor fissures.
  - Because fluid fills not only the airspaces but also the bronchi themselves, usually no air bronchograms are seen in pulmonary alveolar edema.
  - Classically, **pulmonary edema clears rapidly** after treatment (<48 hours).
- **Aspiration** (see also Chapter 7)
  - Aspiration tends to affect whatever part of the lung is most dependent at the time the patient aspirates, and its manifestations depend on the substance(s) aspirated (Fig. 3-7).
  - For most bedridden patients, aspiration usually occurs in either the **lower lobes** or the **posterior portions of the upper lobes.**
  - Because of the course and caliber of the right main bronchus, **aspiration occurs more often in the right lower lobe** than the left lower lobe.

Box 3-1 Classification of Parenchymal Lung Diseases

Airspace Diseases

Acute

Pneumonia

Pulmonary alveolar edema

Hemorrhage

Aspiration

Near-drowning

Chronic

Bronchoalveolar cell carcinoma

Alveolar cell proteinosis

Sarcoidosis

Lymphoma

Interstitial Diseases

Reticular

Idiopathic pulmonary fibrosis

Pulmonary interstitial edema

Rheumatoid lung

Scleroderma

Sarcoid

Nodular

Bronchogenic carcinoma

Metastases

Silicosis

Miliary tuberculosis

Sarcoid

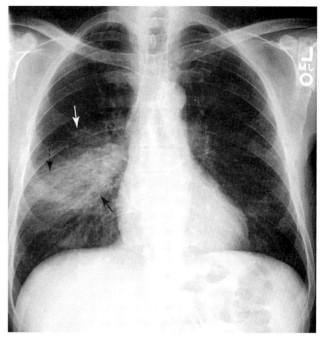

Figure 3-2 Right lower lobe pneumonia. An area of increased opacification is in the right midlung field (*solid black arrow*) that has indistinct margins (*solid white arrow*) characteristic of airspace disease. The minor fissure (*dotted black arrow*) appears to bisect the disease, locating this pneumonia in the superior segment of the right lower lobe. The right heart border and the right hemidiaphragm are still visible because the disease is not in anatomical contact with either of those structures.

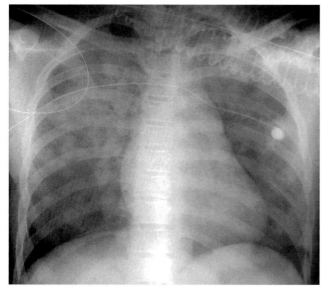

Figure 3-1 Diffuse airspace disease of pulmonary alveolar edema. Opacities throughout both lungs primarily involve the upper lobes, which can be described as fluffy, hazy, or cloudlike and are confluent and poorly marginated, all pointing to airspace disease. This is a typical example of pulmonary alveolar edema (due to a heroin overdose in this patient).

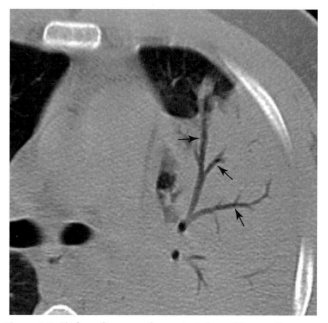

Figure 3-3 Air bronchograms demonstrated on CT scan. Numerous black, branching structures (*solid black arrows*) represent air that is now visible inside the bronchi because the surrounding airspaces are filled with inflammatory exudate in this patient with an obstructive pneumonia from a bronchogenic carcinoma. Normally, on conventional radiographs, air inside bronchi is not visible because the bronchial walls are very thin, they contain air, and they are surrounded by air.

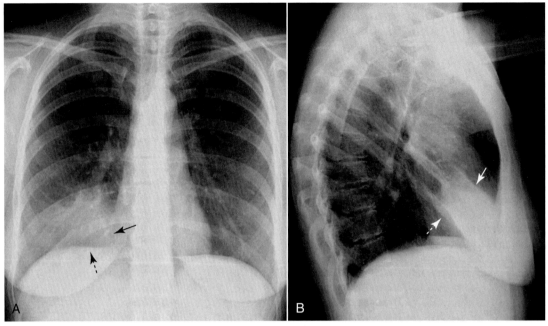

Figure 3-4 Silhouette sign, right middle lobe pneumonia. A, Fluffy, indistinctly marginated airspace disease is seen to the right of the heart. It obscures the right heart border (*solid black arrow*) but not the right hemidiaphragm (*dotted black arrow*). This is called the **silhouette sign** and establishes that the disease (1) is in contact with the right heart border (which lies anteriorly in the chest) and (2) is the same radiographic density as the heart (fluid or soft tissue). Pneumonia fills the airspaces with an inflammatory exudate of fluid density. **B,** The area of the consolidation is indeed anterior, located in the right middle lobe, which is bound by the major fissure below (*dotted white arrow*) and the minor fissure above (*solid white arrow*).

Box 3-2 Characteristics of Airspace Disease

Produces opacities in the lung that can be described as fluffy, cloudlike, and hazy.

The opacities tend to be confluent, merging into one another.

The margins of airspace disease are fuzzy and indistinct.

Air bronchograms or the silhouette sign may be present.

- What is aspirated and whether it becomes infected will determine the radiographic appearance of aspiration and how quickly the airspace disease resolves.
  - **Aspiration of** bland (neutralized) gastric juice or **water usually clears rapidly,** within 24 to 48 hours, whereas aspiration that becomes infected can take weeks to resolve.

CHARACTERISTICS OF INTERSTITIAL LUNG DISEASE

- The lung's interstitium consists of connective tissue, lymphatics, blood vessels, and bronchi. These are the structures that surround and support the airspaces.
- Interstitial lung disease is sometimes referred to as *infiltrative lung disease*.

Interstitial lung disease produces what can be thought of as **discrete "particles" of disease** that develop in the abundant interstitial network of the lung (Fig. 3-8).

- These "particles" of disease can be further characterized as having **three patterns of presentation:**

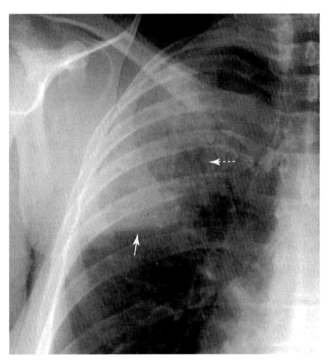

Figure 3-5 Right upper lobe pneumococcal pneumonia. Close-up view of the right upper lobe demonstrates confluent airspace disease with air bronchograms (*dotted white arrow*). The inferior margin of the pneumonia is more sharply demarcated because it is in contact with the minor fissure (*solid white arrow*). This patient had *Streptococcus pneumoniae* cultured from the sputum.

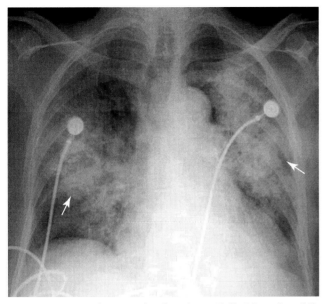

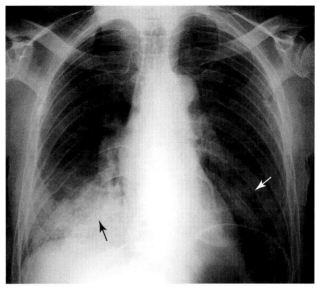

Figure 3-6 Acute pulmonary alveolar edema. Fluffy, bilateral, perihilar airspace disease with indistinct margins, sometimes described as having a **bat-wing** or **angel-wing** configuration, is present (*solid white arrows*). No air bronchograms are seen. The heart is enlarged. This represents pulmonary alveolar edema secondary to congestive heart failure.

Figure 3-7 Aspiration, right and left lower lobes. An area of opacification in the right lower lobe is fluffy and confluent with indistinct margins characteristic of airspace disease (*solid black arrow*). To a much lesser extent, a similar density is seen in the left lower lobe (*solid white arrow*). The bibasilar distribution of this disease should raise the suspicion of aspiration as an etiology. This patient had a recent stroke and aspiration was demonstrated on a video swallowing study.

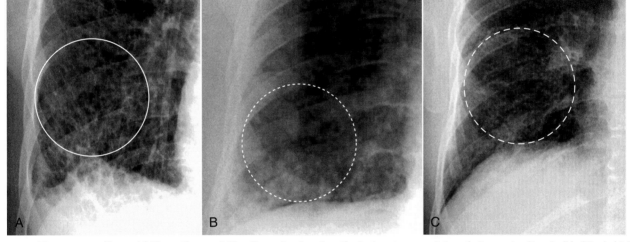

Figure 3-8 The patterns of interstitial lung disease. A, The disease is primarily **reticular** in nature, consisting of crisscrossing lines (*solid white circle*). This patient had advanced sarcoidosis. **B,** The disease is predominantly **nodular** (*dotted white circle*). The patient was known to have thyroid carcinoma, and these nodules represent innumerable small metastatic foci in the lungs. **C,** Interstitial disease of the lung, **reticulonodular**. Most interstitial diseases of the lung have a mixture of both a reticular (lines) and nodular (dots) pattern, as does this case, which is a close-up view of the right lower lobe in another patient with sarcoidosis. The disease (*dashed white circle*) consists of both an intersecting, lacy network of lines and small nodules.

- **Reticular interstitial disease** appears as a network of lines (see Fig. 3-8A).
- **Nodular interstitial disease** appears as an assortment of dots (see Fig. 3-8B).
- **Reticulonodular interstitial disease** contains both lines and dots (see Fig. 3-8C).
- These "particles" or "packets" of interstitial disease tend to be **inhomogeneous**, separated from each other by visible areas of normally aerated lung.
- The **margins of "particles" of interstitial lung disease are sharper** than the margins of airspace disease that tend to be indistinct.

- Interstitial lung disease **can be focal** (as in a solitary pulmonary nodule) **or diffusely distributed** in the lungs (Fig. 3-9).
- **Usually no air bronchograms are present**, as there may be with airspace disease.

⚠️ **Pitfall:** Sometimes, so much interstitial disease is present that the overlapping elements of disease may superimpose and mimic airspace disease on conventional chest radiographs. Remember that conventional radiographs are two-dimensional representations of three-dimensional objects (humans) so all of the densities in the lung, for

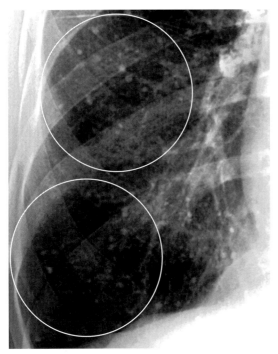

Figure 3-9 Varicella pneumonia. Innumerable calcified granulomas occur in the lung interstitium, here seen as small, discrete nodules in the right lung (*white circles*). This patient had a history of varicella (chicken pox) pneumonia years earlier. Varicella pneumonia clears with multiple small calcified granulomas remaining.

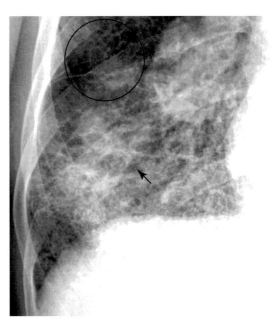

Figure 3-10 The edge of the lesion. Notice how a portion of this disease appears confluent, like airspace disease (*solid black arrow*). Always look at the peripheral margins of parenchymal lung disease to best determine the nature of the "packets" of abnormality and to help in differentiating airspace disease from interstitial disease. At the periphery of this disease (*black circle*), this is more clearly seen to be reticular interstitial disease.

example, are superimposed on themselves on any one projection. This may make the tiny packets of interstitial disease seem coalescent and more like airspace disease.

- **Solutions:** Look at the periphery of such confluent shadows in the lung to help in determining whether they are, in fact, caused by airspace disease or a superimposition of numerous reticular and nodular densities (Fig. 3-10).
- Obtain a CT scan of the chest.
- The characteristics of interstitial lung disease are summarized in Box 3-3.

SOME CAUSES OF INTERSTITIAL LUNG DISEASE

- Just as with the airspace pattern, there are many diseases that produce an interstitial pattern in the lung. Several will be discussed briefly here. They are roughly divided into those diseases that are predominantly reticular and those that are predominantly nodular.

➡ Keep in mind that **many diseases have patterns that overlap and many interstitial lung diseases have** mixtures of both reticular and nodular changes (reticulonodular disease).

Predominantly Reticular Interstitial Lung Diseases

- **Pulmonary interstitial edema**
  - Pulmonary interstitial edema can occur because of increased capillary pressure (congestive heart failure),

---

Box 3-3 Characteristics of Interstitial Lung Disease
Interstitial disease has discrete reticular, nodular, or reticulonodular patterns.
"Packets" of disease are separated by normal-appearing, aerated lung.
Margins of "packets" of interstitial disease are usually sharp and discrete.
Disease may be focal or diffusely distributed in the lungs.
Usually no air bronchograms are present.

increased capillary permeability (allergic reactions), or decreased fluid absorption (lymphangitic blockage from metastatic disease).
- Considered the precursor of alveolar edema, pulmonary interstitial edema classically manifests **four key radiologic findings**: fluid in the fissures (major and minor), peribronchial cuffing (from fluid in the walls of bronchioles), pleural effusions, and Kerley B lines.
- Classically, the patient may have few physical findings in the lungs (rales) even though their chest radiograph demonstrates considerable pulmonary interstitial edema, because almost all of the fluid is in the interstitium of the lung rather than in the airspaces.
- With appropriate therapy, pulmonary interstitial edema usually clears rapidly (<48 hours) (Fig. 3-11).
- **Idiopathic pulmonary fibrosis**
  - A disease of unknown etiology, usually occurring in older men who develop cough and shortness of breath.
  - The early stage is a milder form known as *desquamative interstitial pneumonia (DIP)* and its findings are usually seen best on high-resolution CT scans of the chest.

- Later in the disease, it is called *usual interstitial pneumonia (UIP),* and there is marked thickening of the interstitium, bronchiectasis, and a pattern of cystic changes in the lung called *honeycombing*.
- UIP is also best demonstrated on high-resolution CT scans of the chest.
- Conventional radiographs of the chest may show a **fine** or, later in the disease, a **coarse** reticular pattern that is

bilaterally symmetrical, most prominent at the **bases, subpleural** in location and frequently associated with **volume loss**.
- Idiopathic pulmonary fibrosis is considered the end-stage disease along the spectrum of these interstitial pneumonias (Fig. 3-12).

■ **Rheumatoid lung**
- Rheumatoid lung disease is found in some patients with rheumatoid arthritis.
- The three most common manifestations of rheumatoid lung disease are (in order of decreasing frequency) **pleural effusions, interstitial lung disease,** and **nodules** in the lung called *necrobiotic nodules.*
- **Pleural effusions** are usually **unilateral** and characteristically remain unchanged in appearance for long periods of time.
- Rheumatoid interstitial lung disease is usually **reticular,** can be seen diffusely throughout the lung, but is usually **most prominent at the lung bases**.
- Necrobiotic nodules are identical to subcutaneous rheumatoid nodules and occur **mostly at the lung bases** near the **periphery of the lung; cavitation is frequent.**
- Unlike the joint findings of rheumatoid arthritis, which are more common in women, the thoracic manifestations of rheumatoid arthritis are more common in men (Fig. 3-13).

Predominantly Nodular Interstitial Diseases

■ **Bronchogenic carcinoma** (see Chapter 12)
- Bronchogenic carcinoma has four major cell types: adenocarcinoma, squamous cell carcinoma, small cell carcinoma, and large cell carcinoma.
- Adenocarcinomas, in particular, can present as a solitary peripheral pulmonary nodule.
- As a rule, on conventional chest radiographs, nodules or masses in the lung are more sharply marginated than airspace disease, producing a relatively clear demarcation between the nodule and the surrounding normal lung tissue.

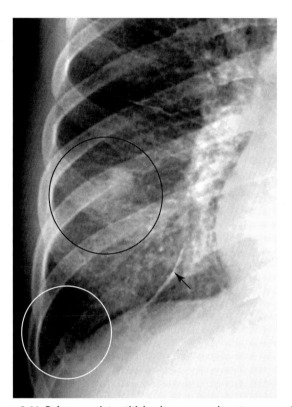

Figure 3-11 Pulmonary interstitial edema secondary to congestive heart failure. A close-up view of the right lung shows an accentuation of the pulmonary interstitial markings (*black circle*). Multiple Kerley B lines (*white circle*) represent fluid in thickened interlobular septa. Fluid is seen in the inferior accessory fissure (*solid black arrow*).

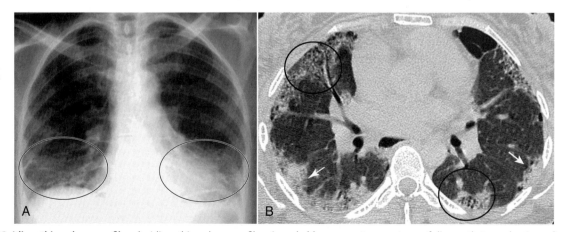

Figure 3-12 Idiopathic pulmonary fibrosis. Idiopathic pulmonary fibrosis probably represents a spectrum of disease that may begin as *desquamative interstitial pneumonia (DIP)* and lead to the findings here of *usual interstitial pneumonia (UIP).* **A,** coarse reticular interstitial markings represent fibrosis, predominantly at the lung bases (*black circles*). **B,** A high-resolution CT scan of the chest shows abnormalities at the lung bases in a subpleural location, the typical distribution for UIP. There are small cystic spaces called **honeycombing** (*black circles*) with hazy densities called **ground-glass opacities** (*solid white arrows*).

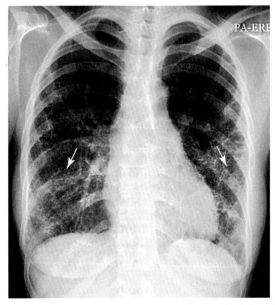

Figure 3-13 Rheumatoid lung. Prominent markings at both lung bases have a predominantly reticular appearance (*solid white arrows*). Bibasilar interstitial disease can be found in numerous diseases including bronchiectasis, asbestosis, desquamative interstitial pneumonia (DIP), scleroderma, and sickle cell disease. This patient was known to have rheumatoid arthritis. Pleural effusion is the most common manifestation of rheumatoid lung disease, and pulmonary fibrosis, usually diffuse but more prominent at the bases, is second most common.

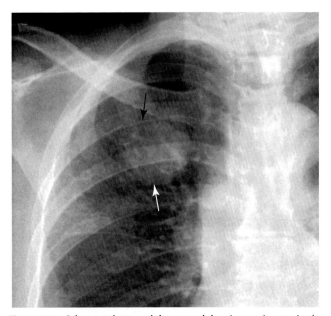

Figure 3-14 Adenocarcinoma, right upper lobe. A mass is seen in the right upper lobe (*solid white arrow*). Its margin is slightly indistinct along the superolateral border (*solid black arrow*). CT scan of the chest confirmed the presence of the mass and also demonstrated paratracheal and right hilar adenopathy. The mass was biopsied and was an adenocarcinoma, primary to the lung. Adenocarcinoma of the lung most commonly presents as a peripheral nodule.

- CT scans may demonstrate spiculation or irregularity of the lung nodule that may not be apparent on conventional radiographs (Fig. 3-14).
- **Metastases to the lung**
  - Metastases to the lung can be divided into three categories depending on the pattern of disease demonstrated

in the lung: hematogenous, lymphangitic and direct extension.

- **Hematogenous metastases** arrive via the bloodstream and usually produce two or more nodules in the lungs, sometimes called *cannonball metastases* because of their **large, round appearance.**
- Primary tumor sites that classically produce nodular metastases to the lung include breast, colorectal, renal cell, bladder and testicular, head and neck carcinomas, soft tissue sarcomas, and malignant melanoma (Fig. 3-15A).
- The second form of tumor dissemination is **lymphangitic spread.** The pathogenesis of lymphangitic spread to the lungs is somewhat controversial but most likely involves blood-borne spread to the pulmonary capillaries and then invasion of adjacent lymphatics. An alternative means of lymphangitic spread is obstruction of central lymphatics usually in the hila with retrograde dissemination through the lymphatics in the lung.
- Regardless of the mode of transmission, lymphangitic spread to the lung tends to **resemble pulmonary interstitial edema** from congestive heart failure, except, unlike congestive heart failure, it tends to be **localized to a segment or involve only one lung.**
- Primary tumor sites that classically produce the lymphangitic pattern of metastases to the lung include breast, lung, stomach, pancreatic, and, infrequently, prostate carcinoma.
  - Findings include: Kerley lines, fluid in the fissures, and pleural effusions (Fig. 3-15B).
- **Direct extension** is the least common form of tumor spread to the lungs because the pleura is surprisingly resistant to the spread of malignancy through direct violation of its layers.
  - Direct extension would most likely produce a **localized subpleural mass** in the lung, frequently with **adjacent rib destruction** (Fig. 3-15C).

Mixed Reticular and Nodular Interstitial Disease (Reticulonodular Disease)

- **Sarcoidosis**
  - In addition to the **bilateral hilar** and **right paratracheal adenopathy** characteristic of this disease, about half of patients with thoracic sarcoid also demonstrate **interstitial lung disease.**
  - The interstitial lung disease is frequently a mixture of both **reticular** and **nodular** components.
  - There is a progression of disease in sarcoid that tends to start with adenopathy (*Stage I*), proceed to a combination of both interstitial lung disease and adenopathy (*Stage II*), and then progress to a stage in which the adenopathy regresses while the interstitial lung disease remains (*Stage III*).
  - Most patients with parenchymal lung disease will undergo complete resolution of the disease (Fig. 3-16).

WEBLINK

Registered users may obtain more information on Recognizing Airspace Versus Interstitial Lung Disease on StudentConsult.com.

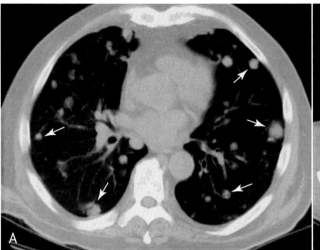

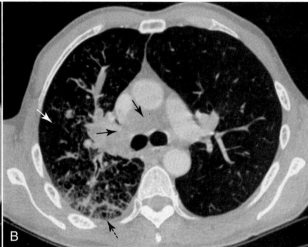

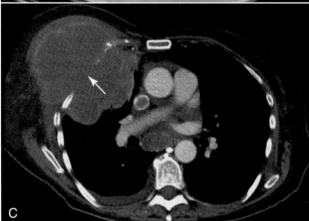

Figure 3-15 Metastases to the lung, CT scans. A, Multiple discrete nodules of varying size are present throughout both lungs (*solid white arrows*). The diagnosis of exclusion, whenever multiple nodules are found in the lungs, is metastatic disease. In this case, the metastases were from colon carcinoma. **B,** The interstitial markings in the right lung are prominent (*solid white arrow*), there are septal lines (*dotted black arrow*) and lymphadenopathy (*solid black arrows*) from lymphangitic spread of a bronchogenic carcinoma. **C,** In this case, the lung cancer has grown through the chest wall (*solid white arrow*) and invaded it by direct extension. The pleura usually serves as a strong barrier to the direct spread of tumor.

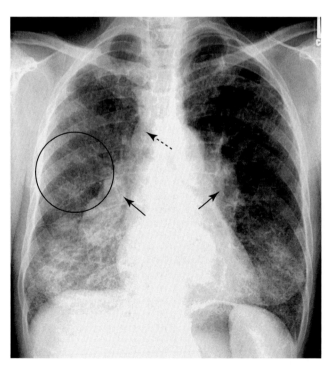

Figure 3-16 Sarcoidosis. A frontal radiograph of the chest reveals bilateral hilar (*solid black arrows*) and right paratracheal adenopathy (*dotted black arrow*), a classical distribution for the adenopathy in sarcoidosis. In addition, the patient has diffuse, bilateral interstitial lung disease (*black circle*) that is reticulonodular in nature. In some patients with this stage of disease, the adenopathy regresses while the interstitial disease remains. In the overwhelming majority of patients with sarcoid, the disease completely resolves.

TAKE-HOME POINTS

Recognizing Airspace Versus Interstitial Lung Disease

Parenchymal lung disease can be divided into airspace (alveolar) and interstitial (infiltrative) patterns.

Recognizing the pattern of disease can help in reaching the correct diagnosis.

Characteristics of airspace disease include fluffy, confluent densities that are indistinctly marginated and may demonstrate air bronchograms.

Characteristics of interstitial lung disease include discrete "particles" or "packets" of disease with distinct margins that tend to occur in a pattern of lines (reticular), dots (nodular), or very frequently a combination of lines and dots (reticulonodular).

Examples of airspace disease include pulmonary alveolar edema, pneumonia, and aspiration.

Examples of interstitial lung disease include pulmonary interstitial edema, pulmonary fibrosis, metastases to the lung, bronchogenic carcinoma, sarcoidosis, and rheumatoid lung.

An **air bronchogram** is typically a sign of airspace disease and occurs when something other than air (such as inflammatory exudate or blood) surrounds the bronchus, allowing the air inside the bronchus to become visible.

When two objects of the same radiographic density are in contact with each other, the normal edge or margin between them will disappear. The disappearance of the margin between these two structures is called the **silhouette sign** and is useful throughout radiology in identifying either the location or the density of the abnormality in question.

Chapter 4

Recognizing the Causes of an Opacified Hemithorax

- Mr. Smith, age 73, presents to the Emergency Department very short of breath. His frontal chest radiograph is shown in Figure 4-1.
- As you can see, Mr. Smith's right hemithorax is almost completely opaque.
  - Mr. Smith's treatment will vary greatly depending on whether he has *atelectasis* (which may require emergent bronchoscopy), a large *effusion* (which may require emergent thoracentesis), or *pneumonia* (which would require starting antibiotics).
  - To be able to treat him correctly, you have to know what is producing the opacification and that question is answered on the radiograph if you know how to approach the problem.
- **There are three major causes of an opacified hemithorax** (plus one other that is less common):
  - **Atelectasis of the entire lung**
  - **A very large pleural effusion**
  - **Pneumonia of an entire lung**
  - And a fourth cause: **pneumonectomy**—removal of an entire lung

ATELECTASIS OF THE ENTIRE LUNG

- **Atelectasis of an entire lung** usually results from **complete obstruction of the right or left main bronchus.**
  - With bronchial obstruction, no air can enter the lung. The remaining air in the lung is absorbed into the bloodstream through the pulmonary capillary system.
  - This leads to **loss of volume** of the affected lung.
- In an older individual, an **obstructing neoplasm**, like a bronchogenic carcinoma, might cause atelectasis. In younger individuals, **asthma** may produce mucous plugs that obstruct the bronchi or a **foreign body** may have been aspirated. Critically ill patients also develop atelectasis from **mucous plugs.**
- **In obstructive atelectasis**, even though there is volume loss within the affected lung, **the visceral and parietal pleura almost never separate from each other.**
  - That is an important fact about atelectasis and is sometimes confusing to beginners who try to picture atelectasis and a pneumothorax as both producing collapse of a lung without understanding why they look completely different (Fig. 4-2 and Table 4-1).
  - Because the visceral and parietal pleura do not separate from each other in atelectasis, mobile structures in the thorax are "pulled" toward the side of the atelectasis producing a *shift* (movement) of certain mobile thoracic structures **toward the side of opacification.**

- The most visible mobile structures in the thorax are the **heart**, the **trachea**, and the **hemidiaphragms**.
- **In obstructive atelectasis, one or all of these structures will shift toward the side of opacification (toward side of volume loss)** (Fig. 4-3).
- Table 4-2 summarizes the movement of the mobile structures in the thorax in patients with atelectasis.

MASSIVE PLEURAL EFFUSION

- If fluid, whether blood, an exudate, or a transudate, fills the pleural space so as to opacify almost the entire hemithorax, then the **fluid acts like a mass** compressing the underlying lung tissue.
- When enough pleural fluid accumulates, the **large effusion "pushes" mobile structures away, and the heart and trachea shift away from the side of opacification** (Fig. 4-4).
- Massive pleural effusions are frequently the result of malignancy, either in the form of a **bronchogenic carcinoma** or secondary to **metastases to the pleura** from a distant organ. Trauma can produce a **hemothorax** and **tuberculosis** is notorious for causing large, clinically silent effusions. The effusions from **congestive heart failure**, while very common, are most often *bilateral* (but asymmetrical) and they rarely grow large enough to occupy an entire hemithorax.

> ⚠️ At times, there may be a perfect **balance** between the **push** of a malignant effusion and the **pull** of underlying obstructive atelectasis from the malignancy itself.

- In an adult patient with an opacified hemithorax, no air bronchograms and little or no shift of the mobile thoracic structures, it is important to suspect an obstructing bronchogenic carcinoma, perhaps with metastases to the pleura. A CT scan of the chest will reveal the abnormalities (Fig. 4-5).
- Table 4-3 summarizes the movement of the mobile structures in the thorax in patients with a large pleural effusion.

PNEUMONIA OF AN ENTIRE LUNG

- With pneumonia, inflammatory exudate fills the air spaces causing consolidation and opacification of the lung.
- The hemithorax becomes opaque because the lung no longer contains air, but there is **neither a pull toward** the

side of the pneumonia by volume loss **nor a push away** from the side of the pneumonia by a large effusion.

■ **Neither the heart nor trachea shifts**.
  • **Air bronchograms** may be present (Fig. 4-6).
■ Table 4-4 summarizes the movement of the mobile structures in the thorax in patients with pneumonia of the entire lung.

POSTPNEUMONECTOMY

■ Pneumonectomy means the removal of an entire lung.
  • To perform this procedure, **either the 5th or 6th rib on the affected side is almost always removed**.

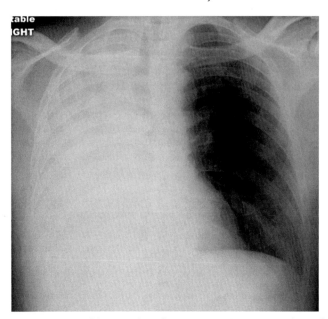

Figure 4-1 Mr. Smith comes into the Emergency Department short of breath. This is his frontal chest radiograph. Would you recommend bronchoscopy for atelectasis, emergent thoracentesis for a large pleural effusion, or a course of antibiotics for his large pneumonia? The answer is on the radiograph (and in this chapter).

• In most cases, **metallic surgical clips will be visible in the region of the hilum** on the pneumonectomized side.
■ For about 24 hours following the surgery, only air occupies the hemithorax from which the lung has been removed (Fig. 4-7).
■ Over the course of the next two weeks, the hemithorax gradually fills with fluid.
■ By about 4 months after surgery, the pneumonectomized hemithorax should be completely opaque.
■ The mobile mediastinal structures gradually shift toward the side of opacification.
■ Eventually, **fibrous tissue forms in the pneumonectomized hemithorax** and in most patients the **entire hemithorax is completely opaque**. The heart and trachea shift toward the side of opacification.

➡ The chest examination looks identical to that of a patient with atelectasis of the entire lung. To tell the difference, look for the missing 5th or 6th rib and look for the surgical clips in the hilum to indicate a pneumonectomy has been performed (Fig. 4-8).

TABLE 4-1 PNEUMOTHORAX VERSUS OBSTRUCTIVE ATELECTASIS

Feature	Pneumothorax	Obstructive Atelectasis
Pleural space	Air in the pleural space separates the visceral from the parietal pleura	The visceral and parietal pleura do not separate from each other
Density	The pneumothorax itself will appear "black" (air density); the hemithorax may appear more lucent than normal	Atelectasis is the absence of air in the lung; the hemithorax will appear more opaque ("whiter") than normal
Shift	The heart or trachea never shift toward the side of a pneumothorax	The heart and trachea almost always shift toward the side of the atelectasis

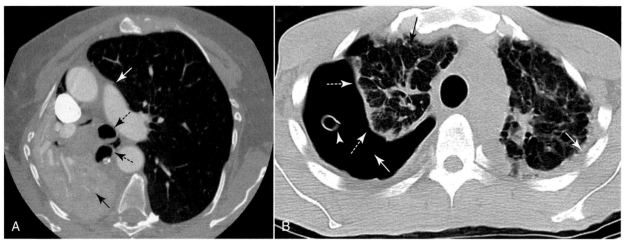

Figure 4-2 Obstructive atelectasis versus a pneumothorax. Two different causes of lung collapse and the difference in their radiologic appearance. **A,** There is atelectasis of the entire right lung (*solid black arrow*) from an obstructing endobronchial lesion. The visceral and parietal pleura remain in contact with each other. Other mobile structures in the mediastinum, such as the trachea and right main bronchus (*dotted black arrows*), shift toward the atelectasis. The left lung overexpands and crosses the midline (*solid white arrow*). **B,** This patient has a large right-sided pneumothorax. Air (*solid white arrow*) interposes between the visceral (*dotted white arrows*) and parietal pleurae, causing the lung to undergo passive atelectasis (*solid black arrow*). A chest tube is seen in the right hemithorax (*arrowhead*) that had been removed from suction.

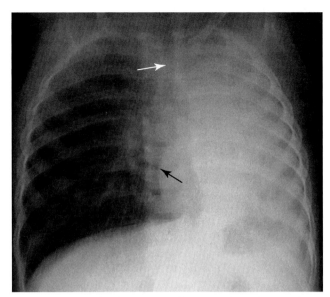

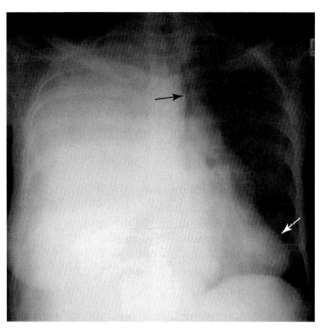

Figure 4-3 Child with wheezing and shortness of breath. Frontal chest radiograph shows opacification of the entire left hemithorax. The heart has shifted toward the left such that the right heart border no longer projects to the right of the spine. The heart now overlies the spine (*solid black arrow*). The trachea (*solid white arrow*) has moved leftward from the midline toward the side of the opacification. These findings are characteristic of atelectasis of the entire lung. The child had asthma. Bronchoscopy was performed and a large mucous plug that was obstructing the left main bronchus was removed.

Figure 4-4 Complete opacification of the right hemithorax. The trachea is deviated to the left (*solid black arrow*) and the apex of the heart is also displaced to the left, close to the lateral chest wall (*solid white arrow*). These findings are characteristic of a large pleural effusion that is producing a mass effect. Almost two liters of serosanguinous fluid were removed at thoracentesis. The fluid contained malignant cells from a primary bronchogenic carcinoma.

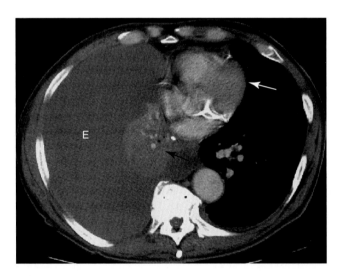

Figure 4-5 Atelectasis and effusion. A balance exists between a large pleural effusion (*E*) and atelectasis of the right lung (*solid black arrow*) so that there is no significant resultant shift of the mobile midline structures. The heart remains in essentially its normal position (*solid white arrow*). This combination of findings is highly suggestive of a central bronchogenic malignancy with a malignant effusion.

TABLE 4-2 RECOGNIZING A "SHIFT" IN ATELECTASIS/PNEUMONECTOMY

Structure	Normal Position	Right-Sided Atelectasis or Pneumonectomy	Left-Sided Atelectasis or Pneumonectomy
Heart	Midline	Heart moves rightward; left heart border may come to lie near left side of spine	Heart moves leftward; right heart border overlaps the spine
Trachea	Midline	Shifts toward right	Shifts toward left
Hemidiaphragm	Right slightly higher than left	Right hemidiaphragm moves upward and may disappear (silhouette sign)	Left hemidiaphragm moves upward and may disappear (silhouette sign)

TABLE 4-3 RECOGNIZING A "SHIFT" IN PLEURAL EFFUSION

Structure	Normal Position	Right-Sided Effusion	Left-Sided Effusion
Heart	Midline	Heart moves leftward; apex may lie near chest wall	Heart moves rightward; more of heart protrudes to right of spine
Trachea	Midline	Shifts toward left	Shifts toward right
Hemidiaphragm	Right higher than left	Right hemidiaphragm disappears on chest radiograph (silhouette sign)	Left hemidiaphragm disappears on chest radiograph (silhouette sign)

TABLE 4-4 RECOGNIZING A "SHIFT" IN PNEUMONIA

Structure	Normal Position	Right-Sided Pneumonia	Left-Sided Pneumonia
Heart	Midline	The heart usually does not shift from its normal position	The heart usually does not shift from its normal position
Trachea	Midline	Midline	Midline
Hemidiaphragm	Right higher than left	Right hemidiaphragm may disappear on chest radiograph (silhouette sign)	Left hemidiaphragm may disappear on chest radiograph (silhouette sign)

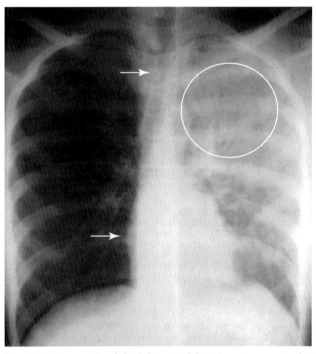

Figure 4-6 Pneumonia of the left upper lobe. There is near-complete opacification of the left hemithorax with no shift of the heart and little shift of the trachea (*solid white arrows*). Air bronchograms are suggested within the upper area of opacification (*circle*). These findings suggest a pneumonia rather than atelectasis or pleural effusion. The patient had *Streptococcus pneumoniae* present in the sputum and improved quickly on antibiotics.

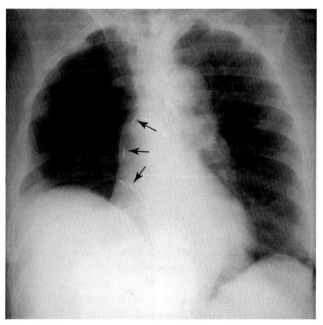

Figure 4-7 Postpneumonectomy day 1, right lung. A pneumonectomy is the removal of the entire lung. This postoperative radiograph was obtained less than 24 hours after this patient underwent a pneumonectomy on the right side for a bronchogenic carcinoma. Surgical clips are in the region of the right hilum (*solid black arrows*), and the right 5th rib has been surgically removed in order to perform the pneumonectomy. Over the next several weeks, the right hemithorax will fill with fluid, and the heart and mediastinal structures will gradually shift toward the side of the pneumonectomy (see Fig. 4-8).

- So let's return to the frontal radiograph of Mr. Smith with the opacified hemithorax, who has been waiting patiently in the Emergency Department while you read this chapter.
  - Now, how would you proceed with his abnormality?
    - You'll notice a shift of the heart and trachea **toward** the side of opacification (Fig. 4-9).
    - This is characteristic of **atelectasis of the entire right lung**.

- Mr. Smith had a CT scan performed, which showed a large mass in the right hilum that was bronchoscopically proven to be bronchogenic carcinoma.

WEBLINK

Registered users may obtain more information on Recognizing the Causes of an Opacified Hemithorax on StudentConsult. com.

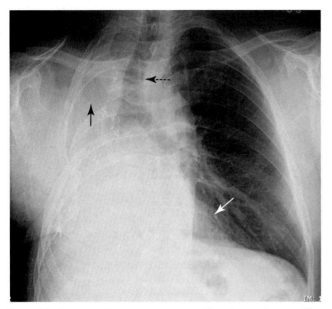

Figure 4-8 One year after pneumonectomy. There is complete opacification of the right hemithorax. The right 5th rib (*solid black arrow*) is surgically absent. The heart (*solid white arrow*) and trachea (*dotted black arrow*) are deviated towards the side of opacification. These signs are characteristic of volume loss. The surgery had been performed one year earlier for a bronchogenic carcinoma. The fluid that gradually filled the right hemithorax immediately following the pneumonectomy has probably fibrosed, leading to a permanent shift towards the pneumonectomized side.

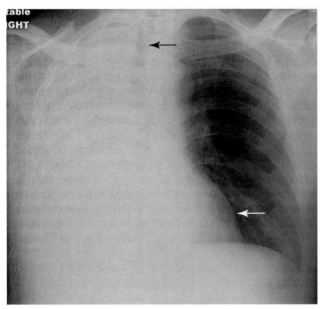

Figure 4-9 Mr. Smith's frontal chest radiograph. The entire right hemithorax is opacified. The trachea has shifted toward the right (*solid black arrow*), and the heart is displaced toward the right as well (*solid white arrow*). Both of these mobile structures have moved toward the side of opacification. These signs are characteristic of atelectasis of the entire right lung and in a patient like Mr. Smith, who is 73, a bronchogenic carcinoma is the most likely diagnosis. An obstructing carcinoma was found at bronchoscopy in the right main bronchus.

TAKE-HOME POINTS

Recognizing the Causes of an Opacified Hemithorax

The differential possibilities for an opacified hemithorax should include atelectasis of the entire lung, a very large pleural effusion, pneumonia of the entire lung, or post-pneumonectomy.

The trachea, heart, and hemidiaphragms are mobile structures that have the capability of moving (*shifting*) if there is either something pushing on them or something pulling them.

With atelectasis, there is a shift **toward** the side of the opacified hemithorax because of volume loss in the affected lung.

With a large pleural effusion, there is a shift **away** from the side of opacification because the large pleural effusion can act as if it were a mass.

With pneumonia of an entire lung, there is usually **no shift**, but air bronchograms may be present.

Occasionally, the shift of a malignant effusion may be balanced by the opposite shift of atelectasis caused by an underlying, obstructing bronchogenic carcinoma so that the hemithorax will be completely opaque but there will be no shift.

In the post-pneumonectomy patient, there is eventually volume loss on the side from which the lung has been removed, and the clues to such surgery may include surgical absence of the 5th or 6th rib on the affected side or metallic surgical clips in the hilum.

Chapter 5

Recognizing Atelectasis

WHAT IS ATELECTASIS?

- Common to all forms of atelectasis is a **loss of volume in some or all of the lung, usually leading to increased density of the lung involved.**
  - The lung normally appears "black" on a chest radiograph because it contains air. When something of fluid or soft tissue density is substituted for that air or when the air in the lung is resorbed (as it can be in atelectasis), that part of the lung becomes whiter (more dense or more opaque).
- Unless mentioned otherwise, statements in this chapter that refer to "atelectasis" are referring to *obstructive atelectasis*. This might be a good time to review the chart from Chapter 4 (see Table 4-1) highlighting the markedly different appearances of the thorax in a large pneumothorax and atelectasis of the entire lung (see Fig. 4-2).

SIGNS OF ATELECTASIS

- **Displacement (shift) of the interlobar fissures** (major and minor) toward the area of atelectasis.
- **Increase in the density of the affected lung** (Fig. 5-1).
- **Displacement (shift) of the mobile structures of the thorax.**
  - The **mobile structures** are those capable of movement due to changes in lung volume.
    - Trachea
      - **Normally midline in location** and centered on the spinous processes of the vertebral bodies (also midline structures) on a nonrotated, frontal chest x-ray. **A slight rightward deviation of the trachea is always present at the site of the left-sided aortic knob.**
      - With atelectasis, especially of the upper lobes, the trachea may shift toward the side of the volume loss (Fig. 5-2).
    - Heart
      - **At least 1 cm of the right heart border normally projects to the right of the spine** on a nonrotated, frontal radiograph.
      - With atelectasis, especially of the lower lobes, the heart may shift to one side or the other.
        - When the heart shifts toward the left, the right heart border will overlap the spine (Fig. 5-3).
        - When the heart shifts toward the right, the left heart border will approach the midline (Fig. 5-4).
    - Hemidiaphragm
      - The **right hemidiaphragm is almost always higher than the left** by about half the interspace

distance between two adjacent ribs. In about 10% of normal people, the left hemidiaphragm is higher than the right.
      - In the presence of atelectasis, especially of the lower lobes, the hemidiaphragm on the affected side will usually be displaced upward (Fig. 5-5).
- **Overinflation of the unaffected ipsilateral lobes or the contralateral lung.**
  - The greater the volume loss and the more chronic its presence, the more the lung on the side **opposite** the atelectasis or the **unaffected lobe(s) in the ipsilateral lung** will attempt to **overinflate** to compensate for the volume loss.
  - This may be noticeable on the lateral projection by an **increase in the size of the retrosternal clear space** and on the frontal projection by **extension of the overinflated contralateral lung across the midline** (Fig. 5-6).
- The signs of atelectasis are summarized in Box 5-1.

TYPES OF ATELECTASIS

- **Subsegmental atelectasis** (also called *discoid atelectasis* or *platelike atelectasis*) (Fig. 5-7)
  - **Subsegmental atelectasis produces linear densities of varying thickness usually parallel to the diaphragm,** most commonly **at the lung bases**.
    - It does not produce a sufficient amount of volume loss to cause a shift of the mobile thoracic structures.
  - It occurs **mostly in patients who are "splinting,"** i.e., not taking a deep breath, such as **postoperative patients** or patients with **pleuritic chest pain**.
  - **Subsegmental atelectasis is not due to bronchial obstruction.**
    - It is most likely related to **deactivation of surfactant**, which leads to collapse of airspaces in a nonsegmental or nonlobar distribution.
  - On a single study, without prior examinations for comparison, subsegmental atelectasis and **chronic, linear scarring can look identical.** Subsegmental atelectasis **typically disappears within a matter of days** with resumption of normal deep breathing whereas **scarring remains**.
- Compressive atelectasis
  - Loss of volume due to **passive compression of the lung** can be caused by:
    - A poor inspiratory effort in which passive atelectasis of the lung is seen at the bases (Fig. 5-8).
    - A **large pleural effusion, large pneumothorax,** or a **space-occupying lesion** (such as a large mass in the lung).

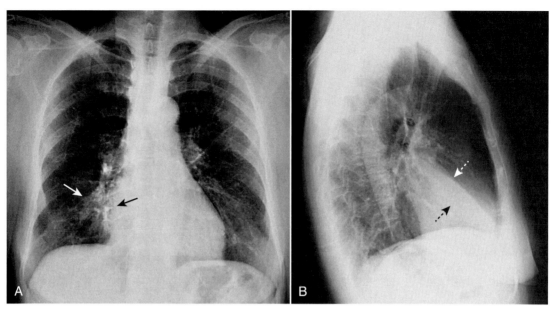

Figure 5-1 Right middle lobe atelectasis. Frontal **(A)** and lateral **(B)** views of the chest show an area of increased density (*solid white arrow*), which is silhouetting the normal right heart border (*solid black arrow*) indicating its anterior location in the right middle lobe. On the lateral view **(B)**, the minor fissure is displaced downward (*dotted white arrow*) and the major fissure is displaced slightly upward (*dotted black arrow*). Note the anterior location of the middle lobe.

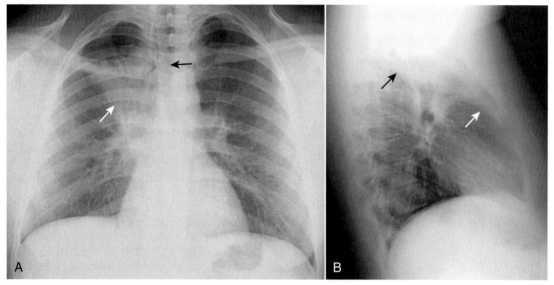

Figure 5-2 Right upper lobe atelectasis. A fan-shaped area of increased density is seen on the frontal projection **(A)** representing the airless right upper lobe. The minor fissure is displaced upward (*solid white arrow*). The trachea is shifted to the right (*solid black arrow*). The lateral **(B)** demonstrates a similar wedge-shaped density near the apex of the lung. The minor fissure (*solid white arrow*) is pulled upward and the major fissure is pulled forward (*solid black arrow*). This is a child who had asthma leading to formation of a mucous plug, which obstructed the right upper lobe bronchus.

- When caused by a poor inspiratory effort, passive atelectasis may mimic airspace disease at the bases.

 Pitfall: Be suspicious of compressive atelectasis if the patient has taken less than an 8 posterior-rib breath.

- **Solution:** Check the lateral projection for confirmation of the presence of real airspace disease at the base.
- When caused by a large effusion or pneumothorax, the loss of volume associated with compressive atelectasis may balance the increased volume produced by either fluid (as in pleural effusion) or air (as in pneumothorax).

- In an adult patient with an **opacified hemithorax, no air bronchograms and little or no shift of the mobile thoracic structures**, it is important to **suspect an obstructing bronchogenic carcinoma**, perhaps with metastases to the pleura (Fig. 5-9).
- **Round atelectasis**
  - This form of compressive atelectasis is **usually seen at the periphery of the lung base** and develops from a **combination of prior pleural disease** (such as from asbestos exposure or tuberculosis) **and the formation of a pleural effusion that produces adjacent compressive atelectasis.**

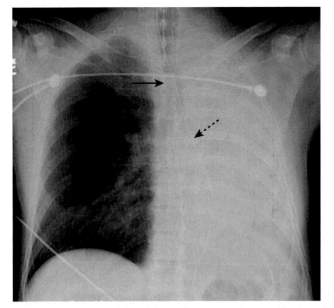

Figure 5-3 Atelectasis of the left lung. There is complete opacification of the left hemithorax with shift of the trachea (*solid black arrow*) and the esophagus (marked here by a nasogastric tube, *dotted black arrow*) toward the side of the atelectasis. The right heart border, which should project about a centimeter to the right of the spine, has been pulled to the left side and is no longer visible. The patient had an obstructing bronchogenic carcinoma in the left main bronchus.

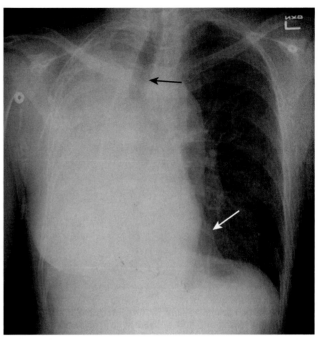

Figure 5-4 Atelectasis of the right lung. There is complete opacification of the right hemithorax with shift of the trachea (*solid black arrow*) toward the side of the atelectasis. The left heart border is displaced far to the right and now almost overlaps the spine (*solid white arrow*). This patient had an endobronchial metastasis in the right main bronchus from her left-sided breast cancer. Did you notice the left breast was surgically absent?

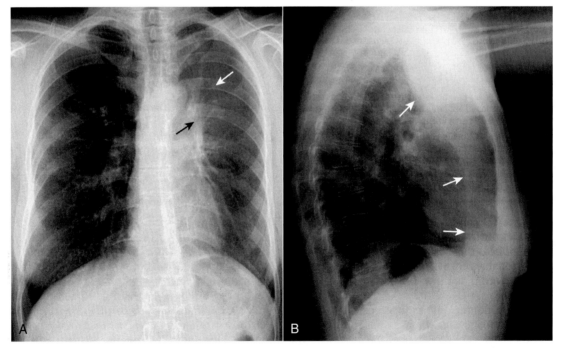

Figure 5-5 Left upper lobe atelectasis. On the frontal projection **(A)**, there is a hazy density surrounding the left hilum (*solid white arrow*) and there is a soft tissue mass in the left hilum (*solid black arrow*). Notice how the left hemidiaphragm has been pulled up to the same level as the right. The lateral projection **(B)** shows a bandlike zone of increased density (*solid white arrows*) representing the atelectatic left upper lobe sharply demarcated by the major fissure, which has been pulled anteriorly. The patient had a squamous cell carcinoma of the left upper lobe bronchus that was producing complete obstruction of that bronchus.

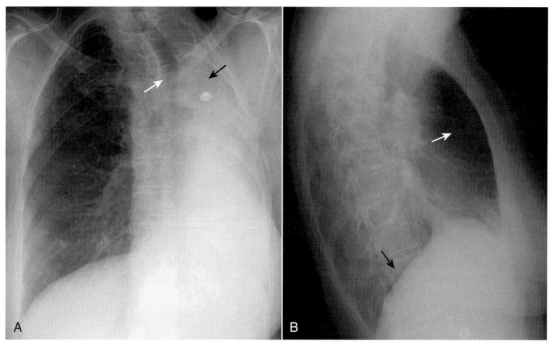

Figure 5-6 Left-sided pneumonectomy. Complete opacification of the left hemithorax **(A)** is most likely from a fibrothorax produced following complete removal of the lung. There is associated marked volume loss with shift of the trachea to the left (*solid white arrow*). The left 5th rib was surgically removed during the pneumonectomy (*solid black arrow*). The right lung has herniated across the midline in an attempt to "fill-up" the left hemithorax, which is seen by the increased lucency behind the sternum in **(B)** (*solid white arrow*). Notice that because only the right hemithorax has an aerated lung remaining, only the right hemidiaphragm is visible on the lateral projection (*solid black arrow*). The left hemidiaphragm has been silhouetted by the airless hemithorax above it.

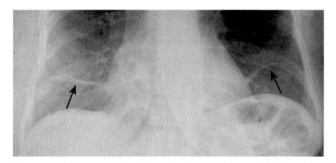

Figure 5-7 Subsegmental atelectasis. Close-up view of the lung bases demonstrates several linear densities extending across all segments of the lower lobes, paralleling the diaphragm (*solid black arrows*). This is a characteristic appearance of *subsegmental atelectasis,* sometimes also called *discoid atelectasis* or *platelike atelectasis.* The patient was postoperative from abdominal surgery and was unable to take a deep breath. The atelectasis disappeared within a few days after surgery.

Box 5-1 Signs of Atelectasis

Displacement of the major or minor fissure*

Increased density of the atelectatic portion of lung

Shift of the mobile structures in the thorax, i.e., the heart, trachea, and/or hemidiaphragms*

Compensatory overinflation of the unaffected segments, lobes, or lung

*Toward the atelectasis.

- When the pleural effusion recedes, the underlying pleural disease leads to a portion of the **atelectatic lung becoming "trapped."** This **produces a masslike lesion** that can be confused for a tumor.
- On CT scan of the chest, the bronchovascular markings characteristically lead from the *round atelectasis* back to the hilum producing a *comet-tail appearance* (Fig. 5-10).

- Obstructive atelectasis (see Fig. 5-3)
  - Obstructive atelectasis is associated with the **resorption of air from the alveoli,** through the pulmonary capillary bed, **distal to an obstructing lesion** of the bronchial tree.
    - The rate at which air is absorbed and the lung collapses depends on its gas content when occluded. It takes about **18-24 hours for an entire lung to collapse** with the patient breathing room air but **less than an hour** with the patient breathing near 100% oxygen.
  - The **affected segment, lobe, or lung collapses** and becomes more opaque (whiter) because it contains no air. The **collapse leads to volume loss** in the affected segment/lobe/lung.
  - Because the visceral and parietal pleura invariably remain in contact with each other as the lung loses volume, the **mobile structures of the thorax are *pulled toward* the area of atelectasis.**
- The types of atelectasis are summarized in Table 5-1.

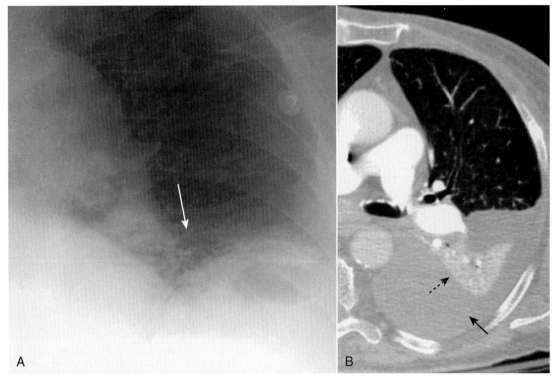

Figure 5-8 Compressive (passive) atelectasis. Passive compression of the lung can occur either from a poor inspiratory effort **(A),** which is manifest as increased density at the lung bases (*solid white arrow*) or secondary to a large pleural effusion or pneumothorax **(B).** Axial CT scan of the chest showing only the left hemithorax **(B)** demonstrates a large left pleural effusion (*solid black arrow*). The left lower lobe (*dotted black arrow*) is atelectatic, having been compressed by the pleural fluid surrounding it.

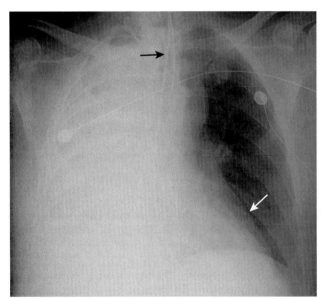

Figure 5-9 Atelectasis and effusion in balance, an ominous combination. There is complete opacification of the right hemithorax. There are neither air bronchograms to suggest pneumonia nor any shift of the trachea (*solid black arrow*) or heart (*solid white arrow*). The absence of any shift suggests the possibility of atelectasis and pleural effusion in balance, a combination that should raise suspicion for a central bronchogenic carcinoma (producing obstructive atelectasis) with metastases (producing a large pleural effusion).

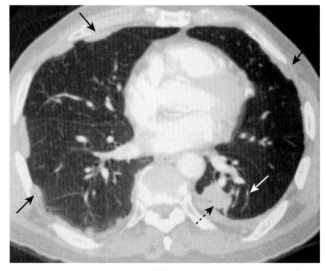

Figure 5-10 Round atelectasis, left lower lobe. There is a masslike density in the left lower lobe (*dotted black arrow*). The patient has underlying pleural disease in the form of pleural plaques from asbestos exposure (*solid black arrows*). There are comet-tail shaped bronchovascular markings that emanate from the "mass" and extend back to the hilum (*solid white arrow*). This combination of findings is characteristic of round atelectasis and should not be mistaken for a tumor.

Recognizing Atelectasis

TABLE 5-1 TYPES OF ATELECTASIS

Type	Associated With	Remarks
Subsegmental atelectasis	Splinting, especially in postoperative patients and those with pleuritic chest pain	May be related to deactivation of surfactant; does not usually lead to volume loss; disappears in days
Compressive atelectasis	Passive external compression of the lung from poor inspiration, pneumothorax, or pleural effusion	Volume loss of compressive atelectasis can balance volume increase from effusion or pneumothorax resulting in no shift; round atelectasis is a form of compressive atelectasis
Obstructive atelectasis	Obstruction of a bronchus from malignancy or mucus plugging	Visceral and parietal pleura maintain contact; mobile structures in the thorax are pulled toward the atelectasis

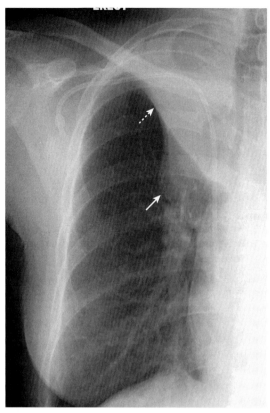

Figure 5-11 **Right upper lobe atelectasis and hilar mass:** *S sign of Golden.* There is a soft tissue mass in the right hilum (*solid white arrow*). There is opacification of the right upper lobe from atelectasis. The minor fissure is displaced upward toward the area of increased density (*dotted white arrow*), indicating right upper lobe volume loss. The shape of the curved edge formed by the mass and the elevated minor fissure is called the *S sign of Golden.* The patient had a large squamous cell carcinoma obstructing the right upper lobe bronchus.

PATTERNS OF COLLAPSE IN LOBAR ATELECTASIS

- Obstructive atelectasis produces **consistently recognizable patterns of collapse** depending on the location of the atelectatic segment or lobe and the degree to which such factors as collateral airflow between lobes and obstructive pneumonia allow the affected lobe to collapse.
- In general, lobes collapse in a fanlike configuration with the **base** of the fan-shaped triangle **anchored at the pleural surface and the apex of the triangle anchored at the hilum**.
- Other unaffected lobes will undergo compensatory hyperinflation in an attempt to "fill" the affected hemithorax, and this hyperinflation may limit the amount of shift of the mobile chest structures.

⚠ **Pitfall:** The **more atelectatic a lobe or segment becomes** (that is, the smaller its volume), the **less visible it becomes on the chest radiograph**. This can lead to the false assumption of improvement when, in fact, the atelectasis is worsening.

- **Solution:** This can usually be resolved with a careful analysis of the study to check for the degree of displacement of the interlobar fissures or hemidiaphragms or with a CT scan of the chest.
- **Right upper lobe atelectasis** (see Fig. 5-2)
  - On the frontal radiograph:
    - There is an upward shift of the minor fissure.
    - There is a rightward shift of the trachea.
  - On the lateral radiograph:
    - There is an upward shift of the minor fissure and a forward shift of the major fissure.
  - If right upper lobe atelectasis is produced by a large enough mass in the right hilum, the combination of the hilar mass and the upward shift of the minor fissure produces a characteristic appearance on the frontal radiograph named the *S sign of Golden* (Fig. 5-11).
- **Left upper lobe atelectasis** (see Fig. 5-5)

- On the frontal radiograph:
  - There is a hazy area of increased density around the left hilum.
  - There is a leftward shift of the trachea.
  - There may be elevation with "**tenting**" (**peaking**) of the left hemidiaphragm.
  - Compensatory overinflation of the lower lobe may cause the superior segment of the left lower lobe to extend to the apex of the thorax on the affected side.
- On the lateral radiograph:
  - There is forward displacement of the major fissure, and the opacified upper lobe forms a band of increased density running roughly parallel to the sternum.
- **Lower lobe atelectasis** (Fig. 5-12)
  - On the frontal radiograph:
    - Both the right and left lower lobes collapse to form a triangular density that extends from its apex at the hilum to its base at the medial portion of the affected hemidiaphragm.
    - Elevation of the hemidiaphragm is seen on the affected side.
    - The heart may shift toward the side of the volume loss.
    - On the right (only), there is a downward shift of the minor fissure.

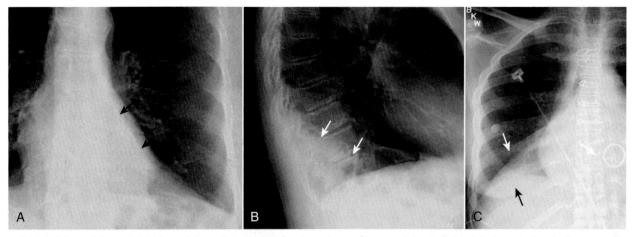

Figure 5-12 Left lower lobe and right lower lobe atelectasis. A, A fan-shaped area of increased density behind the heart is sharply demarcated by the medially displaced major fissure (*solid black arrows*) representing the characteristic appearance of left lower lobe atelectasis. **B,** On the lateral view, the major fissure (*solid white arrows*) is displaced posteriorly. The small triangular density in the posterior costophrenic sulcus is in the characteristic location for left lower lobe atelectasis on the lateral projection. **C,** In a different patient there is a fan-shaped triangular density in the right lower lobe bounded superiorly by the major fissure (*solid white arrow*). Notice how the unaerated lower lobe silhouettes the right hemidiaphragm (*solid black arrow*).

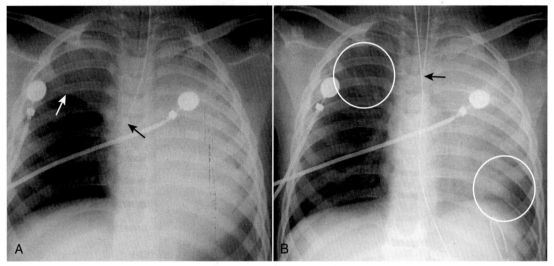

Figure 5-13 Right upper lobe and left lung atelectasis from an endotracheal tube. A, The tip of the endotracheal tube extends beyond the carina into the bronchus intermedius (*solid black arrow*), which aerates only the right middle and lower lobes. The right upper lobe and entire left lung are opaque from atelectasis. The minor fissure is elevated (*solid white arrow*). **B,** One hour later, the tip of the endotracheal tube has been retracted above the carina (*solid black arrow*) and the right upper lobe and a portion of the left lower lobe are again aerated (*white circles*).

- On the lateral radiograph:
  - There is both downward and posterior displacement of the major fissure until the completely collapsed lower lobe forms a small triangular density at the posterior costophrenic angle.

 In the critically-ill patient, atelectasis occurs most frequently in the left lower lobe.

  - **Always check that the left hemidiaphragm is seen in its entire extent** through the heart since **left lower lobe atelectasis will manifest by disappearance (silhouetting) of all or part of the left hemidiaphragm** (see Fig. 5-12).
- **Right middle lobe atelectasis** (see Fig. 5-1)
  - On the frontal radiograph:
    - There is a triangular density with its base silhouetting the right heart border and its apex pointing toward the lateral chest wall.
    - The minor fissure is displaced downward.

- On the lateral radiograph:
  - There is a triangular density with its base directed anteriorly and its apex at the hilum.
  - The minor fissure may be displaced inferiorly and the major fissure superiorly.
- **Endotracheal tube too low** (Fig. 5-13)
  - If the tip of an endotracheal tube enters the **right lower lobe bronchus**, only the right lower lobe tends to be aerated and remain expanded. Within a short time, atelectasis of the entire left lung and the right upper and middle lobes will develop.
  - Once the tip of the endotracheal tube is withdrawn above the carina, the atelectasis usually clears quite rapidly.
- **Atelectasis of the entire lung** (see Figs. 5-3 and 5-4)
  - On the frontal radiograph:
    - There is opacification of the atelectatic lung due to loss of air.
    - The **hemidiaphragm** on the side of the atelectasis will be **silhouetted** by the nonaerated lung above it.

TABLE 5-2 MOST COMMON CAUSES OF OBSTRUCTIVE ATELECTASIS

Cause	Remarks
Tumors	Includes bronchogenic carcinoma (especially squamous cell), endobronchial metastases, and carcinoid tumors
Mucous plug	Especially in bedridden individuals; postoperative patients; those with asthma, cystic fibrosis
Foreign body aspiration	Especially peanuts; toys; following a traumatic intubation
Inflammation	As in scarring caused by tuberculosis

- There is a shift of all of the mobile structures of the thorax is toward the side of the atelectatic lung.
- On the lateral radiograph:
  - The **hemidiaphragm on the side of the atelectasis will be silhouetted by the nonaerated lung above it**. Look closely and you'll see **only one hemidiaphragm** on the lateral exposure, instead of two.

HOW ATELECTASIS RESOLVES

- Depending in part on the rapidity with which the segment, lobe, or lung became atelectatic, atelectasis has the capacity to **resolve within hours or last for many days once the obstruction has been removed**.
- Slowly-resolving lobar or whole-lung atelectasis may manifest patchy areas of airspace disease surrounded by progressively increasing zones of aerated lung until the atelectasis has completely cleared.
- The most common causes of obstructive atelectasis are summarized in Table 5-2.

WEBLINK

Registered users may obtain more information on Recognizing Atelectasis on StudentConsult.com.

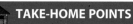

TAKE-HOME POINTS

Recognizing Atelectasis

Volume loss is common to all forms of atelectasis, but the radiographic appearance of atelectasis will differ depending on the type of atelectasis.

The three most commonly observed types of atelectasis are subsegmental atelectasis (also known as discoid or platelike atelectasis), compressive or passive atelectasis, and obstructive atelectasis.

Subsegmental atelectasis usually occurs in patients who are not taking a deep breath (splinting) and produces horizontal linear densities, usually at the lung bases.

Compressive atelectasis occurs passively when the lung is collapsed by a poor inspiration (at the bases), or from a large, adjacent pleural effusion or pneumothorax. When the underlying abnormality is removed, the lung usually expands.

Round atelectasis is a type of passive atelectasis in which the lung does not re-expand when a pleural effusion recedes, usually due to pre-existing pleural disease. Round atelectasis may produce a masslike lesion that can mimic a tumor on chest radiographs.

Obstructive atelectasis occurs distal to an occluding lesion of the bronchial tree because of reabsorption of the air in the distal airspaces via the pulmonary capillary bed.

Obstructive atelectasis produces consistently recognizable patterns of collapse based on the assumptions that the visceral and parietal pleura invariably remain in contact with each other and every lobe of the lung is anchored at or near the hilum.

Signs of obstructive atelectasis include displacement of the fissures, increased density of the affected lung, shift of the mobile structures of the thorax toward the atelectasis, and compensatory overinflation of the unaffected ipsilateral or contralateral lung.

Atelectasis tends to resolve quickly if it occurs acutely; the more chronic the process, the longer it usually takes to resolve.

Chapter 6

Recognizing a Pleural Effusion

NORMAL ANATOMY AND PHYSIOLOGY OF THE PLEURAL SPACE

- Normal anatomy
  - The **parietal pleura lines the inside of the thoracic cage** and the **visceral pleura adheres to the surface of the lung** parenchyma, including its interface with the mediastinum and diaphragm (see Chapter 2, *The Normal Frontal Chest Radiograph*). The **enfolds of the visceral pleura form the interlobar fissures**—the **major (oblique)** and **minor (horizontal)** on the right, only the major on the left. The space between the visceral and parietal pleura, i.e., the *pleural space*, is a potential space normally containing only about 2-5 mL of pleural fluid.
- Normal physiology
  - Normally, several hundred milliliters of pleural fluid are produced and reabsorbed each day. **Fluid is produced primarily at the parietal pleura** from the pulmonary capillary bed and is **resorbed at the visceral pleura and by lymphatic drainage through the parietal pleura**.

CAUSES OF PLEURAL EFFUSIONS

- Fluid accumulates in the pleural space when the rate at which the fluid forms exceeds the rate by which it is cleared.
  - **The rate of formation may be increased by**:
    - Increasing hydrostatic pressure, as in left heart failure.
    - Decreasing colloid osmotic pressure, as in hypoproteinemia.
    - **Increasing capillary permeability**, as can occur in toxic disruption of the capillary membrane in pneumonia or hypersensitivity reactions.
  - **The rate of resorption can decrease** by:
    - Decreased absorption of fluid by lymphatics, either from lymphangitic blockade by tumor or from increased venous pressure, which decreases the rate of fluid transport via the thoracic duct.
    - **Decreased pressure in the pleural space**, as in atelectasis of the lung due to bronchial obstruction.
- Pleural effusions **can also form when there is transport of peritoneal fluid from the abdominal cavity** through the diaphragm or via lymphatics from a subdiaphragmatic process (Table 6-1).

TYPES OF PLEURAL EFFUSIONS

- Pleural effusions are **divided into exudates or transudates**, depending on their **protein content** and their **lactate dehydrogenase (LDH) concentrations**.

- **Transudates** tend to form when there is **increased capillary hydrostatic pressure or decreased osmotic pressure**, such as occurs in:
  - **Congestive heart failure**, primarily left heart failure, which is the most common cause of a transudative pleural effusion
  - **Hypoalbuminemia**
  - **Cirrhosis**
  - **Nephrotic syndrome**
- Exudates
  - **Most common cause of an exudative pleural effusion is malignancy.**
  - **Empyema**—an exudate containing pus
  - **Hemothorax**—has a fluid hematocrit >50% blood hematocrit
  - **Chylothorax**—contains increased triglycerides or cholesterol

SIDE SPECIFICITY OF PLEURAL EFFUSIONS

- Certain diseases tend to produce pleural effusions on one side or the other, or bilaterally.
- Diseases that usually produce **bilateral effusions**:
  - Congestive heart failure
    - Usually about the same amount of fluid in each hemithorax.
    - If **markedly** different amounts are in each hemithorax, suspect a **parapneumonic effusion** or **malignancy** on the side with the greater volume of fluid.
  - **Lupus erythematosus**—usually bilateral, but when unilateral, the effusions are usually left-sided.
- Diseases that can produce effusions on either side (but are usually unilateral):
  - **Tuberculosis** and other exudative effusions associated with infectious agents, including viruses
  - **Pulmonary thromboembolic disease**
  - **Trauma**
- Diseases that usually produce **left-sided effusions**:
  - **Pancreatitis**
  - **Distal thoracic duct obstruction**
  - **Dressler syndrome** (Box 6-1, Fig. 6-1)
- Diseases that usually produce **right-sided effusions**:
  - **Abdominal disease related to the liver or ovaries**—some ovarian tumors can be associated with a right pleural effusion and ascites (*Meigs syndrome*)
  - **Rheumatoid arthritis**—the effusion can remain unchanged for years
  - **Proximal thoracic duct obstruction**

RECOGNIZING THE DIFFERENT APPEARANCES OF PLEURAL EFFUSIONS

■ Forces that influence the appearance of pleural fluid on a chest radiograph depend on the position of the patient, the force of gravity, the amount of fluid and the degree of elastic recoil of the lung.

■ The descriptions that follow, unless otherwise indicated, assume the patient is in the upright position.

TABLE 6-1 SOME CAUSES OF PLEURAL EFFUSIONS

Cause	Examples
Excess formation of fluid	Congestive heart failure Hyponatremia Parapneumonic effusions Hypersensitivity reactions
Decreased resorption of fluid	Lymphangitic blockade from tumor Elevated central venous pressure Decreased intrapleural pressure
Transport from peritoneal cavity	Ascites

Box 6-1 Dressler Syndrome

Postpericardiotomy/postmyocardial infarction syndrome

Typically occurs 2-3 weeks after a transmural myocardial infarct producing a left pleural effusion, pericardial effusion, and patchy airspace disease at the left lung base

Associated with chest pain and fever, it usually responds to high-dose aspirin or steroids

---

Subpulmonic Effusions

■ It is believed that **almost all pleural effusions first collect in a subpulmonic location beneath the lung** between the parietal pleura lining the superior surface of the diaphragm and the visceral pleura under the lower lobe.

■ If the effusion remains entirely subpulmonic in location, it can be difficult to detect on conventional radiographs except for contour alterations in what appears to be the hemidiaphragm but is actually the fluid-lung interface beneath the lung.

■ The different appearances of subpulmonic effusions are summarized in Table 6-2 (Figs. 6-2 and 6-3).

➡ Subpulmonic does not mean loculated.

• Most **subpulmonic effusions flow freely** as the patient changes position.

Blunting of the Costophrenic Angles

■ As the subpulmonic effusion grows in size, it first fills and *blunts* the **posterior costophrenic sulcus**, visible on the lateral view of the chest (Fig. 6-4).
  • This occurs with approximately **75 mL of fluid**.

■ **When the effusion reaches about 300 mL in size, it blunts the lateral costophrenic angle**, visible on the frontal chest radiograph (Fig. 6-5).

⚠ **Pitfall:** Pleural thickening caused by fibrosis can also produce blunting of the costophrenic angle.

• **Solutions:** Scarring sometimes produces a characteristic *ski-slope appearance* of blunting, unlike the meniscoid appearance of a pleural effusion (Fig. 6-6).

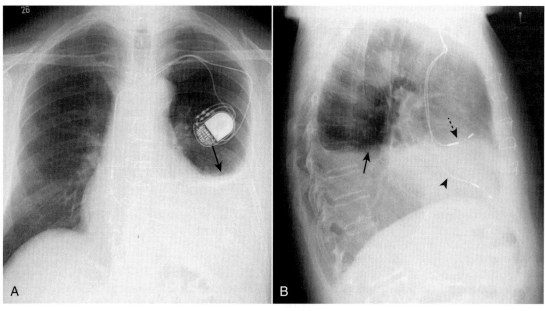

Figure 6-1 Dressler syndrome (postpericardiotomy/postmyocardial infarction syndrome). A left pleural effusion **(A)** is present (*solid black arrows*). This syndrome typically occurs 2 to 3 weeks after a transmural myocardial infarct. It also can occur following pericardiotomy such as occurs in patients undergoing coronary artery bypass surgery, as in this case. The combination of chest pain and fever, left pleural effusion, patchy left lower lobe airspace disease, and pericardial effusion several weeks following a myocardial infarction or open-heart surgery should suggest the syndrome. It usually responds to high-dose aspirin or steroids. This patient has a dual lead pacemaker in place and, on the lateral projection **(B),** the leads are seen in the region of the right atrium (*dotted black arrow*) and right ventricle (*arrowhead*).

TABLE 6-2 RECOGNIZING A SUBPULMONIC EFFUSION

Right-Sided Findings (Fig. 6-2)		Left-Sided Findings (Fig. 6-3)	
Frontal View	**Lateral View**	**Frontal View**	**Lateral View**
The highest point of the apparent hemidiaphragm* is displaced more laterally than the highest point of a normal hemidiaphragm would be. These are more difficult to recognize than left-sided subpulmonic effusions because the liver is the same density as the pleural fluid above it.	Posteriorly, the apparent hemidiaphragm has a curved arc, but as it meets the junction with the major fissure, the apparent hemidiaphragm* assumes a flat edge that drops sharply to the anterior chest wall.	The distance between the stomach bubble and the apparent left hemidiaphragm is increased (should normally be only about 1 cm from top of stomach bubble to bottom of aerated left lower lobe). The highest point of the apparent hemidiaphragm* is displaced more laterally than the highest point of a normal hemidiaphragm would be.	Posteriorly, the apparent hemidiaphragm has a curved arc, but as it meets the junction with the major fissure, the apparent hemidiaphragm* assumes a flat edge that drops sharply to the anterior chest wall.

Apparent hemidiaphragm is the term used because the shadow being cast is actually from the subpulmonic fluid interfacing with the lung. The actual hemidiaphragm is invisible, silhouetted by the soft tissue in the abdomen below it and the pleural fluid above it.

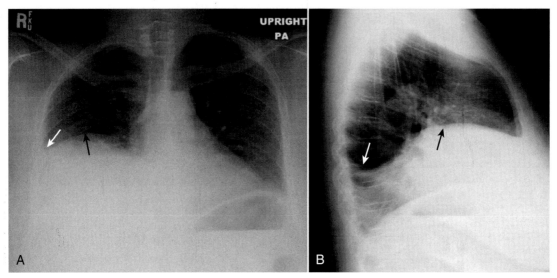

Figure 6-2 Right-sided subpulmonic effusion. In the frontal projection **(A)**, the apparent right hemidiaphragm appears to be elevated (*solid black arrow*). This edge does not represent the actual right hemidiaphragm, which has been rendered invisible by the pleural fluid that has accumulated above it, but the interface between the effusion and the base of the lung (thus the term "apparent hemidiaphragm"). There is blunting of the right costophrenic sulcus (*solid white arrow*). On the lateral projection **(B)**, there is blunting of the posterior costophrenic sulcus (*solid white arrow*). The apparent hemidiaphragm is rounded posteriorly but then changes its contour as the effusion interfaces with the major fissure on the left side (*solid black arrow*).

- **Pleural thickening will not change in location** with a change in patient position, as most effusions will.

The Meniscus Sign

- Because of the natural elastic recoil of the lungs, **pleural fluid appears to rise higher along the lateral margin of the thorax than it does medially** in the frontal projection. This produces a characteristic *meniscus* shape to the effusion.
- In the lateral projection, the fluid assumes a U-shape ascending equally high both anteriorly and posteriorly (Fig. 6-7).
  - Identifying an abnormal lung density that demonstrates a meniscoid shape is strongly suggestive of a pleural effusion.
- Effect of patient positioning on the appearance of pleural fluid:
  - In the **upright position**, pleural fluid falls to the base of the thoracic cavity due to the force of gravity.

- In the **supine position**, the same free-flowing effusion will layer along the posterior pleural space and produce a homogeneous "haze" over the entire hemithorax when viewed *en face* (Fig. 6-8).
- When the patient is **semirecumbent**, pleural fluid will form a triangular density of varying thickness at the lung base with the apex, or thinnest part, of the triangle ascending to varying heights, depending on how recumbent the patient is and how much fluid is present.

⚠ **Pitfall:** Depending on the patient's degree of recumbence, the upper lung fields may appear clearer if the patient is upright and the fluid settles to the base of the thorax or denser (whiter) as the patient becomes more recumbent and the effusion begins to layer posteriorly. This change in appearance can occur with the same volume of pleural fluid redistributed because of patient positioning.

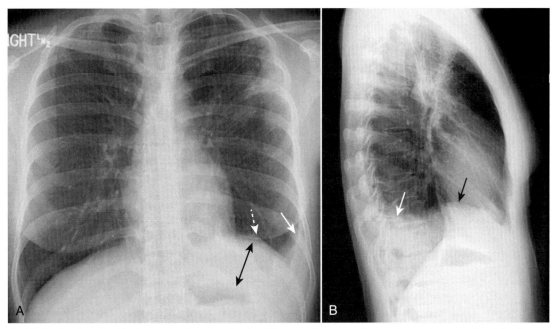

Figure 6-3 **Left-sided subpulmonic effusion.** In the frontal projection **(A),** more than 1 cm distance is seen between the air in the stomach and the apparent left hemidiaphragm (*double black arrow*). The edge between the aerated lung and the *dotted white arrow* does not represent the actual left hemidiaphragm, which has been rendered invisible by the pleural fluid that has accumulated above it, but the interface between the effusion and the base of the lung. There is blunting of the left costophrenic sulcus (*solid white arrow*) on both projections. On the lateral projection **(B),** the apparent hemidiaphragm is rounded posteriorly but then changes its contour as the effusion interfaces with the major fissure (*solid black arrow*).

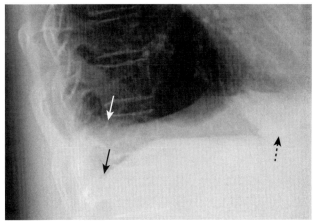

Figure 6-4 **Blunting of the right posterior costophrenic sulcus on the lateral projection.** When approximately 75 mL of fluid has accumulated in the pleural space, the fluid will typically blunt the posterior costophrenic sulcus (angle) first (*solid white arrow*). This can be visualized only on the lateral projection. A normal, sharp posterior costophrenic angle is visible on the opposite side (*solid black arrow*). Notice how the normal left hemidiaphragm is silhouetted by the heart anteriorly (*dotted black arrow*) indicating that is the left hemidiaphragm. The pleural effusion is on the right side.

- **Solution:** In the best of all worlds, each portable chest radiograph would be exposed with the patient in the same position.
- ■ **The lateral decubitus view of the chest**
  - The effect of patient positioning on the location of pleural fluid can be used for diagnostic advantage by having the patient lie on the side containing the effusion while taking a chest exposure using an x-ray beam directed horizontally.
  - If the patient lies on the right side, it is called a *right lateral decubitus.* If he lies on the left side, it is called a *left lateral decubitus* view of the chest.
  - Decubitus views can be used to:
    - Confirm the presence of a pleural effusion.
    - Determine whether a pleural effusion flows freely in the pleural space or not, an important factor to know before attempting to drain pleural fluid.
    - "Uncover" a portion of the underlying lung hidden by the effusion.
  - If a pleural effusion can flow freely in the pleural space, the fluid will produce a characteristic **bandlike area of increased density along the inner margin of the chest cage on the dependent side of the body**.

  ⇨ With a **right lateral decubitus view of the chest,** the patient's right side will be dependent and a **right pleural effusion will layer** along the dependent surface. With a **left lateral decubitus view of the chest,** the patient's left side will be dependent and a **left pleural effusion will layer** along the dependent surface (Fig. 6-9).

  - Pleural fluid **may not flow freely** in the pleural space **if adhesions are present** that might impede the free flow of the fluid (see "Loculated Effusions").

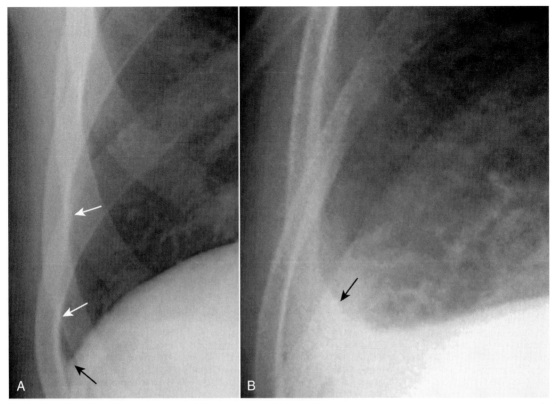

Figure 6-5 Normal and blunted right lateral costophrenic angle. The hemidiaphragm usually makes a sharp and acute angle as it meets the lateral chest wall on the frontal projection **(A)** to produce the lateral costophrenic sulcus (*solid black arrow*). Notice how normally aerated lung extends to the inner margin of each of the ribs (*solid white arrows*). When an effusion reaches about 300 mL in volume **(B),** the lateral costophrenic sulcus loses its acute angulation and becomes **blunted** (*solid black arrow*).

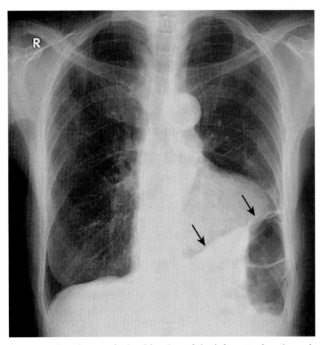

Figure 6-6 Scarring producing blunting of the left costophrenic angle. Scarring from such things as previous infection, surgery, or blood in the pleural space sometimes produces a characteristic "ski-slope appearance" of blunting (*solid black arrows*), unlike the meniscoid appearance of a pleural effusion. This fibrosis would not change in appearance or location with a change in the patient's position, as free-flowing pleural fluid would.

- **Decubitus views** of the chest **can demonstrate effusions as small as 15-20 mL** but CT scans of the chest have largely supplanted decubitus views in detecting very small amounts of pleural fluid.

⚠️ **Pitfall:** Don't order a lateral decubitus view of the chest if the entire hemithorax is opacified since there can be no change in the position of the fluid and the underlying lung will be no more visible in the decubitus position than it was with the patient upright. CT scan of the chest is a better means of evaluating the underlying lung if the hemithorax is opacified.

Opacified Hemithorax

- When **the hemithorax of an adult contains about 2 L of fluid, the entire hemithorax will be opacified** (Fig. 6-10).
- As fluid fills the pleural space, the lung tends to undergo passive collapse (atelectasis) (see Chapter 5).
- **Large effusions are sufficiently opaque** on conventional chest radiographs **so as to mask whatever disease may be present in the lung** enveloped by them. **CT is the modality usually employed** to visualize the underlying lung.
- **Large effusions** act like a mass and **displace the heart and trachea away** from the **side of opacification** (see Fig. 6-10).

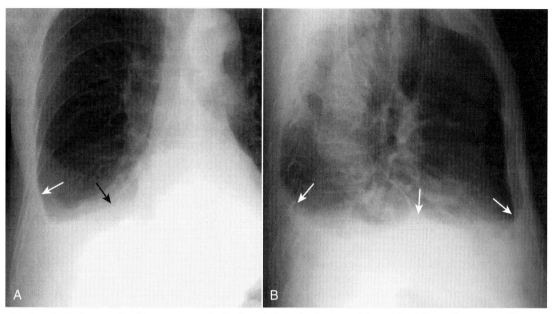

Figure 6-7 **Right pleural effusion, meniscoid appearance.** On the frontal projection in the upright position **(A),** an effusion typically ascends more laterally (*solid white arrow*) than it does medially (*solid black arrow*) because of factors affecting the natural elastic recoil of the lung. On the lateral projection **(B)** the fluid ascends about the same amount anteriorly and posteriorly, forming a U-shaped, meniscoid density (*solid white arrows*).

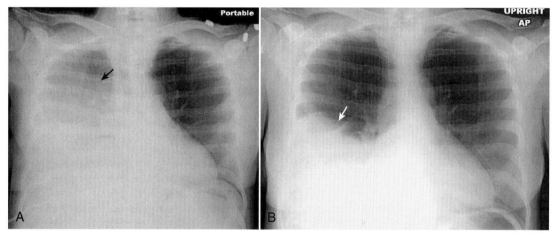

Figure 6-8 **Effect of patient positioning on the appearance of a pleural effusion.** In the recumbent position **(A),** the right-sided effusion layers along the posterior pleural surface and produces a "haze" over the entire hemithorax that is densest at the base and less dense toward the apex of the lung (*solid black arrow*). In the same patient x-rayed a few minutes later in a more upright position **(B),** pleural fluid falls to the base of the thoracic cavity due to the force of gravity (*solid white arrow*). This simple change in position can produce the mistaken impression that an effusion has improved (or worsened if the supine study follows the upright examination) when there has actually been no change in the amount of pleural fluid. Ideally, the patient should be x-rayed in the same position each time for a meaningful comparison.

- For more on the opacified hemithorax, go to Chapter 4, *Recognizing the Causes of an Opacified Hemithorax.*

LOCULATED EFFUSIONS

- **Adhesions in the pleural space**, caused most often by old empyema or hemothorax, **may limit the normal mobility of a pleural effusion**, so that it remains in the same location no matter what position the patient assumes.
- **Imaging findings**
  - Loculated effusions **can be suspected when an effusion has an unusual shape or location in the thorax**, e.g.,

the effusion defies gravity by remaining at the apex of the lung even though the patient is upright (Fig. 6-11).

- **Loculation of pleural fluid has therapeutic importance** since such collections tend to be traversed by multiple adhesions that make it difficult to drain the noncommunicating pockets of fluid with a single pleural drainage tube in the same way free-flowing effusions can be drained.

Fissural Pseudotumors

- *Pseudotumors* (also called *vanishing tumors*) are **sharply marginated collections of pleural fluid** contained between

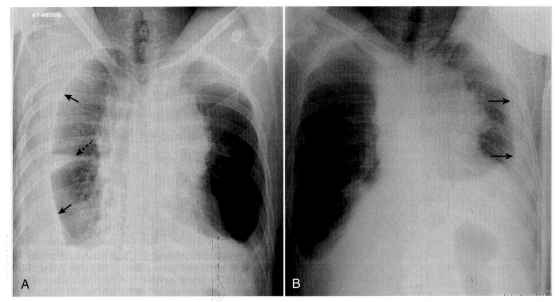

Figure 6-9 Decubitus views of the chest. A, A right lateral decubitus view of the chest. The film is exposed with the patient lying on the right side on the examining table while a horizontal x-ray beam is directed posteroanteriorly (PA). Because the patient's right side is dependent, any free-flowing pleural fluid will layer along the right side (*solid black arrows*), forming a bandlike density. Notice how the fluid flows into the minor fissure (*dotted black arrow*). **B,** A left lateral decubitus view of the chest. When the same patient lies on the table with the left side down, free fluid on the left side layers along the left lateral chest wall (*solid black arrows*). This patient has pleural effusions from lymphoma.

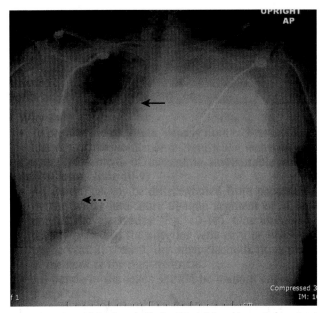

Figure 6-10 Large left pleural effusion. The left hemithorax is completely opacified, and the mobile mediastinal structures such as the trachea (*solid black arrow*) and the heart (*dotted black arrow*) have **shifted away** from the side of opacification. This is characteristic of a large pleural effusion, which acts like a mass. In most adults, about 2 L of fluid is required to fill or almost fill the entire hemithorax such as this.

the layers of an **interlobar pulmonary fissure** or in a subpleural location just beneath the fissure.

- They are **transudates** that **almost always occur in patients with congestive heart failure (CHF)**.
- The imaging findings of a pseudotumor are characteristic so that they should not be mistaken for an actual tumor (from which they derive their name).
  - They are **lenticular in shape**, most often occur in the **minor fissure (75%)** and frequently have **pointed ends**

on each side where they insinuate into the fissure, much like the shape of a lemon. They **do not tend to flow freely** with a change in patient positioning.

- They **disappear when the underlying condition (usually CHF) is treated**, but they **tend to recur in the same location** each time the patient's failure recurs (Fig. 6-12).

Laminar Effusions

- A laminar effusion is a form of pleural effusion in which the fluid assumes **a thin, bandlike density along the lateral chest wall, especially near the costophrenic angle**. Unlike a usual pleural effusion, the lateral costophrenic angle tends to maintain its acute angle with a laminar effusion.
- Laminar effusions are **almost always the result of** elevated left atrial pressure, as in **CHF** or secondary to **lymphangitic spread of malignancy**. They are **usually not free-flowing**.
- They can be recognized by the band of increased density that separates the air-filled lung from the inside margin of the ribs at the lung base on the frontal chest radiograph.
  - In normal subjects, aerated lung should extend to the inside of each contiguous rib (Fig. 6-13).

Hydropneumothorax

- The presence of **both** air in the pleural space (pneumothorax) **and** abnormal amounts of fluid in the pleural space (pleural effusion or hydrothorax) is called a *hydropneumothorax*.
- Some of the more common causes of a hydropneumothorax are **trauma**, **surgery**, or a **recent tap to remove pleural fluid** in which air enters the pleural space.
  - *Bronchopleural fistula*, an abnormal and relatively uncommon connection between the bronchial tree and

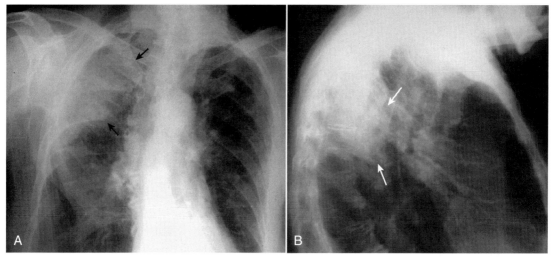

Figure 6-11 **Loculated pleural effusion in frontal (A) and lateral (B) projections.** A pleural-based soft tissue density in the right upper lung field represents a loculated pleural effusion (*solid black arrows* in **A** and *solid white arrows* in **B**). Loculated effusions can be suspected when an effusion has an unusual shape or location in the thorax; for example, the effusion defies gravity by remaining at the apex of the lung even though the patient is upright.

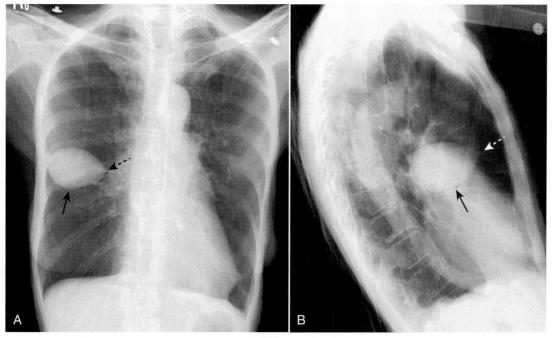

Figure 6-12 **Pseudotumor in the minor fissure, frontal (A) and lateral (B) projection.** A sharply marginated collection of pleural fluid contained between the layers of the minor fissure produces a characteristic lenticular shape (*solid black arrows* in **A** and **B**) that frequently has pointed ends on each side where it insinuates into the fissure so that pseudotumors look like a lemon on frontal **(A)** or lateral **(B)** chest radiographs (*dotted black arrow* on **A** and *dotted white arrow* on **B**). Pseudotumors almost always occur in patients with congestive heart failure and, although the pseudotumors disappear when the underlying condition is treated, they frequently return each time the patient's failure recurs.

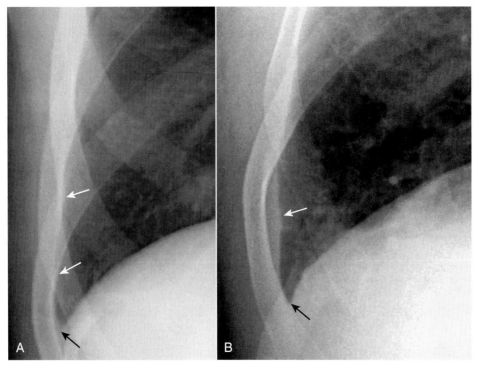

Figure 6-13 Normal patient versus laminar pleural effusion. In **A,** which is a normal patient, notice how normally aerated lung extends to the inner margin of each of the ribs (*solid white arrows*). The costophrenic sulcus is sharp (*closed black arrow*). In **B,** a thin band of increased density extends superiorly from the lung base (*solid white arrow*) but does not appear to cause blunting of the costophrenic angle (*solid black arrow*). This is the appearance of a **laminar pleural effusion** that is most often associated with either congestive heart failure or lymphangitic spread of malignancy in the lung. This patient was in congestive heart failure.

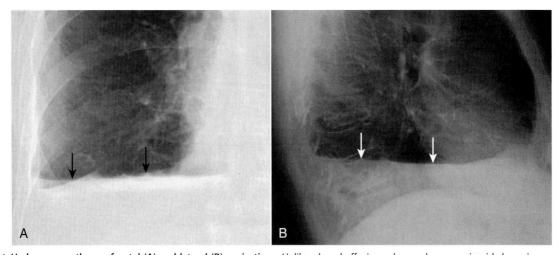

Figure 6-14 Hydropneumothorax, frontal (A) and lateral (B) projections. Unlike pleural effusions alone, whose meniscoid shape is governed by the elastic recoil of the lung, hydropneumothorax produces an air-fluid level in the hemithorax (*solid black arrows* in **A** and *solid white arrows* in **B**) marked by a straight edge and a sharp, air-over-fluid interface when the exposure is made with a horizontal x-ray beam. Surgery, trauma, a recent thoracentesis to remove pleural fluid, and bronchopleural fistulae are among the causes of a hydropneumothorax. This person was stabbed in the right side. This actually represents a hemopneumothorax, but conventional radiography is unable to distinguish between blood and any other fluid. A pleural tap might be necessary to better define the pleural fluid.

the pleural space most often due to tumor, surgery or infection, can also produce both air and fluid in the pleural space.

- Unlike pleural effusion alone, whose mensicoid shape is governed by the elastic recoil of the lung, a **hydropneumothorax produces an air-fluid level in the hemithorax** marked by a straight edge and a sharp, air-over-fluid interface when the exposure is made with a horizontal x-ray beam (Fig. 6-14).
- CT is frequently necessary to distinguish between some presentations of hydropneumothorax and a **lung abscess**, both of which may have a similar appearance on conventional chest radiographs.

WEBLINK

Registered users may obtain more information on Recognizing a Pleural Effusion on StudentConsult.com.

 TAKE-HOME POINTS

Recognizing a Pleural Effusion

Pleural effusions collect in the potential space between the visceral and parietal pleura and are either transudates or exudates depending on their protein content and LDH concentration.

There are normally a few milliliters of fluid in the pleural space; about 75 mL are required to blunt the posterior costophrenic sulcus (seen on the lateral view) and about 200-300 mL to blunt the lateral costophrenic sulcus (seen on the frontal view); approximately 2 L of fluid will cause opacification of the entire hemithorax in an adult.

Whether an effusion is unilateral or bilateral, mostly right-sided or mostly left-sided, can be an important clue as to its etiology.

Most pleural effusions begin life collecting in the pleural space between the hemidiaphragm and the base of the lung; these are called **subpulmonic effusions**.

As the amount of fluid increases, it forms a **meniscus** shape on the upright frontal chest radiograph due to the natural elastic recoil properties of the lung.

Very large pleural effusions act like a mass and characteristically produce a shift of the mobile mediastinal structures (e.g., the heart) away from the side of the effusion.

In the absence of pleural adhesions, effusions will flow freely and change location with a change in the patient's position; with pleural adhesions (usually from old infection or hemothorax) the fluid may assume unusual appearances or occur in atypical locations; such effusions are said to be **loculated**.

A **pseudotumor** is a type of effusion that occurs in the fissures of the lung (mostly the minor fissure) and is most frequently secondary to congestive heart failure; it clears when the underlying failure is treated.

Laminar effusions are best recognized at the lung base just above the costophrenic angles on the frontal projection and most often occur as a result of either congestive heart failure or lymphangitic spread of malignancy.

A **hydropneumothorax** consists of both air and increased fluid in the pleural space and is recognizable on an upright view of the chest by a straight, air-fluid interface rather than the typical meniscus shape of pleural fluid alone.

Chapter 7

Recognizing Pneumonia

GENERAL CONSIDERATIONS

- Pneumonia can be defined as **consolidation of lung produced by inflammatory exudate, usually as a result of an infectious agent.**
- **Most pneumonias produce airspace disease, either lobar or segmental.**
- Other **pneumonias demonstrate interstitial disease,** and others produce findings in both the airspaces and the interstitium.
- Most microorganisms that produce pneumonia are **spread to the lungs via the tracheobronchial tree, either through inhalation or aspiration** of the organisms.
- In some instances, microorganisms are spread via the bloodstream and in even fewer cases, by direct extension.
- Because many different microorganisms can produce similar imaging findings in the lungs, it is **difficult to identify with certainty the causative organism from the radiographic presentation alone.**
  - However, **certain patterns** of disease are **very suggestive** of a particular causative organism (Table 7-1).
  - Some use the term "infiltrate" synonymously with pneumonia, although many diseases, from amyloid to pulmonary fibrosis, can infiltrate the lung

GENERAL CHARACTERISTICS OF PNEUMONIA

- Because **pneumonia** fills the involved airspaces or interstitial tissues with some form of fluid or inflammatory exudate, pneumonias **appear denser (whiter) than the surrounding, normally aerated lung.**
- **Pneumonia may contain air bronchograms** if the bronchi themselves are not filled with inflammatory exudate or fluid (see Fig. 3-3).
- Air bronchograms are **much more likely to be visible when the pneumonia involves the central portion** of the lung near the hilum. Near the periphery of the lung, the bronchi are usually too small to be visible (Fig. 7-1).
- Remember that anything of fluid or soft tissue density that replaces the normal gas in the airspaces may also produce this sign, so **an air bronchogram is not specific for pneumonia** (see Chapter 3, *Recognizing Airspace versus Interstitial Lung Disease*).
- Pneumonia that involves the airspaces **appears fluffy** and its **margins are indistinct.**
  - **Where pneumonia abuts a pleural surface,** such as an interlobar fissure or the chest wall, **it will be sharply marginated.**
- **Interstitial pneumonia,** on the other hand, may produce prominence of the interstitial markings in the affected part

of the lung or may spread to adjacent airways and resemble airspace disease.
- Except for the presence of air bronchograms, airspace **pneumonia is usually homogeneous in density** (Fig. 7-2).
- In some types of pneumonia (i.e., bronchopneumonia), **the bronchi, as well as the airspaces, contain inflammatory exudate.** This can lead to **atelectasis associated with the pneumonia.**
  - Box 7-1 summarizes the keys to recognizing pneumonia.

PATTERNS OF PNEUMONIA

- Pneumonias may be distributed in the lung in several patterns described as *lobar*, *segmental*, *interstitial*, *round*, and *cavitary* (Table 7-2).
- Remember, these are terms that simply describe the distribution of the disease in the lungs; they aren't diagnostic of pneumonia because many other diseases can produce the same patterns of disease distribution in the lung.

Lobar Pneumonia

- The **prototypical lobar pneumonia is pneumococcal pneumonia** caused by *Streptococcus pneumoniae* (Fig. 7-3).
- Although we are calling it lobar pneumonia, the patient may present before the disease involves the entire lobe. In its most classic form, the disease fills most or all of a lobe of the lung.
- Because lobes are bound by interlobar fissures, **one or more of the margins of a lobar pneumonia may be sharply marginated.**
- Where the disease is not bound by a fissure, it will have an **indistinct and irregular margin.**
- Lobar pneumonias almost always produce a *silhouette sign* where they come in contact with the heart, aorta, or diaphragm, and they almost always contain *air bronchograms* if they involve the central portions of the lung.

Segmental Pneumonia (Bronchopneumonia)

- The **prototypical bronchopneumonia is caused by *Staphylococcus aureus*.** Many gram-negative bacteria, such as *Pseudomonas aeruginosa*, can produce the same picture.
- Brochopneumonias are spread centrifugally via the tracheobronchial tree to **many foci in the lung at the same time.** Therefore **they frequently involve several segments** of the lung simultaneously.

TABLE 7-1 PATTERNS THAT MIGHT SUGGEST A CAUSATIVE ORGANISM

Pattern of Disease	Likely Causative Organism
Upper lobe cavitary pneumonia with spread to the opposite lower lobe	*Mycobacterium* tuberculosis (TB)
Upper lobe lobar pneumonia with bulging interlobar fissure	*Klebsiella pneumoniae*
Lower lobe cavitary pneumonia	*Pseudomonas aeruginosa* or anaerobic organisms (*Bacteroides*)
Perihilar interstitial disease or perihilar airspace disease	*Pneumocystis carinii (jiroveci)*
Thin-walled upper lobe cavity	*Coccidioides* (Coccidiomycosis), TB
Airspace disease with effusion	*Streptococci, staphylococci,* TB
Diffuse nodules	*Histoplasma, Coccidioides, Mycobacterium tuberculosis* (histoplasmosis, coccidiomycosis, TB)
Soft-tissue, fingerlike shadows in upper lobes	*Aspergillus* (allergic bronchopulmonary aspergillosis)
Solitary pulmonary nodule	*Cryptococcus* (cryptococcosis)
Spherical soft-tissue mass in a thin-walled upper lobe cavity	*Aspergillus* (aspergilloma)

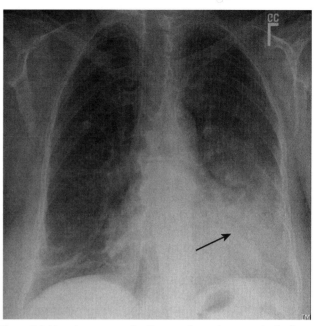

Figure 7-2 Lingular pneumonia. Airspace disease is present in the lingular segments of the left upper lobe. The disease is of homogeneous density. The disease is in contact with the left lateral border of the heart, which is "silhouetted" by the fluid density of the consolidated upper lobe in contact with the soft tissue density of the heart (*solid black arrow*).

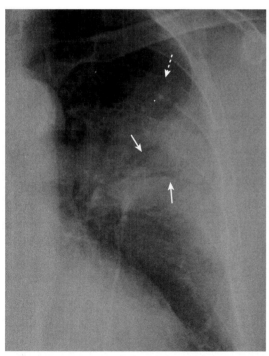

Figure 7-1 Left upper lobe pneumonia. Several black, branching structures are seen in this upper lobe pneumonia (*solid white arrows*) that represent typical **air bronchograms** seen centrally in airspace disease in this patient with pneumococcal pneumonia. The disease is homogeneous in density, except for the presence of the air bronchograms. Because this is airspace disease, its outer edges are poorly marginated and fluffy (*dotted white arrow*).

Box 7-1 Recognizing a Pneumonia—Key Signs

More opaque than surrounding normal lung.

In airspace disease, the margins may be fluffy and indistinct except where they abut a pleural surface like the interlobar fissures where the margin will be sharp.

Interstitial pneumonias will cause a prominence of the interstitial tissues of the lung in the affected area; in some cases, the disease can spread to the alveoli and resemble airspace disease.

Pneumonia tends to be homogeneous in density.

Lobar pneumonias may contain air bronchograms.

Segmental pneumonias may be associated with atelectasis in the affected portion of the lung.

TABLE 7-2 PATTERNS OF APPEARANCE OF PNEUMONIAS

Pattern	Characteristics
Lobar	Homogeneous consolidation of affected lobe with air bronchogram
Segmental (bronchopneumonia)	Patchy airspace disease frequently involving several segments simultaneously; no air bronchogram; atelectasis may be associated
Interstitial	Reticular interstitial disease usually diffusely spread throughout the lungs early in the disease process; frequently progresses to airspace disease
Round	Spherically shaped pneumonia usually seen in the lower lobes of children that may resemble a mass
Cavitary	Produced by numerous microorganisms, chief among them being *Mycobacterium tuberculosis*

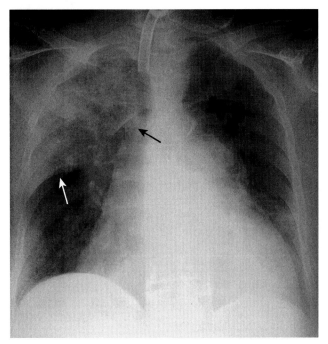

Figure 7-3 Right upper lobe pneumococcal pneumonia. Airspace disease is visible in the right upper lobe and occupies all of that lobe. Because lobes are bounded by interlobar fissures, in this case the minor or horizontal fissure (*solid white arrow*) produces a sharp margin on the inferior aspect of the pneumonia. Where the disease contacts the ascending aorta (*solid black arrow*), the border of the aorta is silhouetted by the fluid-density of the pneumonia.

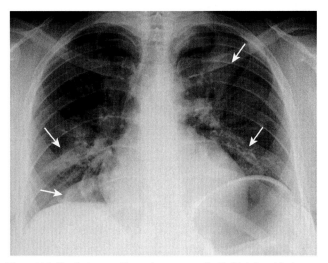

Figure 7-4 Staphylococcal bronchopneumonia. Multiple irregularly marginated patches of airspace disease are present in both lungs (*solid white arrows*). This is a characteristic distribution and appearance of bronchopneumonia. The disease is spread centrifugally via the tracheobronchial tree to many foci in the lung at the same time so it frequently involves several segments. Because lung segments are not bound by fissures, the margins of segmental pneumonias tend to be fluffy and indistinct. No air bronchograms are present because inflammatory exudate fills the bronchi as well as the airspaces around them.

- Because lung segments are not bound by fissures, all of the **margins of segmental pneumonias tend to be fluffy and indistinct** (Fig. 7-4).
- Unlike lobar pneumonia, **segmental bronchopneumonias produce exudate that fills the bronchi.**
  - Therefore, **air bronchograms are usually not present,** and frequently some **volume loss (atelectasis)** is associated with bronchopneumonia.

Interstitial Pneumonia

- The **prototypes for interstitial pneumonia are viral pneumonia,** *Mycoplasma pneumoniae,* and **Pneumocystis pneumonia** in patients with AIDS.
- Interstitial pneumonias **tend to involve the airway walls and alveolar septa** and may produce, especially early in their course, a **fine, reticular pattern in the lungs.**
- Most **interstitial pneumonias eventually spread to the adjacent alveoli** and produce patchy or confluent airspace disease, **making the original interstitial nature of the pneumonia impossible to recognize** radiographically.

 Pneumocystis carinii (jiroveci) pneumonia (PCP)

- PCP is the **most common** clinically recognized infection in patients with acquired immunodeficiency syndrome (AIDS).
- It classically presents as a **perihilar, reticular interstitial pneumonia** or as **airspace disease that may mimic the central distribution pattern of pulmonary edema** (Fig. 7-5).

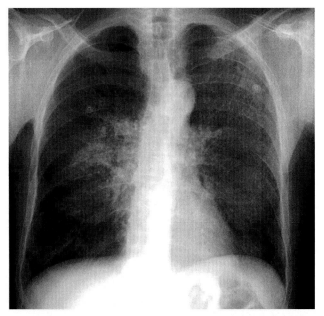

Figure 7-5 *Pneumocystis carinii* (jiroveci) pneumonia (PCP). Diffuse interstitial lung disease is seen, which is primarily reticular in nature. Without the additional history that this patient had acquired immunodeficiency syndrome (AIDS), this could be mistaken for pulmonary interstitial edema or a chronic, fibrotic process such as sarcoidosis. No pleural effusions are present, as might be expected with pulmonary interstitial edema, and there is no evidence of hilar adenopathy, as might occur in sarcoid.

- Other presentations, such as unilateral airspace disease or widespread, patchy airspace disease, are less common.
- There are usually **no pleural effusions** and **no hilar adenopathy.**
- Opportunistic infections **usually occur with CD4 counts under 200** per cubic mL of blood.

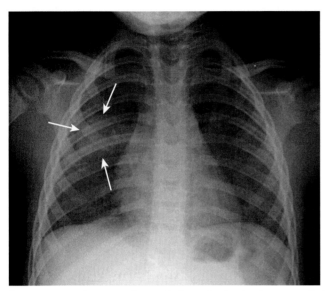

Figure 7-6 **Round pneumonia.** A soft tissue density that has a rounded appearance (*solid white arrows*) is seen in the right midlung field. The patient is a 10-month-old baby who had a cough and fever. This is a characteristic appearance of a round pneumonia, most common in children and frequently due to either *Haemophilus*, streptococcal, or pneumococcal infection.

Round Pneumonia

- Some pneumonias, mostly in children, can assume a **spherical shape** on chest radiographs.
- These *round pneumonias* are almost always **posterior** in the lungs, usually **in the lower lobes.**
- Causative agents include *Haemophilus influenzae, Streptococcus,* and *Pneumococcus.*
- A round pneumonia could be confused with a tumor mass except that symptoms associated with infection usually accompany the pulmonary findings and tumors are uncommon in children (Fig. 7-6).

Cavitary Pneumonia

 The prototypical organism producing cavitary pneumonia is *Mycobacterium tuberculosis.*

- **Primary tuberculosis (primary TB)**
  - Cavitation is rare in primary TB.
  - Primary TB **affects the upper lobes slightly more than the lower** and produces airspace disease that **may be associated with ipsilateral hilar adenopathy** (especially in children) and **large, often unilateral, pleural effusions** (especially in adults) (Fig. 7-7).
- **Post-primary tuberculosis (reactivation tuberculosis)**
  - Cavitation is common.
  - The cavity is usually **thin-walled** and has a **smooth inner margin** and **no air-fluid level** (Fig. 7-8).
  - Post-primary tuberculosis almost always **affects the apical or posterior segments of the upper lobes or the superior segments of the lower lobes.**
  - **Bilateral upper lobe disease is very common.**
  - **Transbronchial spread** (from one upper lobe to the opposite lower lobe or to another lobe in the lung) **should make you think of infection with *Mycobacterium tuberculosis.***

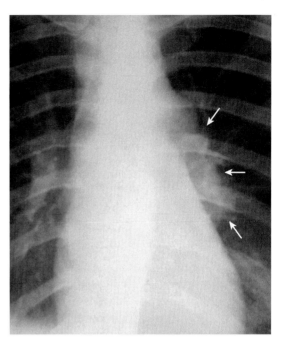

Figure 7-7 **Primary tuberculosis.** There is prominence of the left hilum that is caused by left hilar adenopathy (*solid white arrows*). Unilateral hilar adenopathy may be the only manifestation of primary infection with *Mycobacterium tuberculosis*, especially in children. When it produces pneumonia, primary TB affects the upper lobes slightly more than the lower. It produces airspace disease that may be associated with ipsilateral hilar adenopathy (especially in children) and large, often unilateral, pleural effusions (especially in adults).

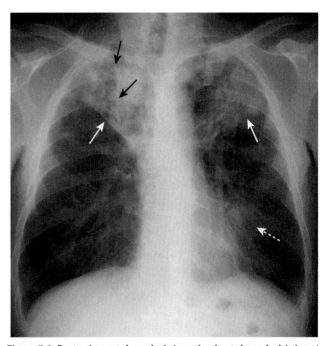

Figure 7-8 **Post-primary tuberculosis (reactivation tuberculosis).** A cavitary pneumonia is present in both upper lobes (*solid white arrows*). Numerous lucencies (cavities) are seen throughout the airspace disease in the right upper lobe (*solid black arrows*). A cavitary upper lobe pneumonia is presumptively TB, until proven otherwise. In addition, airspace disease is seen in the lingula (*dashed white arrow*), another finding suggestive of TB, a disease which can spread via a transbronchial route to the opposite lower lobe or another lobe in the lung.

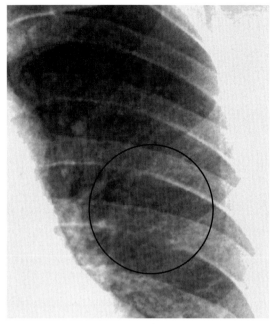

Figure 7-9 Miliary tuberculosis. Innumerable small round nodules are present in this close-up of the left lung in a patient with miliary tuberculosis (*black circle*). At the start of the disease, the nodules are so small they are frequently difficult to detect on conventional radiographs. When they reach about 1 mm or more in size, they begin to become visible. Miliary tuberculosis will clear relatively rapidly with appropriate treatment and does not heal with calcification.

- Healing of post-primary TB usually occurs with fibrosis and retraction.
■ Miliary tuberculosis
  - Considered to be a manifestation of primary TB, although the clinical appearance of miliary TB may not occur for many years after the initial infection.
  - When first visible, the **small nodules measure only about 1 mm in size**; they can grow to 2-3 mm if untreated (Fig. 7-9).
  - **When miliary TB is treated, clearing is usually rapid. Miliary TB seldom,** if ever, **heals with residual calcification**.
■ **Other infectious agents** that produce cavitary disease:
  - **Staphylococcal pneumonia** can cavitate and produce thin-walled *pneumatocoeles*.
  - *Streptococcal* pneumonia, *Klebsiella* pneumonia, **and coccidiomycosis** can also produce cavitating pneumonias.

ASPIRATION

■ There are many causes of aspiration of foreign material into the tracheobronchial tree, among them neurologic disorders (stroke, traumatic brain injury), altered mental status (anesthesia, drug overdose), gastroesophageal reflux, and postoperative changes from head and neck surgery.
■ Aspiration almost always occurs in the **most dependent portions of the lung.**
  - When the person is **upright,** the most dependent portions of the lung will usually be the **lower lobes.**

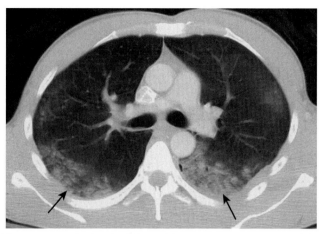

Figure 7-10 Aspiration, both lower lobes. Single, axial CT image of the lungs demonstrates bilateral lower lobe airspace disease in a patient who had aspirated (*solid black arrows*). Aspiration usually affects the most dependent portions of the lung. In the upright position, the lower lobes are affected. In the recumbent position, the superior segments of the lower lobes and the posterior segments of the upper lobes are most involved. Aspiration of water or neutralized gastric acid will usually clear in 24-48 hours depending on the volume aspirated.

TABLE 7-3 THREE PATTERNS OF ACUTE ASPIRATION

Pattern	Characteristics
Bland gastric acid or water	Rapidly appearing and rapidly clearing airspace disease in dependent lobe(s); not a pneumonia
Infected aspirate (aspiration pneumonia)	Usually lower lobes; frequently cavitates and may take months to clear
Unneutralized stomach acid (chemical pneumonitis)	Almost immediate appearance of dependent airspace disease that frequently becomes secondarily infected

- The **right side is more often affected than the left** because of the straighter and wider nature of the right main bronchus.
- When a person is **recumbent,** aspiration usually occurs into the **superior segments of the lower lobes or the posterior segments of the upper lobes.**
- **Acute aspiration** will produce radiographic findings of **airspace disease**.
  - Its location, the rapidity with which it appears, and the group of patients predisposed to aspirate are clues to its etiology (Fig. 7-10).

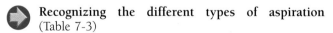 Recognizing the different types of aspiration (Table 7-3)

■ The clinical and radiologic course of aspiration depends on what was aspirated.
  - **Aspiration of bland (neutralized) gastric juices or water**
    - This is technically **not a pneumonia** because it does not involve an infectious agent, is handled by the lungs as if it were pulmonary edema fluid and **classically remains for only a day or two before clearing** through resorption.

- **Aspiration that produces pneumonia due to micro-organisms in the lung**
  - We **routinely aspirate numerous microorganisms present in the normal oropharyngeal flora**, but these microorganisms can develop into pneumonia in some patients such as those who are immunocompromised, elderly, debilitated, or have underlying lung disease.
  - Pneumonia caused by aspiration is usually due to **anaerobic organisms,** such as *Bacteroides.* These organisms produce **lower lobe airspace disease** that **frequently cavitates.** They may take **months to resolve.**
- **Aspiration of unneutralized stomach acid (*Mendelson syndrome*)**
  - When large quantities of unneutralized gastric acid are aspirated, **chemical pneumonitis develops,** producing dependent lobe airspace disease or **pulmonary edema.**
  - The disease may appear quickly, within a few **hours** of the aspiration.
  - Clearing may take **days or longer,** and the chemical pneumonitis is prone to become **secondarily infected.**

radiograph. CT may further localize and characterize the disease as well as demonstrate associated pathology, such as pleural effusions or cavities too small to see on conventional radiographs.
- Sometimes only a frontal radiograph may be available, as with critically ill or debilitated patients who require a portable bedside examination.
- Nevertheless, it is still frequently **possible to localize the pneumonia using only the frontal radiograph** by analyzing which structure's edges are obscured by the disease (i.e., the silhouette sign) (Table 7-4).
- **Silhouette sign** (see also Chapter 3 under "Characteristics of Airspace Disease")
  - If two objects of the **same** radiographic density **touch** each other, then the **edge between them disappears** (see Fig. 7-2).
    - The silhouette sign is valuable in localizing and identifying tissue types throughout the body, not just the chest.
- The *spine sign* (Fig. 7-11)
  - On the lateral chest radiograph, the **thoracic spine normally appears to get darker (blacker) as you survey it from the shoulder girdle to the diaphragm.**

LOCALIZING PNEUMONIA

- An antibiotic will travel to every lobe of the lung without regard for which lobe actually harbors the pneumonia. But determining the location of a pneumonia may provide clues as to the causative organism (e.g., upper lobes, think of TB) and the presence of associated pathology (e.g., lower lobes, think of recurrent aspiration).
- **On conventional radiographs,** it is always **best to localize disease using two views taken at 90° to each other** (*orthogonal views*) like a frontal and lateral chest

TABLE 7-4 USING THE SILHOUETTE SIGN ON THE FRONTAL CHEST RADIOGRAPH

Structure That Is No Longer Visible	Disease Location
Ascending aorta	Right upper lobe
Right heart border	Right middle lobe
Right hemidiaphragm	Right lower lobe
Descending aorta	Left upper or lower lobe
Left heart border	Lingula of left upper lobe
Left hemidiaphragm	Left lower lobe

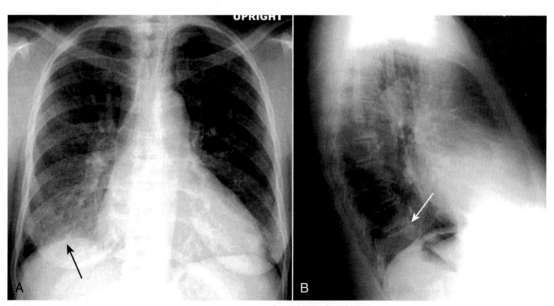

Figure 7-11 The spine sign. Frontal **(A)** and lateral **(B)** views of the chest demonstrate airspace disease on the lateral projection **(B)** in the right lower lobe that may not be immediately apparent on the frontal projection (you can see the pneumonia in the right lower lobe in **(A)** (*solid black arrow*). Normally, the thoracic spine appears to get "blacker" as you view it from the neck to the diaphragm because there is less tissue for the x-ray beam to traverse just above the diaphragm than in the region of the shoulder girdle (see also Fig. 2-3). In this case, a right lower lobe pneumonia superimposed on the lower spine in the lateral view (*solid white arrow*) makes the spine appear "whiter" (more dense) just above the diaphragm. This is called the **spine sign.**

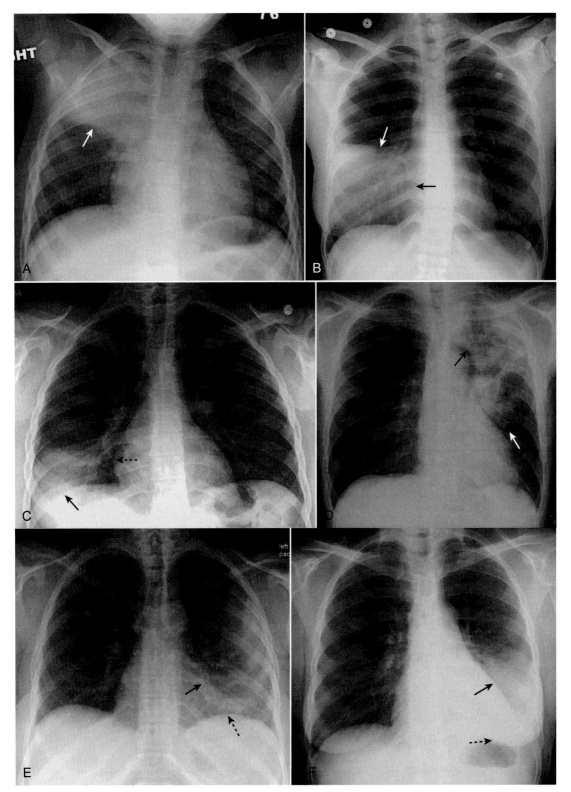

Figure 7-12 Composite appearances of lobar pneumonias. A, Right upper lobe. The disease obscures (silhouettes) the ascending aorta. Where it abuts the minor fissure, it produces a sharp margin (*white arrow*). **B,** Right middle lobe. The disease silhouettes the right heart border (*solid black arrow*). Where it abuts the minor fissure, it produces a sharp margin (*solid white arrow*). **C,** Right lower lobe. The disease silhouettes the right hemidiaphragm (*solid black arrow*). It spares the right heart border (*dotted black arrow*). **D,** Left upper lobe. The disease is poorly marginated (*solid white arrow*) and obscures the aortic knob (*solid black arrow*). **E,** Lingula. The disease silhouettes the left heart border (*solid black arrow*) but spares the left hemidiaphragm (*dotted black arrow*). **F,** Left lower lobe. The disease obscures the left hemidiaphragm (*dotted black arrow*) but spares the left heart border (*solid black arrow*).

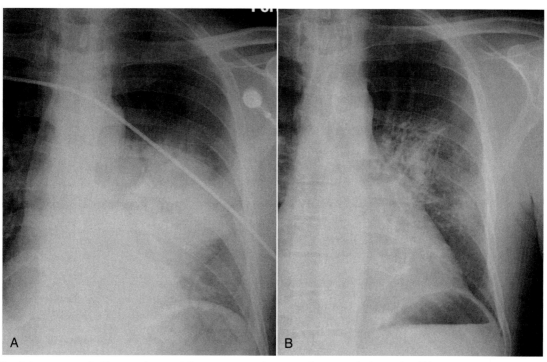

A   B

Figure 7-13 Resolving pneumonia. Pneumonia, especially pneumococcal pneumonia, can resolve in 2-3 days if the organism is sensitive to the antibiotic administered. Most pneumonias, like that in the lingula in radiographs taken four days apart shown in **(A)** and **(B)**, typically resolve from within (vacuolize), gradually disappearing in a patchy fashion over days or weeks. If a pneumonia does not resolve in weeks, you should consider the presence of an underlying obstructing lesion, such as a neoplasm, that is preventing adequate drainage from that portion of the lung.

- This is because the x-ray beam normally needs to penetrate more tissue (more bones, more muscle) around the shoulders than it does just above the diaphragm, where it needs to pass through only the heart and aerated lungs.
- **When disease** of soft tissue or fluid density **involves the posterior portion of the lower lobe**, more of the x-ray beam will be absorbed by the new, added density, and **the spine will appear to become "whiter" (more opaque) just above the posterior costophrenic sulcus.**
  - This is called the *spine sign* and it provides another way to localize disease in the lungs.
- The **lower lobe disease may not be apparent on the frontal projection** if the disease falls below the plane of the highest point of the affected side's hemidiaphragm. Therefore, the *spine sign* **may indicate** the presence of lower lobe disease, like lower lobe pneumonia, **which may be otherwise invisible on the frontal projection.**
- Figure 7-12 is a composite of the characteristic appearances of lobar pneumonia as seen on a frontal chest radiograph.

HOW PNEUMONIA RESOLVES

- Pneumonia, especially pneumococcal pneumonia, can resolve in 2-3 days if the organism is sensitive to the antibiotic administered.
- **Most pneumonias typically resolve from within** (vacuolize), gradually disappearing in a patchy fashion over days or weeks (Fig. 7-13).
- If a pneumonia **does not** resolve in several weeks, consider the presence of an underlying **obstructing lesion**, such as

a **neoplasm,** that is preventing adequate drainage from that portion of the lung. A CT scan of the chest may help to demonstrate the obstructing lesion.

WEBLINK

Registered users may obtain more information on Recognizing Pneumonia on StudentConsult.com.

TAKE-HOME POINTS

Recognizing Pneumonia

Pneumonia is more opaque than the surrounding normal lung; its margins may be fluffy and indistinct except for where it abuts a pleural margin; it tends to be homogeneous in density; it may contain air bronchograms; it may be associated with atelectasis.

Although there is considerable overlap in the patterns of pneumonia that different organisms produce, some appearances are highly suggestive of particular etiologies.

Lobar pneumonia (prototype: pneumococcal pneumonia) tends to be homogeneous, occupies most or all of a lobe, has air bronchograms centrally and produces the silhouette sign.

Segmental pneumonia (prototype: staphylococcal pneumonia) tends to be multifocal, does not have air bronchograms, and can be associated with volume loss because the bronchi are also filled with inflammatory exudate.

Interstitial pneumonia (prototype: viral pneumonia or PCP) tends to involve the airway walls and alveolar septa and may produce, especially early in the course, a fine, reticular pattern in the lungs; later in the course, it produces airspace disease.

Round pneumonia (prototype: haemophilus) usually occurs in children in the lower lobes posteriorly and can resemble a mass, the clue being that masses in children are uncommon.

Cavitary pneumonia (prototype: tuberculosis) has lucent cavities produced by lung necrosis as its hallmark; post-primary tuberculosis usually involves the upper lobes; it can spread via a transbronchial route that can infect the opposite lower lobe or another lobe in the same lung.

Aspiration occurs in the most dependent portion of the lung at the time of the aspiration, usually the lower lobes or the posterior segments of the upper lobes; aspiration can be bland and clear quickly, can be infected and take months to clear, or may be from a chemical pneumonitis which can take weeks to clear.

Pneumonia can be localized by using the silhouette sign and the spine sign as aids.

Pneumonias frequently resolve by "breaking up" so that they contain patchy areas of newly aerated lung within the confines of the previous pneumonia (**vacuolization**).

Chapter 8

Recognizing Pneumothorax, Pneumomediastinum, Pneumopericardium, and Subcutaneous Emphysema

RECOGNIZING A PNEUMOTHORAX

- A **pneumothorax occurs when air enters the pleural space.**
  - When this occurs, the negative pressure normally present in the pleural space rises higher than the intralveolar pressure and the lung collapses.
  - The parietal pleura remains in contact with the inner surface of the chest wall, but the visceral pleura retracts toward the hilum with the collapsing lung.
    - The **visceral pleura becomes visible as a thin, white line** outlined by air on both sides, marking the outer border of the lung and indicating the presence of the pneumothorax. The visible visceral pleura is called the *visceral pleural white line* or simply the *visceral pleural line*.

 You **must be able to identify the visceral pleural line** (Fig. 8-1) to make the definitive diagnosis of a pneumothorax!

- Even as the lung collapses, it tends to maintain its usual lunglike shape so that the curvature of **the visceral pleural line parallels the curvature of the chest wall**; that is, the visceral pleural line is **convex outward toward the chest wall** (Fig. 8-2).
  - Most other linear densities that mimic a pneumothorax do not demonstrate this spatial relationship with the chest wall.
- There is usually, but not always, an **absence of lung markings peripheral to the visceral pleural line.**

 Pitfall: Pleural adhesions may keep part, but not all, of the visceral pleura adherent to the parietal pleura, even in the presence of a pneumothorax (Fig. 8-3).

- On conventional radiographs, it may be possible to visualize lung markings in front or in back of the pneumothorax and to overlook the presence of a pneumothorax because lung markings appear to extend to the chest wall.
  - **Absence of lung markings alone is not sufficient for the diagnosis of pneumothorax nor is the presence of lung markings distal to the visceral pleural line sufficient to eliminate the possibility of a pneumothorax.**
- The **presence of an air-fluid interface in the pleural space** is, by definition, an indication that a pneumothorax is present (see Fig. 6-14).

- For more about recognizing a hydropneumothorax, see Chapter 6, *Recognizing a Pleural Effusion.*
- In the supine position, air in a relatively large pneumothorax may collect anteriorly and inferiorly in the thorax and manifest itself by **displacing the costophrenic sulcus inferiorly** while, at the same time, producing **increased lucency of that costophrenic sulcus.**
  - This is called the *deep sulcus sign* and it is presumptive evidence for the presence of a pneumothorax on a supine chest radiograph (Fig. 8-4).
- The key signs for recognizing a pneumothorax are summarized in Box 8-1

RECOGNIZING THE PITFALLS IN OVERDIAGNOSING A PNEUMOTHORAX

- Several pitfalls can lead to the mistaken diagnosis of a pneumothorax.

 Pitfall 1: Absence of lung markings mistaken for a pneumothorax.

- The simple absence of lung markings is not sufficient to warrant the diagnosis of a pneumothorax as other diseases produce such a finding.
- These diseases include:
  - **Bullous disease of the lung** (Fig. 8-5)
  - **Large cysts in the lung**
  - **Pulmonary embolism,** which can lead to a lack of perfusion and hence a decrease in the number of vessels visible in a particular part of the lung (*Westermark sign of oligemia*).
- In none of these diseases would the treatment ordinarily include the insertion of a chest tube. In fact, insertion of a chest tube into a bulla might actually **produce** an intractable pneumothorax.
  - **Solution:** Look at the contour of the structure you believe is the visceral pleural line. Unlike the margin of a bulla, the **visceral pleural line** will be **convex outward** toward the chest wall and will **parallel the curve of the chest wall** (Fig. 8-6).

 Pitfall 2: Mistaking a skin fold for a pneumothorax.

- When the patient lies directly on the radiographic cassette (as for a portable supine radiograph), a fold of the patient's skin may become trapped between the patient's back and the surface of the cassette.
- This can produce an *edge* in the expected position of the visceral pleural line which **may, in fact, parallel the** **chest wall** just as you would expect the visceral pleural line in a pneumothorax (Fig. 8-7).
  - **Solution:** Unlike the thin, white line of the visceral pleura, **skin folds produce a relatively thick, white band of density**.

⚠ **Pitfall 3: Mistaking the medial border of the scapula for a pneumothorax.**

- Ordinarily, the patient is positioned for an upright frontal chest radiograph in such a way that the scapulae are

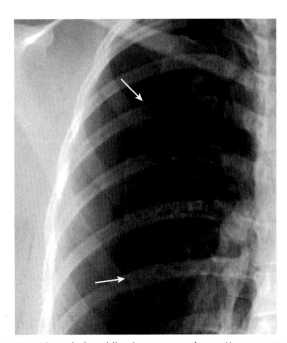

Figure 8-1 Visceral pleural line in a pneumothorax. You must see the visceral pleural line to make the definitive diagnosis of a pneumothorax (*solid white arrows*). The visceral and parietal pleurae are normally not visible, both normally lying adjacent to the lateral chest wall. When air enters the pleural space, the visceral pleura retracts toward the hilum along with the collapsing lung and becomes visible as a very thin, white line with air outlining it on either side. Notice how the contour of the pneumothorax parallels the curvature of the adjacent chest wall.

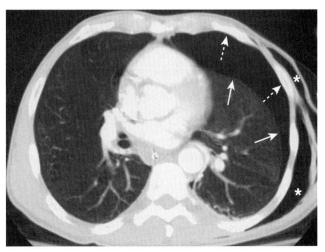

Figure 8-2 Pneumothorax seen on CT. As the lung collapses, it tends to maintain its usual shape so that the curve of the visceral pleural line (*solid white arrows*) parallels the curve of the chest wall (*dotted white arrows*). This is important in differentiating a pneumothorax from artifacts or other diseases that can mimic a pneumothorax. As it collapses, the lung on the side of the pneumothorax also tends to remain lucent until the lung loses almost all of its normal volume, at which point it appears opaque. This patient also has subcutaneous emphysema—air in the soft tissues—of the left lateral chest wall (*white stars*). The patient had suffered a stab wound.

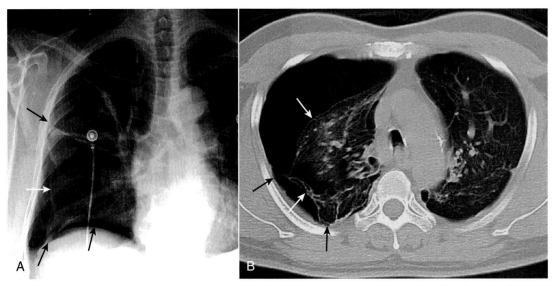

Figure 8-3 Pneumothorax with pleural adhesions. Lung markings may be visible on a conventional radiograph of the chest, **distal** to the visceral pleural line if pleural adhesions are present. In **(A),** a pneumothorax (*solid white arrows*) is prevented from collapsing the lung by pleural adhesions (*solid black arrows*). On a CT scan **(B),** the pleural adhesions (*solid black arrows*) are seen tethering the lung (*solid white arrows*) to the parietal pleura. Adhesions most frequently result from prior infection or blood in the pleural space.

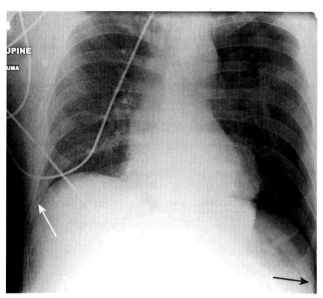

Figure 8-4 Deep sulcus sign. In the supine position, air in a relatively large pneumothorax may collect anteriorly and inferiorly in the thorax and manifest itself by displacing the costophrenic sulcus inferiorly while, at the same time, producing increased lucency of that sulcus (*solid black arrow*). This is called the *deep sulcus sign* and is an indication of a pneumothorax on a supine radiograph. Notice how much lower the left costophrenic sulcus appears than the right sulcus (*solid white arrow*).

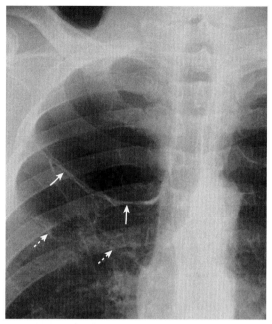

Figure 8-5 Bullous disease, right upper lobe. A thin, white line is visible on this close-up of the right upper lobe (*solid white arrows*) and no lung markings are seen peripheral to it. Unlike the visceral pleural line of a pneumothorax, this white line is convex *away* from the chest wall and does not parallel the curve of the chest wall. This is the classical appearance of a bulla in a patient with emphysema. It is important to differentiate between a pneumothorax and a bulla because inadvertently placing a chest tube into a bulla will almost always **produce** a pneumothorax which may be difficult to re-expand. The walls of several bullae are visible in this patient (*dotted white arrows*). On rare occasions, the bullae can grow so large as to render the hemithorax seemingly devoid of visible lung tissue (***vanishing lung syndrome***).

Box 8-1 Recognizing a Pneumothorax—Signs to Look For

Visualization of the visceral pleural line—a must for the diagnosis

Convex curve of the visceral pleural line paralleling the contour of the chest wall

Absence of lung markings distal to the visceral pleural line (most times)

The *deep sulcus sign* of an inferiorly displaced costophrenic angle seen on a supine chest

The presence of an air-fluid interface in the pleural space

---

retracted lateral to the outer margin of the rib cage, thus preventing the medial borders of the scapulae from overlapping the lung fields.

- With supine radiographs, the **medial borders of the scapulae may superimpose on the upper lobes and mimic the visceral pleural line** of a pneumothorax (Fig. 8-8).
  - **Solution:** Before you diagnose a pneumothorax because you think you see the visceral pleural line, make sure you can **trace the outlines of the scapula** on the side in question and identify its medial border as being separate from the suspected pneumothorax.

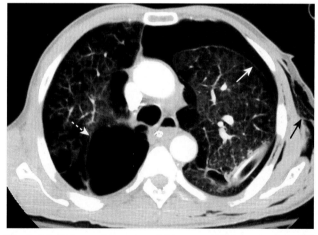

Figure 8-6 Bullous disease on right; pneumothorax on left. This axial section from a chest CT demonstrates the different appearances of bullous disease, seen on the right with its border convex *away* from the chest wall (*dotted white arrow*), and a pneumothorax seen here on the left with its border convex ***toward*** and paralleling the chest wall (*solid white arrow*). This patient also has subcutaneous emphysema on the left (*solid black arrow*).

TYPES OF PNEUMOTHORACES

- Pneumothoraces can be categorized as ***primary***, i.e., occurring in what appears to have been normal lung (***spontaneous pneumothorax*** being an example), or ***secondary***, i.e., those that occur in diseased lung (as in ***emphysema***).
- They have also been classified based on the presence or absence of a **"shift" of the mobile mediastinal structures, like the heart and trachea.**

- **Simple pneumothorax**: the mediastinal structures usually do not shift (Fig. 8-9).
- **Tension pneumothorax**: the mediastinal structures often shift away from the side of the pneumothorax associated with cardiopulmonary compromise (Fig. 8-10).

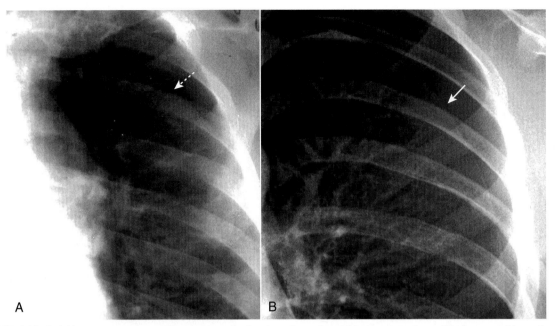

Figure 8-7 Skin fold mimicking a pneumothorax. When patients lie directly on the radiographic cassette as they might for a portable, supine radiograph, a fold of the patient's skin may become trapped between the patient's back and the surface of the cassette. This can produce an *edge* (*dotted white arrow*) in the expected position of a pneumothorax, and that edge may parallel the chest wall just as you would expect a pneumothorax to do **(A).** Unlike the thin, white line of the visceral pleura in a different patient with a pneumothorax (*solid white arrow*—in **B**), skin folds produce relatively thick, white bands of density. A skin fold is an *edge*; the visceral pleura produces a *line*.

- Progressive loss of air into the pleural space through a one-way, check-valve mechanism may cause a shift of the heart and mediastinal structures **away** from the side of the pneumothorax. The air may be entering through a rent in the parietal pleura, visceral pleura, or from the tracheobronchial tree.
  - The continuously **increasing intrathoracic pressure may lead to cardiopulmonary compromise** by **impairing venous return to the heart**.
  - Besides a shift of the mobile mediastinal structures away from the side of the pneumothorax, there may be **inversion of the hemidiaphragm** (especially on the left side) and **flattening of the heart contour on the side under tension**.
- Tension pneumothoraces are associated with a shift of the mediastinal structures away from the side of the pneumothorax; simple pneumothoraces are not associated with any shift. The heart or mediastinal structures **never shift toward** the side of a pneumothorax.
- The question "**How large is the pneumothorax?**" is common but the actual issue is "Does this patient require a chest tube to drain the pneumothorax?" Box 8-2 summarizes the answer.

CAUSES OF A PNEUMOTHORAX

- **Spontaneous**
  - Spontaneous pneumothoraces are common and often develop from **rupture of an apical, subpleural bleb** or bulla. They **characteristically occur in tall, thin males between 20 and 40 years of age**.

- **Traumatic**
  - **The most common** cause of a pneumothorax, either accidental or iatrogenic
    - Through the chest wall, e.g., stab wound
    - Internal, e.g., rupture of a bronchus from a motor vehicle collision
    - Iatrogenic, e.g., following transbronchial biopsy
- **Diseases that decrease lung compliance**
  - Chronic fibrotic diseases, e.g., eosinophilic granuloma
- **Diseases that stiffen the lung**, e.g., hyaline membrane disease in infants
- **Rupture of an alveolus or bronchiole**, e.g., asthma

OTHER WAYS TO DIAGNOSE A PNEUMOTHORAX

- **CT of the chest**
  - CT of the chest has essentially replaced expiratory and decubitus views of the chest if there is a strong clinical suspicion of a pneumothorax that is not demonstrated on conventional radiographs (Fig. 8-11).
  - **CT is able to detect extremely small amounts of air in the pleural space.**
- **Expiratory chest x-rays**
  - Based on the theory that the **volume of air in the lung will normally decrease** on expiration, but the **size of a pneumothorax will not**, small pneumothoraces not visible on an inspiratory radiograph may become visible on a radiograph exposed in **full expiration**. Routine expiratory views are no longer recommended for the detection of pneumothoraces.

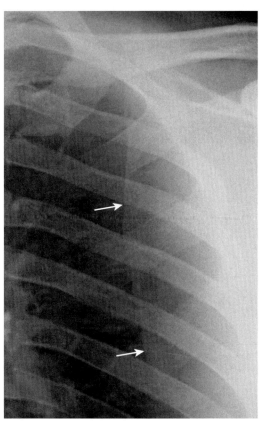

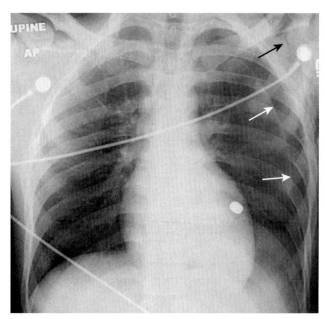

Figure 8-9 Pneumothorax with no shift. A large left-sided pneumothorax (*solid white arrows*) demonstrates no shift of the heart or trachea to the right. Subcutaneous emphysema is seen in the region of the left shoulder (*solid black arrow*). Can you detect why the patient had all of these findings? Yes, that's a bullet superimposed on the heart (but on CT it was posterior to the heart in the left lower lobe).

Figure 8-8 Scapular edge mimicking a pneumothorax. The patient is usually positioned for an upright frontal chest radiograph in such a way that the medial edges of the scapulae are retracted lateral to the outer edges of the rib cage, thus reducing the risk that the scapulae will produce superimposed densities on the chest. On supine radiographs, the medial border of the scapula (*solid white arrows*) will frequently superimpose on the upper lung field and may mimic the visceral pleural line of a pneumothorax. Before you diagnose a pneumothorax, make sure you can identify the medial border of the scapula as being separate from the suspected pneumothorax.

- **Decubitus chest x-rays**
  - Because air rises to the highest point, lateral decubitus films of the chest with the affected side "up" and the x-ray beam directed horizontally (parallel to the floor) may detect a small pneumothorax not seen in the supine position. This method may be helpful in demonstrating a pneumothorax in an infant.
- **Delayed films** are sometimes obtained about **6 hours after a penetrating injury** to the chest in patients in whom no pneumothorax is visible on the initial examination because of the occasional appearance of a delayed traumatic pneumothorax.

PULMONARY INTERSTITIAL EMPHYSEMA

- When the pressure or volume in the alveolus becomes sufficiently elevated, the **alveolus may rupture**.
- This extraalveolar air may take one of two paths:
  - If the alveolus is in close proximity to a pleural surface, the **air may burst outward into the pleural space and create a pneumothorax**.
  - Alternatively, the air can **track backward along the bronchovascular bundles in the lung to the**

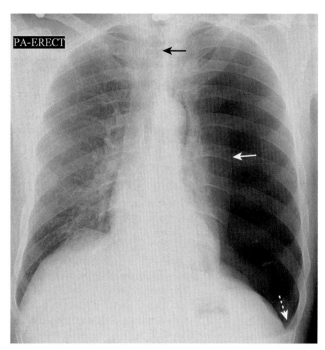

Figure 8-10 Large left-sided tension pneumothorax. Progressive loss of air into the pleural space through a one-way check-valve mechanism may cause a shift of the heart and mediastinal structures away from the side of the pneumothorax and lead to cardiopulmonary compromise by impairing venous return to the heart. In this patient with a spontaneous pneumothorax, the left lung is almost totally collapsed (*solid white arrow*) and the trachea (*solid black arrow*) and heart have shifted to the right. The left hemidiaphragm is depressed because of the elevated left intrathoracic pressure (*dotted white arrow*).

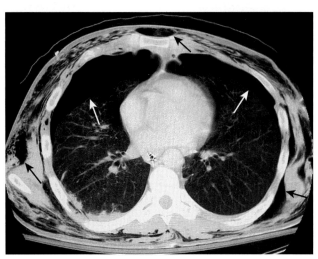

Figure 8-11 Bilateral pneumothoraces. Conventional radiography is the initial modality used for detecting pneumothorax, but smaller pneumothoraces may be visible only on CT scans of the chest. This patient has bilateral pneumothoraces (*solid white arrows*). Air will rise to the highest point (the patient is supine in the CT scanner). Extensive subcutaneous emphysema also is present (*solid black arrows*); it developed because of an "air leak" from a chest tube that had been inserted earlier.

mediastinum, then into the neck and out to the subcutaneous tissues of the chest and abdominal wall. The air can eventually track downward into the abdomen as well as retroperitoneum.

- The air that tracks backward towards the hilum does so along **the perivascular connective tissue of the lung** forming **small, cystic collections** of extra-alveolar air which **dissect retrograde through the bronchovascular sheaths to the hila.**
  - While the extra-alveolar air is confined to the interstitial network of the lung, it is called *pulmonary interstitial emphysema* or *perivascular interstitial emphysema (PIE).*
- Presumably because of the looser connective tissue in the lungs of children and young adults, **pulmonary interstitial emphysema is more likely to occur in those under the age of 40.**
  - **Assisted, mechanical ventilation increases the risk of developing pulmonary interstitial emphysema,** and its formation **heralds a significant risk for the imminent appearance of a pneumothorax,** frequently within a matter of a few hours or days.
  - Other causes of increased intraalveolar pressure and rupture include asthma and barotrauma.

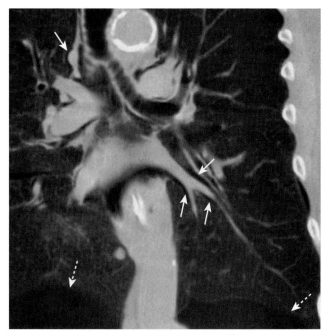

Figure 8-12 Pulmonary interstitial emphysema. This coronal reformatted CT scan of the chest demonstrates air (*solid white arrows*) surrounding the pulmonary arteries (white branching structures) in the lung. This air arose from a ruptured alveolus in a patient with asthma and is tracking back to the hilum where it also produced pneumomediastinum and subcutaneous emphysema. The patient also has bilateral, basilar pneumothoraces (*dotted white arrows*).

- **Pulmonary interstitial emphysema may not be recognizable** on conventional radiographs because the **air collections are small** and a **considerable amount of coexisting disease** is usually present in the lung that obscures it. It may, however, be more visible on CT scans of the chest (Fig. 8-12).

⚠️ **Pitfall:** In infants with hyaline membrane disease (respiratory distress syndrome), pulmonary interstitial emphysema may lead to the appearance of *pseudoclearing* of the lungs (which can appear less dense overall from the formation of the innumerable small air pockets) but its presence actually portends more serious complications.

RECOGNIZING PNEUMOMEDIASTINUM

- When intra-alveolar pressure rises sufficiently to rupture the alveolus, air can **track backward along the bronchovascular bundles in the lung** to the mediastinum.
- About **1 in 3 patients with pulmonary interstitial emphysema will develop pneumomediastinum** (most will develop a pneumothorax).
- **Pneumomediastinum may also develop when an air-containing mediastinal viscus,** such as the esophagus or tracheobronchial tree, **is perforated.**
  - **Rupture of the distal esophagus,** usually the left posterolateral wall, can occur with increased intra-esophageal pressure from retching or vomiting in *Boerhaave syndrome.*
  - **Rupture of the tracheobronchial tree** is most often **secondary to significant trauma,** either **iatrogenic,**

such as during a traumatic **intubation**, or **accidental**, such as from a penetrating wound or severe blunt trauma.

 Radiographic findings of pneumomediastinum:

- **Linear, streaklike lucency associated with a thin, white line paralleling the left heart border.**
- **Streaky air outlining the great vessels** (aorta, superior vena cava, carotid arteries).
- Linear streaks of **air parallel to the spine in the upper thorax extending into the neck** and surrounding the esophagus and trachea (Fig. 8-13).
- *Continuous diaphragm sign*
  - With pneumomediastinum, **air can outline the central portion of the diaphragm** beneath the heart, producing an unbroken superior surface of the diaphragm which extends from one lateral chest wall to the other (Fig. 8-14).

RECOGNIZING PNEUMOPERICARDIUM

- **Pneumopericardium is usually due to direct penetrating injuries to the pericardium, either caused iatrogenically** (during cardiac surgery) **or accidentally** (from penetrating trauma).
  - Pneumopericardium not related to a penetrating injury is more **common in pediatric patients** than adults and may develop in neonates with hyaline membrane disease.
- It is **rare for air in the pleural space to enter the pericardium**, except in those who have a pericardial defect, such as a surgical "window" incised in the pericardium which allows free exchange between the pleural and pericardial spaces.

 Pneumopericardium produces a **continuous** band of **lucency that encircles the heart**, bound by the

parietal pericardial layer **which extends no higher than the root of the great vessels** (corresponding to the level of the main pulmonary artery) (Fig. 8-15).

- Pneumomediastinum, in contrast, will extend above the root of the great vessels into the uppermost thorax.

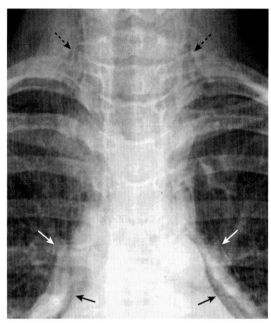

Figure 8-13 Pneumomediastinum, pneumopericardium and subcutaneous emphysema. This patient with asthma developed spontaneous pneumomediastinum, most likely from rupture of an alveolus followed by formation of pulmonary interstitial emphysema. The air tracked back to the hila, then into the mediastinum where it produced streaky white, linear densities (*solid white arrows*) extending to the neck. Subcutaneous emphysema (*dotted black arrows*) is present in the neck. In adults, air does not usually enter the pericardium except by direct penetration, so it is somewhat unusual that this patient also developed pneumopericardium (*solid black arrows*). Notice how the air in the pericardial space does not extend above the reflections of the aorta and pulmonary artery, unlike pneumomediastinum which does extend above the great vessels.

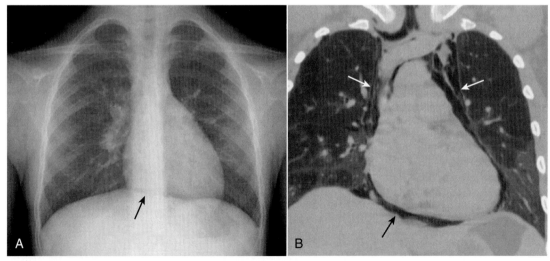

Figure 8-14 Continuous diaphragm sign of pneumomediastinum. With pneumomediastinum, air can outline the central portion of the diaphragm beneath the heart, producing an unbroken diaphragmatic contour that extends from one lateral chest wall to the other (*solid black arrow* on conventional radiograph **A**). This is called the ***continuous diaphragm sign***. Normally, the diaphragm is not visible in the center of the chest because no air is in the mediastinum and the soft tissue density of the heart rests upon and silhouettes the soft tissue density of the diaphragm in its central portion. In **(B)**, a coronal reformatted CT scan of the chest in another patient shows pneumomediastinum outlining the central portion of the diaphragm (*solid black arrow*) and the remainder of the pneumomediastinum extending superior to the great vessels (*solid white arrows*).

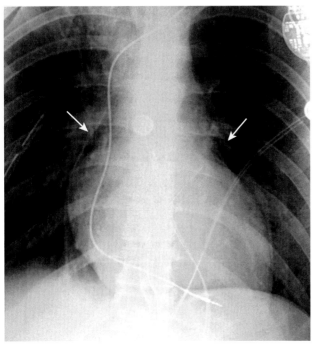

Figure 8-15 Pneumopericardium. This patient underwent a procedure to produce a pericardial window for recurrent pericardial effusions. Postoperatively, there is a pneumopericardium shown by the visible parietal pericardium (*solid white arrows*) outlining air around the heart in the pericardial space. Notice how the air does not extend above the reflection of the aorta and main pulmonary artery. Pneumopericardium in adults usually occurs from direct violation of the pericardium by trauma.

- CT is usually necessary to demonstrate the findings of pneumopericardium.

RECOGNIZING SUBCUTANEOUS EMPHYSEMA

- **Air can extend into the soft tissues of the neck, chest and abdominal walls** from the mediastinum, or it can dissect in the subcutaneous tissues from a thoracotomy drainage tube or a penetrating injury to the chest wall.
- **Air dissecting along muscle bundles** produces a **characteristic comblike, striated appearance** that superimposes on the underlying lung, often making it difficult to evaluate the lungs by conventional radiography (Fig. 8-16).
- Although dramatic radiographically, **subcutaneous emphysema usually produces no serious clinical effects by itself**.
- Depending on the volume of subcutaneous air present, it may require **several days** to **a week** or longer for the air to reabsorb.

WEBLINK

Registered users may obtain more information on Recognizing Pneumothorax, Pneumomediastinum, Pneumopericardium, and Subcutaneous Emphysema on StudentConsult.com.

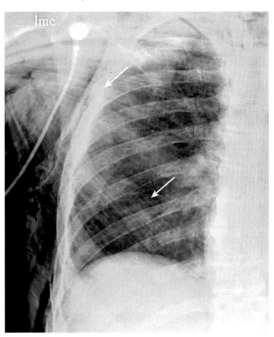

Figure 8-16 Subcutaneous emphysema. Air can extend into the subcutaneous tissues of the neck, chest, and abdominal walls from the mediastinum, or it can dissect in the soft tissues from a thoracotomy drainage tube or a penetrating injury to the chest wall. Air dissecting along muscle bundles produces a characteristic comblike, striated appearance (*solid white arrows*). Although dramatic radiographically, subcutaneous emphysema usually produces no serious clinical effects by itself.

 TAKE-HOME POINTS

Recognizing Pneumothorax, Pneumomediastinum, Pneumopericardium, and Subcutaneous Emphysema

There is normally no air in the pleural space; air in the pleural space is called a **pneumothorax**.

You must identify the visceral pleural white line to diagnose a pneumothorax.

Beware of the pitfalls that resemble pneumothoraces: bullae, skin folds, and the medial border of the scapula.

Simple pneumothoraces are those with no shift of the heart or mobile mediastinal structures; most pneumothoraces are simple.

Tension pneumothoraces (usually associated with cardiorespiratory compromise) produce a shift of the heart and mediastinal structures **away** from the side of the pneumothorax by virtue of a check-valve mechanism that allows air to enter the pleural space but not leave.

Most pneumothoraces are traumatic in etiology, either accidental or idiopathic.

Conventional chest radiographs are poor at estimating the size of a pneumothorax; CT is better; the most important assessment to be made is the clinical status of the patient.

Besides the conventional upright chest radiograph, other ways to diagnose a pneumothorax include: expiratory exposures, decubitus views, and delayed images. CT remains the most sensitive test for detecting small pneumothoraces.

Spontaneous pneumothoraces most often occur as a result of rupture of a small apical, sub-pleural bleb; they most often occur in younger men.

Pulmonary interstitial emphysema results from an increase in the intralveolar pressure that leads to rupture of an alveolus and dissection of air back towards the hila along the bronchovascular bundles; it is frequently difficult to visualize.

Pneumomediastinum can occur when air tracks back to the mediastinum from a ruptured alveolus or from perforation of an air-containing viscus such as the esophagus or trachea; it can produce the *continuous diaphragm sign* on a frontal chest radiograph.

Pneumopericardium usually is due to direct penetration of the pericardium rather than dissection of air from a pneumomediastinum; it can be difficult to differentiate from a pneumomediastinum. A key is that pneumopericardium does not extend above the roots of the great vessels, whereas pneumomediastinum does.

Air dissecting into the neck and chest wall can produce **subcutaneous emphysema**, which, because of its superimposition on the lungs, can make evaluation of the underlying lung more difficult. By itself, it is usually of no clinical significance and usually clears in a few days, depending on its volume.

Chapter 9

Recognizing Adult Heart Disease

We'll begin with an assessment of heart size, then describe the normal and abnormal contours of the heart on the frontal radiograph, and finally illustrate some imaging findings in common cardiac diseases.

RECOGNIZING AN ENLARGED CARDIAC SILHOUETTE

- The cardiac silhouette can appear enlarged for three main reasons:
  - The heart is enlarged (**cardiomegaly**).
  - A **pericardial effusion** mimics the appearance of cardiomegaly on conventional radiographs.
  - An **extracardiac** factor produces apparent cardiac enlargement.

You can estimate the size of the cardiac silhouette on the frontal chest radiograph using the *cardiothoracic ratio*, which is a measurement of the **widest transverse diameter of the heart** compared to the **widest internal diameter of the rib cage** (from inside of rib to inside of rib at the level of the diaphragm) (Fig. 9-1).

- In most normal adults at full inspiration, the cardiothoracic ratio is **less than 50%**. That is, the size of the heart is usually less than half of the internal diameter of the thoracic rib cage.

PERICARDIAL EFFUSION

- Normally, there are 15-50 mL of fluid in the pericardial space between the parietal and visceral pericardial layers.
- Abnormal accumulations of fluid begin in the **dependent portions of the pericardial space**, which, in the supine position, is **posterior to the left ventricle** (Fig. 9-2A).
- As the pericardial effusion increases in size, it tends to accumulate more **along the right heart border** until it fills the pericardial space and **encircles the heart** (Fig. 9-2B).
- CT scans can demonstrate small pericardial effusions, although pericardial ultrasonography is usually the imaging study of first choice. Conventional radiographs are poor at defining a pericardial effusion.
- Some of the causes of pericardial effusions are outlined in Box 9-1.

EXTRACARDIAC CAUSES OF APPARENT CARDIAC ENLARGEMENT

 Although the cardiothoracic ratio provides a handy way of assessing heart size, it does have its pitfalls.

- Sometimes, there is an **extracardiac** cause of apparent cardiac enlargement that may cause the cardiothoracic ratio to appear greater than 50%, **while the heart itself may actually be normal in size.**
- The extracardiac causes of apparent cardiomegaly are outlined in Table 9-1. Magnification of the heart produced by projection, usually on a supine, portable chest examination, is the most common cause of apparent cardiomegaly.

EFFECT OF PROJECTION ON PERCEPTION OF HEART SIZE

- Because the heart resides **anteriorly** in the chest, **on a posteroanterior (PA) chest radiograph** (the standard frontal chest study in which the x-ray beam enters posteriorly and exits anteriorly where the imaging cassette is positioned), **the heart appears truer to its actual size** because it is nearer the imaging surface.
- **On an anteroposterior (AP) chest radiograph** (the usual bedside, portable chest radiograph in which the x-ray beam enters anteriorly and exits posteriorly where the cassette is positioned), **the heart is slightly magnified** because it is farther from the imaging surface.
- Therefore, **the heart will appear slightly larger on an AP chest radiograph** like a portable chest radiograph **than will the same heart on a PA chest radiograph** (see Fig. 2-17).

IDENTIFYING CARDIAC ENLARGEMENT ON AN ANTEROPOSTERIOR CHEST RADIOGRAPH

- So is it possible to estimate the size of the heart on a portable chest radiograph? Glad you asked, because the answer is "yes."
- If the **left heart border** is **touching the left lateral chest wall**, the heart is **enlarged**.
- If the **left heart border** is **very close to the left chest wall**, the heart is **probably enlarged**.
- If the **heart is borderline enlarged on a portable AP radiograph**, it is probably **normal** in size (Table 9-2).

- A good rule of thumb: If the heart appears enlarged on a well-inspired, portable chest radiograph, it probably is enlarged.

RECOGNIZING CARDIOMEGALY ON THE LATERAL CHEST RADIOGRAPH

- Generally speaking, evaluation of cardiac size is best made on the frontal chest radiograph.
- To evaluate for the presence of enlargement of the cardiac silhouette in the lateral projection, **look at the space posterior to the heart and anterior to the spine at the level of the diaphragm**.
- In a normal person, the **cardiac silhouette will usually not extend posteriorly and project over the spine** (see Fig. 2-2).
- As the **heart enlarges**, whether that enlargement is due to cardiomegaly or pericardial effusion, the **posterior border of the heart may extend to, or overlap, the anterior border of the thoracic spine**. This can be useful as a confirmatory sign of cardiac enlargement first suspected on the frontal projection (Fig. 9-3).

Box 9-1 **Causes of Pericardial Effusion**
Congestive heart failure
Infection (TB, viral)
Metastatic malignancy (lung and breast, especially)
Uremic pericarditis
Collagen-vascular disease (lupus)
Trauma
Postpericardiotomy syndrome

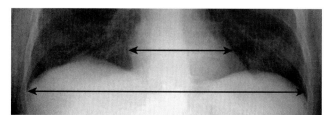

Figure 9-1 The cardiothoracic ratio. To estimate the cardiothoracic ratio, the widest diameter of the heart (*upper double arrow*) is compared to the widest internal diameter of the thoracic cage from the inside of rib to the inside of rib (*lower double arrow*). The widest internal diameter of the thorax is usually at the level of the diaphragm. The cardiothoracic ratio should be less than 50% in most normal adults on a standard PA frontal radiograph taken with an adequate inspiration (about nine posterior ribs showing).

TABLE 9-1 EXTRACARDIAC CAUSES OF APPARENT CARDIOMEGALY

Cause	Reason for Enlarged Appearance
AP portable supine chest—most common cause	Magnification due to AP projection
Suboptimal inspiration	In expiration, the diaphragm moves upward and compresses the heart, making the heart appear larger than it would in full inspiration
	If there are 8 or 9 posterior ribs visible on the frontal chest radiograph, then the inspiration is adequate (see Fig. 2-13)
Obesity, pregnancy, ascites	These conditions prevent an adequate inspiration
Pectus excavatum deformity, a congenital deformity of the lowermost section of the sternum, causes it to bow inward and compress the heart	The heart is compressed between the sternum and the spine
Rotation	Especially when it occurs to the patient's left, rotation may make the heart appear larger
Pericardial effusion	Other imaging modalities (most commonly ultrasound) or electrocardiographic findings will help to identify pericardial fluid

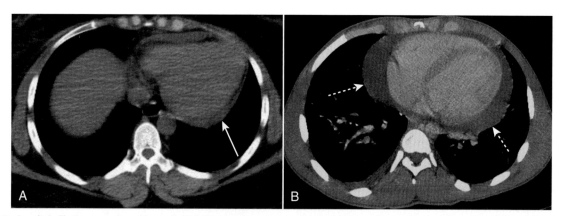

Figure 9-2 Pericardial effusions, small and large. A, Fluid first begins to accumulate in the dependent portions of the pericardial space which is posterior to the left ventricle in the supine position (*solid white arrow*). **B,** As the effusion increases in size, it fills the pericardial space and encircles the heart (*dotted white arrows*). Conventional chest radiographs may show an enlarged cardiac silhouette but cannot differentiate the density of the heart from the effusion.

TABLE 9-2 RECOGNIZING CARDIOMEGALY ON AN AP CHEST RADIOGRAPH

Appearance of Heart on AP Study	Likely Heart Size
Borderline enlarged	Normal size
Significantly enlarged	Enlarged
Touching, or almost touching, the left lateral chest wall	Definitely enlarged

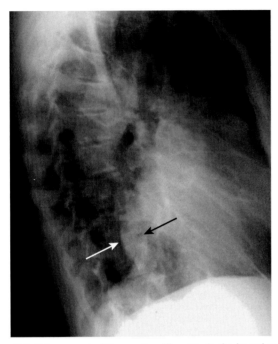

Figure 9-3 Enlargement of the cardiac silhouette in the lateral projection. In most normal patients, the posterior border of the heart does not overlap the thoracic spine. In this patient with cardiomegaly, the posterior border of the heart (*solid white arrow*) overlaps the anterior border of the thoracic spine (*solid black arrow*). Estimation of cardiac size is best made on the frontal projection, but the lateral projection can be used for a confirmatory sign of enlargement of the cardiac silhouette.

RECOGNIZING CARDIOMEGALY IN INFANTS

- Although this chapter focuses primarily on adult cardiac disease, in **newborns and infants** it is important to remember that the **heart will normally appear larger** relative to the size of the thorax than it does in adults. Whereas a cardiothoracic ratio greater than 50% is considered abnormal in adults, the **cardiothoracic ratio may reach up to 65% in infants and still be normal** because newborns cannot take as deep an inspiration as adults can and the relative proportions in the size of their abdomen to chest are not the same as for adults (Fig. 9-4).
- **Any assessment of cardiac enlargement in an infant** should **take into account other factors** such as the appearance of the **pulmonary vasculature** and any **associated clinical signs or symptoms** (e.g., a murmur, tachycardia, or cyanosis).

⚠️ Also, in a child the thymus gland may overlap portions of the heart and sometimes mimic cardiomegaly. The normal thymus may be seen on conventional chest radiographs up to 3 years of age and sometimes may be seen as

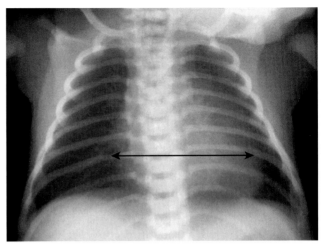

Figure 9-4 Normal infant chest. In the normal infant, the cardiothoracic ratio may be as large as 65% (compared to 50% in adults) (*double arrow*). Any assessment of cardiac enlargement in an infant should also take into account other factors such as the appearance of the pulmonary vasculature and any associated clinical signs or symptoms (such as a murmur, tachycardia, or cyanosis).

late as 8 years of age. The **normal thymus** gland has a somewhat **lobulated** appearance, especially where the ribs indent it (Fig. 9-5).

NORMAL CARDIAC CONTOURS

- The **normal cardiac contours** comprise a series of bumps and indentations visible on the frontal chest radiograph. They are demonstrated in Figure 9-6.

➡️ Key points about the cardiac contours:

- The **ascending aorta** should normally not project farther to the right than the right heart border (i.e., right atrium).
- The **aortic knob** is normally less than 35 mm (measured from the edge of the air-filled trachea) and will normally push the trachea slightly to the right.
- The **normal left atrium** does not contribute to the border of the heart on a nonrotated frontal chest radiograph.
- An **enlarged left atrium** "fills-in" and straightens the normal concavity just inferior to the main pulmonary artery segment and may sometimes be visible on the right side of the heart as well.
- Normally, the **descending aorta** parallels the spine and is barely visible on the frontal radiograph of the chest. When it becomes **tortuous** or **uncoiled**, it swings farther away from the thoracic spine towards the patient's left (Fig. 9-7).

NORMAL PULMONARY VASCULATURE

- Pulmonary vessels produce most of the lines in the lungs visible on a chest radiograph.
- The **main pulmonary artery** segment is usually concave or flat. In younger females it may normally be convex outward.

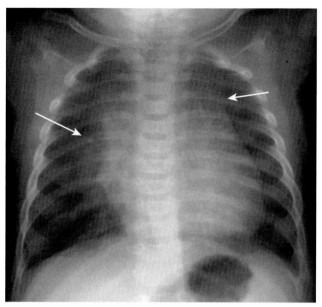

Figure 9-5 Normal thymus gland. The thymus gland may overlap the upper portion of the cardiac silhouette and can be mistaken for cardiomegaly in a child. One aid in identifying the thymus gland is that it is frequently lobulated in appearance (*solid white arrows*). Although the thymus gland will usually involute by age 3, it may still be normally visible in children as old as 8 years of age.

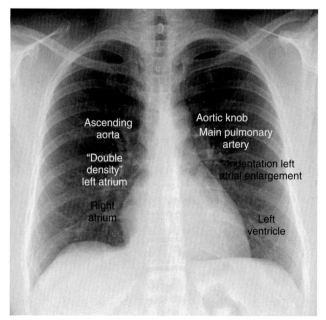

Figure 9-6 Normal cardiac contours seen in the frontal projection. There are seven identifiable cardiac contours on the frontal chest radiograph. On the right side of the heart, the first contour is a low-density, almost straight edge visible just lateral to the trachea reflecting the size of the ascending aorta. Where the contour of the ascending aorta meets the contour of the right atrium, there is usually a slight indentation where the left atrium may appear when it enlarges. The right heart border is formed by the right atrium. On the left, the first contour is the aortic knob, a radiographic structure formed by the foreshortened aortic arch superimposed on a portion of the proximal descending aorta. The next contour below the aortic knob is the main pulmonary artery before it divides into a right and left pulmonary artery. Just below the main pulmonary artery segment there is normally a slight indentation where an enlarged left atrium may appear on the left side of the heart. The left ventricle forms the last contour of the heart on the left. The descending aorta almost disappears with the shadow of the spine.

In the upright position, the blood flow to the bases is normally greater than the flow to the apices because of the effect of gravity. Therefore, the **size** of the vessels at the **base** is normally **larger** than the size of the vessels at the **apex** of the lung.

- Normally, blood vessels branch and taper gradually from central (the hila) to peripheral (near the chest wall) (Fig. 9-8).
- Changes in pressure or flow can alter the normal dynamics of the pulmonary vasculature, some of which are described later in this chapter under "Recognizing Common Cardiac Disorders."

GENERAL PRINCIPLES OF CARDIAC IMAGING

- As you interpret cardiac abnormalities, no matter what modality is being used, the following principles hold true:
  - The **ventricles respond to obstruction** to their outflow **by first undergoing hypertrophy** rather than dilatation. Therefore, the heart may not appear enlarged at first with lesions like **aortic stenosis, coarctation of the aorta, pulmonic stenosis, or systemic hypertension.** When the muscle begins to fail and the heart decompensates, the heart will become enlarged.
  - **Cardiomegaly,** as we usually recognize it, **is primarily produced by ventricular enlargement,** not by isolated enlargement of the atria. Therefore, the heart usually appears normal in size in early **mitral stenosis,** even though the left atrium is enlarged.
  - In general, the most marked chamber enlargement will occur from volume overload rather than pressure overload, so that the largest chambers are usually produced by regurgitant valves rather than stenotic valves. Therefore, the heart will usually be larger with aortic regurgitation rather than aortic stenosis and the left atrium will usually be larger in mitral regurgitation than mitral stenosis (Fig. 9-9).

RECOGNIZING COMMON CARDIAC DISEASES

- In this section, we'll discuss several diseases in more detail.
  - Congestive heart failure and pulmonary edema
    - Cardiogenic versus noncardiogenic pulmonary edema
  - Hypertensive cardiovascular disease
  - Mitral stenosis
  - Pulmonary arterial hypertension
  - Aortic stenosis
  - Cardiomyopathy
  - Thoracic aortic aneurysm and aortic dissection
  - Coronary artery disease

Congestive Heart Failure

- The incidence of congestive heart failure (CHF) has grown rapidly over the last two decades so that CHF is **the most common diagnosis in hospitalized patients over the age of 65.**

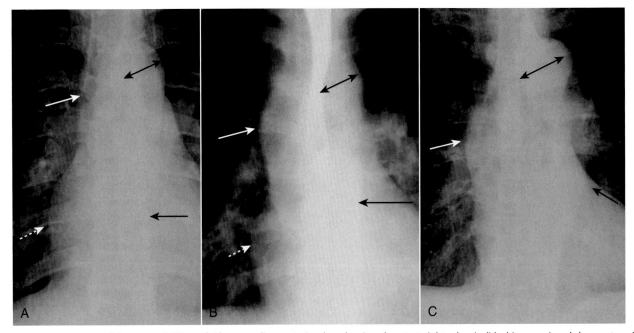

Figure 9-7 Appearances of the aorta. A, Normal. The ascending aorta is a low-density, almost straight edge (*solid white arrow*) and does not project beyond the right heart border (*dotted white arrow*). The aortic knob is not enlarged (*double arrow*), and the descending aorta (*solid black arrow*) almost disappears with the shadow of the thoracic spine. **B, Aortic stenosis.** The ascending aorta is abnormal as it projects convex outward (*solid white arrow*) almost as far as the right heart border (*dotted white arrow*). This is due to *poststenotic dilatation.* The aortic knob (*double arrow*) and descending aorta (*solid black arrow*) remain normal. **C, Hypertension.** Both the ascending (*solid white arrow*) and descending aorta (*solid black arrow*) project too far to the right and left, respectively. The aortic knob is enlarged (*double arrow*).

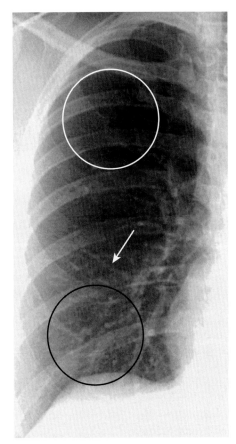

Figure 9-8 Normal pulmonary vasculature. The right lung is shown. The lower lobe vessels (*black circle*) are larger in size than the upper lobe vessels (*white circle*) in the upright position, and all vessels taper gradually from central to peripheral (*white arrow*). Alterations in pulmonary flow or pressure may change these relationships.

- **Causes of CHF**
  - In the United States, the two most common causes of CHF are coronary artery disease and hypertension.
  - Other causes of CHF:
    - **Cardiomyopathy**, such as from longstanding alcohol abuse
    - **Cardiac valvular lesions** like aortic stenosis and mitral stenosis
    - **Arrhythmias**
    - **Hyperthyroidism**
    - **Severe anemia**
    - **Left-to-right shunts**
  - Typically, **CHF** presents with **one of two radiographic patterns: pulmonary interstitial edema** or **pulmonary alveolar edema.** Not every feature of each pattern is always present and often the two patterns overlap.

Pulmonary Interstitial Edema

 Pulmonary interstitial edema has four key radio-graphic signs.

- **Thickening of the interlobular septa**
- **Peribronchial cuffing**
- **Fluid in the fissures**
- **Pleural effusions**
- **Thickening of the interlobular septa: The Kerley B line**
  - The interlobular septae are not detectable on a normal chest radiograph but can become visible if they accumulate excessive fluid, usually at a pulmonary (venous) capillary wedge pressure of about **15 mm Hg**.
  - The thickened septae are called **septal lines** or **Kerley B lines** (named after Peter James Kerley, an Irish neurologist and radiologist).

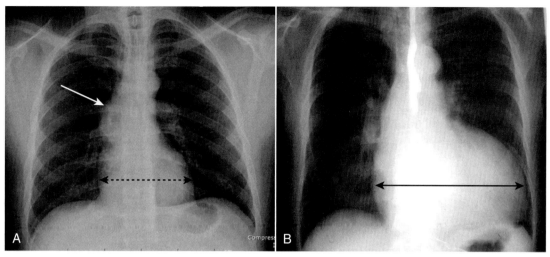

Figure 9-9 Heart size with stenotic versus regurgitant valve. A, Poststenotic dilatation of the ascending aorta (*white arrow*) is present in this patient with aortic stenosis. Notice that the heart is not enlarged because this lesion produces left ventricular hypertrophy (*dotted black double arrow*). **B,** This patient has aortic regurgitation. Note the extremely large heart due to an enlarged left ventricle (*solid black double arrow*). Volume overload will cause a greater increase in chamber size than will increased pressure.

- **Recognizing Kerley B lines**
  - Kerley B lines actually do exist. They will be visible on a frontal radiograph usually **at the lung bases, at or near the costophrenic angles**.
  - They are **very short** (1-2 cm long), **very thin** (about 1 mm), and **horizontal in orientation**, which means they are **perpendicular to the pleural surface**.
  - They **usually extend to and abut the pleural surface** (Fig. 9-10).
  - After repeated episodes of pulmonary interstitial edema, the **septal lines may fibrose** and therefore **remain even after all other signs of pulmonary interstitial edema clear**. These are called **chronic Kerley B lines** and they may be present even if the patient is not clinically in congestive failure.
- **Kerley A lines**
  - Kerley was busy naming other lines seen in CHF besides the "B" line.
  - **Kerley A lines** appear when connective tissue around the bronchoarterial sheaths in the lung distends with fluid. **Kerley A lines extend from the hila for several centimeters (up to 6 cm)** but **do not reach the periphery of the lung** like Kerley B lines do (Fig. 9-11).
  - Once he started, Kerley apparently had trouble stopping and he also described "C" lines, but there is doubt that they exist as separate entities.
- **Peribronchial cuffing**
  - In adults, bronchi may **normally** be visible *en face* in the region of the hila, but their walls are usually too thin and **not visible** more peripherally in the lung.
  - When fluid accumulates in the interstitial tissue around and in the wall of a bronchus, such as in CHF, the **bronchial wall becomes thicker and may appear as a ring-like density that can be seen on-end** in radiographs.
  - When seen on-end, *peribronchial cuffing* appears as numerous, small, ringlike shadows that look like little *doughnuts* (Fig. 9-12).
- **Fluid in the fissures**
  - The major (or horizontal) and minor (or oblique) **fissures may be visible normally** but are almost never

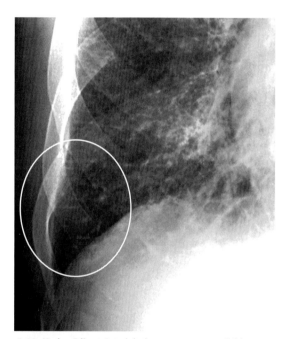

Figure 9-10 Kerley B lines. Interlobular septae are not visible on a normal chest radiograph but can become visible if they accumulate excessive fluid. First described by neurologist/radiologist Peter James Kerley, they are very short (1-2 cm long), very thin (about 1 mm) horizontal lines perpendicular to and abutting the pleural surface (*white oval*).

thicker than a line you could draw with the **point of a sharpened pencil** (Fig. 9-13A).
- **Fluid can collect between the two layers of visceral pleura that form the fissures or in the subpleural space** between the visceral pleura and the lung parenchyma.
- This **fluid** distends the fissure and makes it **thicker**, more **irregular in contour**, and therefore **more visible** than normal (Fig. 9-13B).
- Fluid may also collect in accessory fissures like the *azygous fissure* or *inferior accessory fissure* (Fig. 9-14).

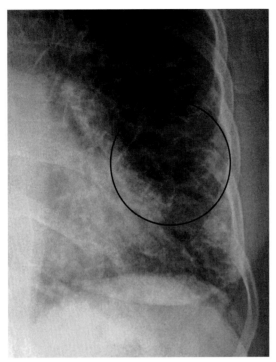

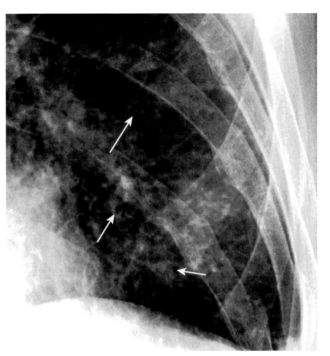

Figure 9-11 Kerley A lines. The A lines (*circle*) appear when connective tissue near the bronchoarterial bundle distends with fluid. They extend from the hila for several centimeters in the midlung and do not reach the periphery of the lung like Kerley B lines do. A network of Kerley lines is produced in the lungs in patients with congestive heart failure producing the "prominence of the pulmonary interstitial markings" seen in that disease.

Figure 9-12 Peribronchial cuffing. Normally the bronchus is invisible when seen on-end in the periphery of the lung. When fluid accumulates in the interstitial tissue around and in the wall of a bronchus as it does in CHF, the bronchial walls become thicker and can appear as ringlike densities when seen on-end (*solid white arrows*). Peribronchial cuffing may not always produce perfectly round circles.

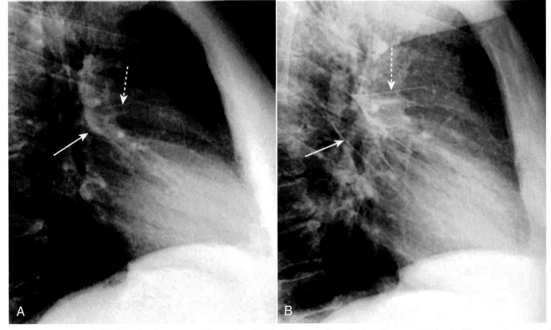

Figure 9-13 Normal fissures and fluid in the fissures. A, The major (*solid white arrow*) and minor fissures (*dashed white arrow*) may be barely visible normally but are almost never thicker than a line you could draw with the point of a sharpened pencil. **B,** Fluid can collect in the fissures in CHF and distend them, making them appear thicker and more irregular in contour and more visible than normal. The major fissure is more prominent (*solid white arrow*) as is the minor fissure (*dashed white arrow*). When the patient's heart failure clears, the fissures will return to normal appearance, but after repeated and prolonged bouts of failure, fibrosis may result in permanent thickening of the fissures.

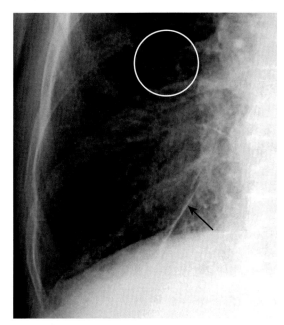

Figure 9-14 Fluid in inferior accessory fissure. In addition to thickening the major and minor fissures, fluid may also distend accessory fissures in the lung. Here, the inferior accessory fissure that separates the medial from the other basilar segments of the lower lobe and is usually barely visible when present is markedly thickened (*solid black arrow*). Peribronchial thickening (*white circle*) is also seen.

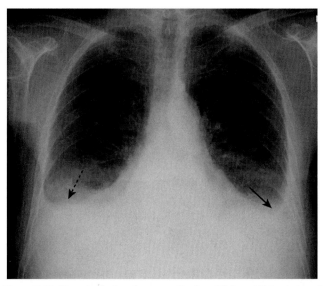

Figure 9-15 Pleural effusions in congestive heart failure. Bilateral pleural effusions (*dotted* and *solid black arrows*) are present in this patient with CHF. Effusions in CHF are most often bilateral but may be asymmetrical, the right side invariably being slightly larger. While a unilateral, left pleural effusion may occur with CHF, a large left effusion should draw suspicion to another possible cause, such as metastatic disease.

- **Pleural effusion**
  - As a result of either increased production or decreased absorption of pleural fluid, fluid in excess of the normal 2-5 mL can collect in the pleural space, typically at a pulmonary capillary wedge pressure of about **20 mm Hg**.
  - **Pleural effusions accompanying CHF are usually bilateral** but can be asymmetric (Fig. 9-15).

Box 9-2 Four Key Findings in Pulmonary Interstitial Edema

Thickening of the interlobular septa—*Kerley B lines*—and fluid in the central connective tissue of the lungs—*Kerley A lines*

Peribronchial cuffing—fluid-thickened bronchial walls visualized *en face*

Fluid in the fissures—opacification and thickening of the interlobar fissures

Pleural effusion—usually bilateral but, when unilateral, usually right-sided

- When **unilateral**, they are **almost always right-sided**.
  - About 15% the time, they can be unilateral and on the left, but if you see a unilateral left pleural effusion, you should think of causes other than CHF, like metastases, tuberculosis, or pulmonary thromboembolic disease.
- At times, pleural fluid accumulates in the form of a **laminar effusion** in which the fluid assumes a **thin, bandlike density along the lateral chest wall, beginning near the costophrenic sulcus**, but often preserving the sulcus itself (see Fig. 6-13).
- For more about pleural effusions, see Chapter 6, *Recognizing Pleural Effusions*.
- The key findings of pulmonary interstitial edema are summarized in Box 9-2.

Pulmonary Alveolar Edema

- When the **pulmonary venous pressure is sufficiently elevated (about 25 mm Hg), fluid spills out of the interstitial tissues** of the lung **into the airspaces**. This results in *pulmonary alveolar edema* (most often shortened to *pulmonary edema* without including "alveolar").

The **radiographic findings** of **pulmonary alveolar edema**:

- **Fluffy, indistinct, patchy airspace densities that are usually centrally located**.
  - The outer third of the lung is frequently spared and the lower lung zones are more affected than the upper.
  - This is called the *bat-wing, angel-wing,* or *butterfly* configuration of pulmonary edema (Fig. 9-16).
- Pleural effusions and fluid in the fissures are commonly found in pulmonary alveolar edema on a cardiogenic basis.
- The key findings in pulmonary alveolar edema are summarized in Box 9-3.
- **What happened to cardiomegaly and cephalization?**
  - While most patients with CHF have an enlarged heart, most patients with an enlarged heart are not in CHF. In any individual, **cardiomegaly itself is not a particularly sensitive indicator for the presence or absence of CHF**.
  - **Cephalization,** defined as redistribution of flow in the lungs such that the upper lobe pulmonary vessels become larger than the lower lobe vessels, is **difficult to identify for most beginners** and is meaningful only if you are

certain the patient was upright at the time of the chest exposure.

- Anyone (even you and me) who undergoes a chest radiograph while supine or semirecumbent (which is the way portable chest radiographs exposed in the intensive care unit are usually performed) will demonstrate cephalization, since gravity will exert the same effect on both the upper and lobe vessels in the supine position.

■ **How pulmonary edema resolves**
- Pulmonary edema generally is both **abrupt in onset** and **quick to clear**—typically in a matter of a few hours to a few days (Fig. 9-17).
- Resolution frequently begins peripherally and moves centrally. Radiologic resolution may lag behind clinical improvement, especially if the patient has large pleural effusions.

Noncardiogenic Pulmonary Edema: General Considerations

■ Although CHF accounts for the majority of the cases of pulmonary edema (*i.e., cardiogenic pulmonary edema*), there are other **noncardiogenic causes of pulmonary edema**.
■ Among the causes of noncardiogenic pulmonary edema is a diverse group of diseases:
- **Increased capillary permeability**—includes all of the various causes of *adult respiratory distress syndrome (ARDS)* such as:
  - Sepsis
  - Uremia
  - Disseminated intravascular coagulopathy
  - Smoke inhalation
  - Near drowning
- **Volume overload**
- **Lymphangitic spread of malignancy**
- Other causes of noncardiogenic pulmonary edema may include:
  - High-altitude pulmonary edema
  - Neurogenic pulmonary edema
  - Reexpansion pulmonary edema (Fig. 9-18)
  - Heroin or other overdoses (see Fig. 3-1)

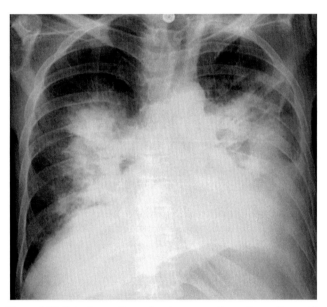

Figure 9-16 Bat-wing pattern of pulmonary edema. The radiographic findings of pulmonary alveolar edema include fluffy, indistinct, patchy airspace densities frequently centrally located and sparing the outer third of the lung. This is called the **bat-wing (angel-wing)** or **butterfly** pattern, and it suggests pulmonary edema versus other airspace diseases such as pneumonia. The patterns of cardiogenic and noncardiogenic pulmonary edema overlap considerably, but the absence of pleural effusions, absence of fluid in the fissures, and the normal-sized heart favor a noncardiogenic cause in this case. The patient was in septic shock from an overwhelming urinary tract infection.

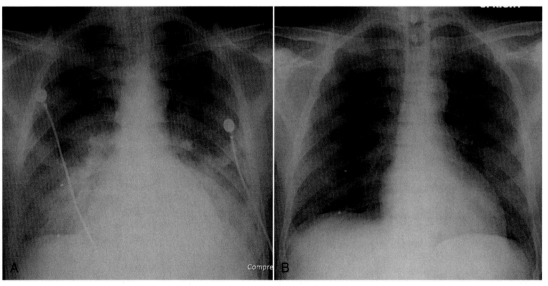

Figure 9-17 Rapidly clearing pulmonary edema. Pulmonary edema generally is both abrupt in its onset and quick to clear. **A,** This patient demonstrates bilateral, perihilar airspace disease with diffuse prominence of the interstitial markings characteristic of pulmonary edema. **B,** Four days later, the lungs are clear. Patients with adult respiratory distress syndrome are not likely to clear this quickly, nor are patients who have coexisting diseases such as renal or hepatic failure or superimposed pneumonia.

Box 9-3 Key Findings in Pulmonary Alveolar Edema

Fluffy, indistinct, patchy airspace densities

Bat-wing or butterfly configuration frequently sparing the outer third of lungs

Pleural effusions are usually present when the edema is cardiogenic in origin

---

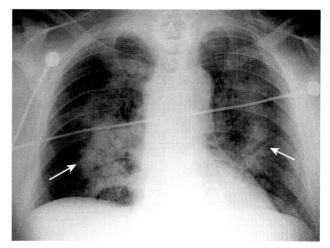

Figure 9-19 Noncardiogenic pulmonary edema. Even though this airspace disease has a perihilar distribution similar to cardiogenic pulmonary edema (*solid white arrows*), there is no pleural fluid, fluid in the fissures or cardiomegaly. In general, noncardiogenic pulmonary edema is less likely to demonstrate pleural effusions and Kerley B lines, more likely to demonstrate a normal pulmonary capillary wedge pressure (PCWP) of less than 12 mm Hg, and more likely to be associated with a normal-sized heart than cardiogenic pulmonary edema.

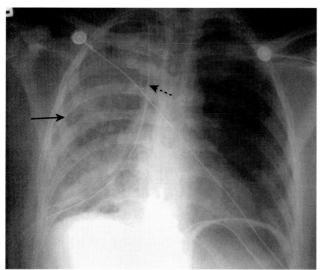

Figure 9-18 Reexpansion pulmonary edema. Unilateral airspace disease affects the entire right lung (*solid black arrow*). In addition, a chest tube (*dotted black arrow*) is seen on the same side. The chest tube was inserted for a large, right-sided, tension pneumothorax that was rapidly reexpanded. Reexpansion pulmonary edema results from the overly rapid expansion of a lung that has typically been chronically collapsed by pneumothorax or a large pleural effusion. Its exact cause is unknown. In general, unilateral pulmonary edema can occur either because of an abnormality on the same side as the pulmonary edema (e.g., prolonged positioning with the affected side dependent) or an abnormality on the opposite side (e.g., large pulmonary embolus occluding flow to the opposite lung).

Noncardiogenic Pulmonary Edema: Imaging Findings

- **Adult respiratory distress syndrome (ARDS)** represents one **form of noncardiogenic pulmonary edema**.
  - Characteristically, **patients with ARDS are radiographically normal for 24-36 hours** after the initial insult. Then, pulmonary abnormalities become evident in the form of **pulmonary interstitial edema** or **patchy airspace disease** or classical bilateral **pulmonary alveolar edema**.
  - Clinically, the **patient demonstrates severe hypoxia, cyanosis, tachypnea, and dyspnea**.
  - Typically, the findings of ARDS stabilize after 5-7 days and begin improving in about two weeks. Complete clearing, when it occurs, may take months.
  - In the later stages of ARDS, a **reticular interstitial pattern may develop**, although the majority of patients who survive tend to have little impairment of lung function.

Differentiating Cardiac from Noncardiac Pulmonary Edema

The **patterns of cardiac (cardiogenic) and noncardiac (noncardiogenic) pulmonary edema overlap considerably**; the patient's **history and clinical picture are key** to establishing the most likely cause of pulmonary edema.

- In general, **noncardiogenic pulmonary edema is**:
  - **Less likely** to demonstrate **pleural effusions** and **Kerley B lines** than cardiogenic pulmonary edema.
  - **More likely** to demonstrate a normal **pulmonary capillary wedge pressure (PCWP)** of less than 12 mm Hg than cardiogenic pulmonary edema.
  - **More likely** to be associated with a **normal-sized heart** (Fig. 9-19).
  - **More likely** to demonstrate airspace disease that is more patchy and peripheral than that in cardiogenic pulmonary edema, but this is highly variable.
  - The key differences between cardiogenic and nocardiogenic pulmonary edema are summarized in Table 9-3.

Hypertensive Cardiovascular Disease

- Chronic elevation of systemic blood pressure leads to left ventricular hypertrophy in about 20% of patients, double that incidence if the patient is obese. Most of the time (90%) the hypertension is *essential* hypertension with no identifiable cause. Heart failure, coronary artery disease, and cardiac arrhythmias are common complications of hypertension.
- Systemic hypertension can lead to left ventricular hypertrophy. Left ventricular hypertrophy occurs at the expense of the lumen, the wall becoming thicker while the lumen becomes smaller.

TABLE 9-3 CARDIOGENIC VERSUS NONCARDIOGENIC PULMONARY EDEMA

Imaging Finding	Cardiogenic	Noncardiogenic
Pleural effusions	Common	Infrequent
Kerley B lines	Common	Infrequent
Heart size	Frequently enlarged	May be normal
Pulmonary capillary wedge pressure	Elevated	Normal

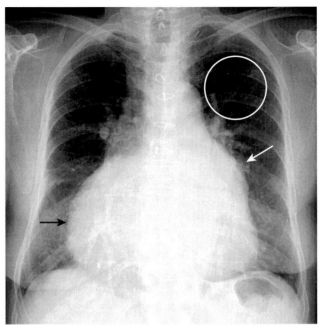

Figure 9-21 Chronic mitral stenosis with tricuspid regurgitation. The left atrium is enlarged (*solid white arrow*). Pulmonary venous hypertension has produced a redistribution of flow in the lungs so that the upper lobe vessels have become more prominent than the lower lobe **(cephalization)** (*white circle*). Due to increased pulmonary vascular resistance and subsequent pulmonary arterial hypertension, the right heart also undergoes changes, eventually including tricuspid regurgitation with enlargement of the right atrium (*solid black arrow*).

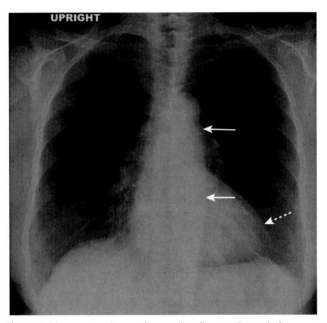

Figure 9-20 Hypertensive cardiovascular disease. Systemic hypertension can lead to hypertrophic cardiomyopathy. The left ventricle (*dotted white arrow*) is only slightly enlarged, but other modalities would demonstrate marked concentric hypertrophy of the left ventricular wall that has occurred at the expense of the lumen. The aorta itself is *uncoiled* (*solid white arrows*) due to increased systemic blood pressure (see also Fig. 9-7C).

- Therefore, **the heart is usually normal or slightly increased in size** early in the disease. It is not until the muscle begins to decompensate that the heart increases dramatically in size.
- **The aorta**, under increased systemic pressure, pivots outward around the aortic valve and the aortic hiatus in the diaphragm and **gradually uncoils**, becoming more prominent in both its ascending and descending portions (Fig. 9-20).
- Prolonged systemic hypertension may eventually lead to CHF.

Mitral Stenosis

- In developed nations, the incidence of mitral stenosis from rheumatic heart disease has declined markedly, but it is still seen in the elderly and in younger individuals from developing countries. The **most common symptoms** are from **left heart failure**: dyspnea on exertion, orthopnea, and paroxysmal nocturnal dyspnea.
- Mitral stenosis leads to obstruction to the outflow of blood from the left atrium and usually becomes symptomatic when the valve area falls below one-third of its normal size. As the left atrial pressure builds, the left atrium enlarges

and the increased pulmonary venous pressure (**pulmonary venous hypertension**) is reflected retrograde into the pulmonary circulation.

- Upper lobe vessels become as large as or more prominent than lower lobe vessels (**cephalization**). Pulmonary venous hypertension eventually leads to CHF. With prolonged elevation of pulmonary venous pressure, physical changes in the pulmonary vasculature may lead to escalating *pulmonary vascular resistance* requiring ever increasing levels of pulmonary arterial pressure.
- Eventually there is **pulmonary arterial hypertension** and right-sided heart failure (Fig. 9-21).

Pulmonary Arterial Hypertension

- The normal mean pulmonary artery pressure is about 15 mm Hg. Pulmonary arterial hypertension may be **idiopathic (primary)** or **secondary** to another disease, usually emphysema. Mitral stenosis is another cause of pulmonary arterial hypertension.
- With primary pulmonary hypertension, the leading cause of death is progressive right heart failure. Secondary pulmonary hypertension shares co-morbidities with the diseases that cause it: emphysema, recurrent pulmonary thromboembolic disease, mitral stenosis, CHF.
- The **hallmark of pulmonary arterial hypertension** is a discrepancy in size between the central pulmonary vasculature (i.e., the main, right, and left pulmonary arteries are large) and the peripheral pulmonary vasculature. This discrepancy is called *pruning*.
- On CT scans, the **main pulmonary artery is normally about the same diameter as the ascending aorta**, but in

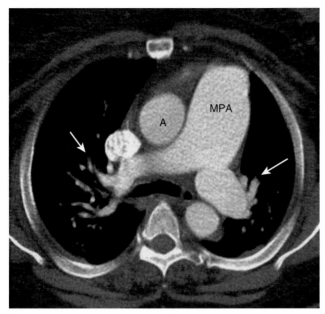

Figure 9-22 Pulmonary arterial hypertension. Normally, the main pulmonary artery (*MPA*) is about the same diameter as the ascending aorta (*A*). In this patient, with pulmonary arterial hypertension, the MPA is much larger than the aorta. There is also a rapid attenuation in the size of the pulmonary arteries (*solid white arrows*) called **pruning,** which is also seen in pulmonary arterial hypertension.

pulmonary arterial hypertension the main pulmonary artery is usually 3 cm or larger in size (Fig. 9-22).

Aortic Stenosis

■ Aortic stenosis may be secondary to a **congenital bicuspid aortic valve**, from **degeneration of a tricuspid valve** or, less frequently, **rheumatic heart disease**.

■ Since left ventricular outflow is obstructed and the ventricles respond to obstruction by undergoing hypertrophy of their walls, the heart is usually normal in size early in the course of the disease.

■ The ascending aorta may be unusually prominent because of *post-stenotic dilatation*, a hallmark of a significantly stenotic lesion in any major artery in which, because of **eddy currents** and **turbulent flow**, intraluminal pressure is increased for several centimeters **distal** to an obstructing lesion (see Fig. 9-9A).

■ Eventually, when the heart begins to decompensate, it will become enlarged and CHF may ensue. The classical triad of symptoms in aortic stenosis includes chest pain, syncope, and shortness of breath.

Cardiomyopathy

■ **Dilated cardiomyopathy**
• Dilated cardiomyopathy is, by definition, a condition in which there is **increased systolic and diastolic volume of the ventricles** associated with a **decreased (<40%) ejection fraction**. It is the **most common** form of **cardiomyopathy** (90%).
• It can be idiopathic (primary) or associated with known diseases such as cardiac ischemia, diabetes, and alcoholism.

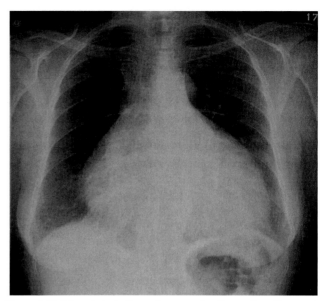

Figure 9-23 Dilated alcoholic cardiomyopathy. The cardiac silhouette is markedly enlarged, primarily as a result of biventricular enlargement. The patient had a long history of alcohol abuse. Dilated cardiomyopathy is frequently associated with congestive heart failure.

• **Decreased contractility and ventricular dilatation are hallmarks** so it is usually characterized by an **enlarged heart**, frequently associated with the imaging signs of **CHF** (Fig. 9-23).
• The diagnosis can usually be made by echocardiography following the initial chest radiograph, in concert with the clinical findings.
• MRI can provide the most accurate and reproducible findings for this disease. Using ECG-gated, cine-magnetic resonance angiography (MRA), **cardiac ejection fraction** and **cardiac dimensions** can be accurately assessed.
• **Radionuclide ventriculography** using small quantities of intravenously injected radioisotope can also determine **ejection fraction** and can be useful in differentiating between **ischemic** and **nonischemic causes of cardiomyopathy**.

■ Hypertrophic cardiomyopathy
• Hypertrophic cardiomyopathy is an abnormality (divided into primary [genetic] and secondary forms). It causes **asymmetric or concentric thickening of the myocardium**, sometimes with obstruction to left ventricular outflow caused by **systolic anterior motion (SAM)** of the anterior **mitral valve leaflet** (in the primary form). It **may lead to sudden cardiac death** and has been implicated as the cause of death in several high-profile athletes.
• In the secondary form, its most common manifestation, it is due to **hypertensive cardiovascular disease,** which produces concentric and diffuse hypertrophy of the left ventricle not associated with left ventricular outflow tract obstruction (see Fig. 9-20).
• The primary form may be diagnosed with echocardiography or ECG-gated MRI of the heart in which the **asymmetric septal hypertrophy (ASH)** may be demonstrated.

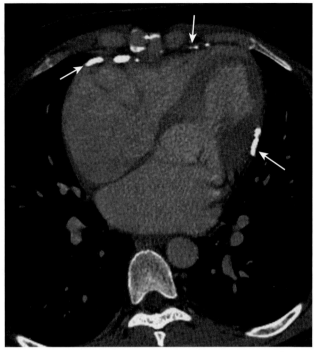

Figure 9-24 Constrictive pericarditis. There is extensive pericardial calcification (*solid white arrows*), most likely post-inflammatory in etiology. Although restrictive cardiomyopathy and constrictive pericarditis can have identical clinical findings, the presence of pericardial calcifications excludes *restrictive cardiomyopathy*. If indicated, pericardiectomy holds the potential for cure for patients with constrictive pericarditis.

- **Restrictive cardiomyopathy**
  - This is a **rare form** of cardiomyopathy characterized by **high diastolic filling pressures of the ventricles** in association with relatively well-preserved systolic function. It is usually secondary to an **infiltrative process** in the myocardium. Such diseases include **amyloid, autoimmune disease, and radiation.** The predominant presenting symptoms are related to **CHF.**
  - While clinically similar to **constrictive pericarditis,** the key difference is that the **pericardium is normal in restrictive cardiomyopathy,** while it is **thickened in constrictive pericarditis.** The importance in differentiating between the two is that constrictive pericarditis, unlike restrictive cardiomyopathy, is surgically curable.
  - In restrictive cardiomyopathy, the **heart is usually not enlarged.** There are pulmonary changes of CHF.
  - MRI can demonstrate the thickness of the pericardium, and if the pericardium is normal in size (<4 mm), constrictive pericarditis can effectively be excluded. If there is pericardial calcification, better seen on CT, restrictive cardiomyopathy can be excluded (Fig. 9-24).

Aortic Aneurysms: General Considerations

- Aneurysms are **defined as enlargement of a vessel greater than 50% of its original size.**
- **Atherosclerosis** is the **most common cause** of a descending thoracic aortic aneurysm. The majority of patients with aortic aneurysms are also hypertensive.
- Most patients with aneurysms are **asymptomatic,** and the aneurysm is **discovered serendipitously.**

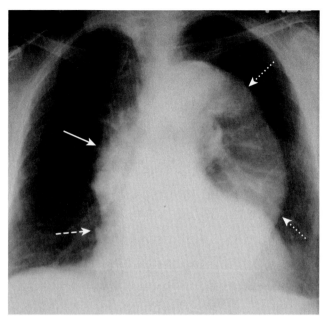

Figure 9-25 Aortic aneurysm. The entire thoracic aorta is enlarged in this 67-year-old man. The ascending aorta (*solid white arrow*) should normally not project farther to the right than the right heart border (*dashed white arrow*) on a nonrotated chest radiograph. The descending thoracic aorta should normally parallel and almost disappear with the thoracic spine; as it becomes larger, it swings farther away from the spine (*dotted white arrows*).

- When an aneurysm of the descending thoracic aorta expands, it may cause pain that classically, but not always, radiates to the back.
- As measured on CT or MRI scans, the **ascending aorta is usually <3.5 cm** in diameter and the **descending aorta is <3 cm.**
- An **aneurysm** of the thoracic aorta is usually defined as a **persistent enlargement of >4 cm.**
- In general, **aneurysms of 5 to 6 cm are at risk to rupture** and will require surgical intervention. The **rate of growth** of an aneurysm is also important in determining the need for surgical intervention and repair. Annual aneurysm growth rates should be <1 cm/year or elective resection is considered.

Recognizing a Thoracic Aortic Aneurysm

- The **appearance** of a thoracic aortic aneurysm **will depend,** in part, **from which portion of the thoracic aorta it arises.**
  - Aneurysms of the **ascending aorta** may extend **anteriorly and to the right.** Aneurysms of the **aortic arch** produce a **middle mediastinal mass.** Aneurysms of the **descending aorta** project **posteriorly, laterally, and to the left** (Fig. 9-25).
- **Contrast-enhanced CT** is the modality **most often used** to diagnose a thoracic aortic aneurysm; MRI is also excellent at demonstrating aneurysms but is usually less available and more expensive.
- On CT, aneurysms can appear as **fusiform (long)** or **saccular (globular)** in shape.
- Their anatomy will be **more readily delineated on CT studies** using iodinated contrast material injected

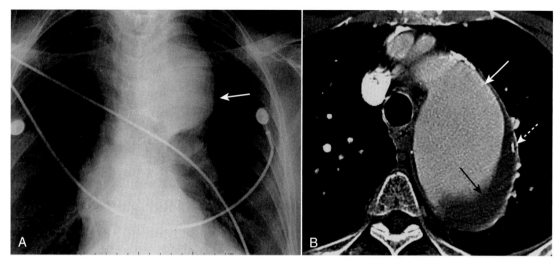

Figure 9-26 Aortic aneurysm, conventional chest radiograph and CT. Close-up view of a frontal radiograph of the chest **(A)** demonstrates a large mediastinal soft tissue mass (*solid white arrow*). This soft tissue density represents a large aneurysm of the proximal descending aorta seen also in the CT scan **(B).** The aneurysm measured 6.7 cm, which placed it at significant risk for rupture. Calcification in the wall of an aneurysm is common (*dotted white arrow*). Contrast material mixes with blood flowing in the lumen of the aorta (*solid white arrow*), but the flowing blood is separated from the intimal calcification by a considerable amount of noncontrast-containing thrombus adherent to the wall (*closed black arrow*).

intravenously as a bolus, but they may be visible on noncontrast (unenhanced) studies as well. Often, both unenhanced and contrast-enhanced CT studies are obtained to fully evaluate the aneurysm and its contained clot.

■ Frequently **calcification is seen in the intima**, which may be **separated** from the **contrast-filled lumen by varying amounts of clot** (Fig. 9-26).

Thoracic Aortic Dissection

■ **Aortic dissections most often originate in the ascending aorta (Stanford type A)** or may involve only the **descending aorta (Stanford type B)**.

■ They result from a tear that allows blood to dissect in the wall for varying lengths of the aorta, usually along the media.

■ In general, **patients with aortic dissection have been hypertensive and may have an underlying condition that can predispose to dissection**, such as cystic medial degeneration, atherosclerosis, Marfan syndrome, Ehlers-Danlos syndrome, trauma, syphilis, or crack cocaine abuse.

■ In many patients, **abrupt onset of ripping or tearing chest pain, which is maximal at its time of origin**, is the characteristic history.

■ **Conventional radiographs** are **not significantly sensitive to be diagnostically reliable**, but they **may point to the diagnosis** when several imaging findings occur together, especially in the proper clinical setting.

  • "Widening of the mediastinum" is a **poor means of establishing the diagnosis** because it is commonly overinterpreted on portable supine radiographs while, on the other hand, it occurs in only about 1 in 4 cases of aortic dissection.

  • **Left pleural effusion** (which **frequently represents a transudate** caused by pleural irritation, although transient hemorrhage from the aorta can also produce a hemothorax) (Fig. 9-27).

  • **Left apical pleural cap** of fluid or blood

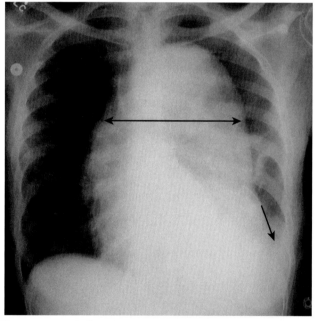

Figure 9-27 Aortic dissection. Conventional radiographs are not sensitive enough to be diagnostically reliable for aortic dissection, but they may point to the diagnosis when several imaging findings are seen together, especially in the proper clinical setting. "Widening of the mediastinum" is frequently not present and is a poor means of establishing the diagnosis, although in this patient the mediastinum is clearly widened by an enlarged aorta (*double black arrow*). Also, a left pleural effusion is present (*solid black arrow*). The combination of a widened mediastinum and a left pleural effusion in a patient with chest pain should alert you to the possibility of an aortic dissection.

  • **Loss of the normal shadow of the aortic knob**
  • **Increased deviation of the trachea or esophagus to the right**

■ **MRI is probably more sensitive** than CT at detecting a dissection, but **CT is usually more readily available**. Transesophageal ultrasound is also used to establish the diagnosis.

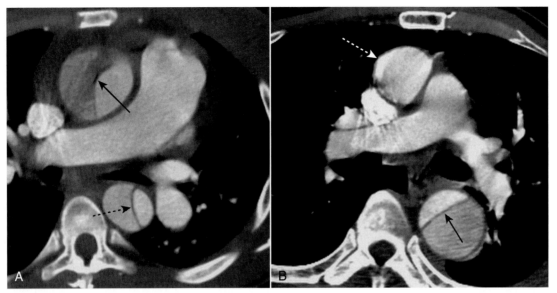

Figure 9-28 Aortic dissections, types A and B. A, An intimal flap is seen to traverse both the ascending (*solid black arrow*) and descending aorta (*dotted black arrow*). This is a Stanford type A dissection. **B,** There is a normal-appearing ascending aorta (*dotted white arrow*) while an intimal flap is noted by the black line traversing the descending aorta (*solid black arrow*). The intimal flap is the characteristic lesion of an aortic dissection. The smaller lumen is usually the true (original) lumen, and the larger, false lumen is actually a channel that has been produced by blood dissecting through the media.

➡ On both **MRI and CT**, the **diagnosis rests on identification** of the **intimal flap** that separates the **true (original)** from the **false lumen** (canal created by the dissection) (Fig. 9-28).

- In general, **type A (ascending aortic) dissections** are treated surgically, whereas type B (descending aortic dissections) are treated medically.

Coronary Artery Disease

- Coronary artery disease is the **leading cause of death worldwide**.
- Varying amounts of atheromatous plaque narrow the coronary artery lumen. Calcium is deposited in the muscular layers of the artery's walls. Vulnerable plaque may rupture and there may be vasospasm or emboli which produce enough stenosis to lead to ischemia and possibly *infarction* of cardiac muscle.
- MRI, CT, and nuclear medicine studies can be used in the evaluation of coronary artery disease.
- MRI can demonstrate **postinfarct scar formation** and **myocardial contractility**. Ventricular **function** can be quantitatively assessed. Some basic terms used in cardiac MRI are listed in Box 9-4 (Figs. 9-29 to 9-32).
- CT is used for imaging of the coronary arteries. It has a very high negative predictive value—a negative test virtually rules out coronary artery disease. One of the major drawbacks in the use of cardiac CT angiography is the relatively high x-ray dose delivered, but changes in equipment and algorithms are reducing this dose considerably. Cardiac CT angiography requires injection of iodinated contrast material.
- CT may also be used in asymptomatic patients for **calcium scoring** in which the calcium found in the coronary arteries is used as a marker for coronary artery disease. The amount

> **Box 9-4 Basic Cardiac MRI Terms**
>
> The three main cardiac imaging planes, called "double oblique" views, are designed to best demonstrate cardiac anatomy. They are:
>
> **Short axis view** (see Fig. 9-29)
>
> **Horizontal long access** (the long axis is the line from the center of the mitral valve to the left ventricular apex), also known as **"four-chamber view"** (see Fig. 9-30)
>
> **Vertical long access,** also known as **"two-chamber view"** (see Fig. 9-31)
>
> **Cardiac function** is usually evaluated using MRI sequences producing **"bright blood"** images because the blood is depicted with increased signal intensity (see Fig. 9-32A).
>
> **Cardiac morphology** is usually evaluated using MRI sequences producing **"black blood"** images. These images are designed to allow for anatomic assessment of the cardiac structures without interference from the bright blood signal (see Fig. 9-32B).
>
> Read more on the basics of MRI in Chapter 20.

of calcium detected on a cardiac CT scan, and calculated by computer, can be a helpful prognostic tool. The findings on cardiac CT are expressed as a calcium score, the higher the score the more extensive the evidence for CAD. Calcium scoring is performed without intravenous contrast (Fig. 9-33).

- CT can also demonstrate complications of myocardial infarction such as ventricular aneurysms and intracardiac clots.
- **Single photon emission computed tomography (SPECT)** is an imaging technique that blends the intravascular injection of a **radioactive isotope** with acquisition of images using a rotating nuclear gamma camera capable of 3-dimensional localization of disease.
  - Stress and resting myocardial perfusion images using SPECT imaging can demonstrate areas of **ischemia**, especially compared to the same study done at rest.

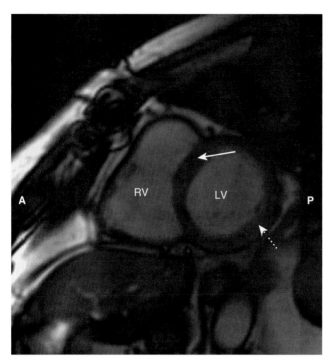

Figure 9-29 Cardiac MRI, short axis view. This is a standard view of the heart using MRI called the **short axis view**. The right ventricle (*RV*) lies anterior to the left ventricle (*LV*), separated by the interventricular septum (*solid white arrow*). Note the wall of the left ventricle (*dotted white arrow*) is normally thicker than the right ventricle. (*A* is anterior and *P* is posterior.)

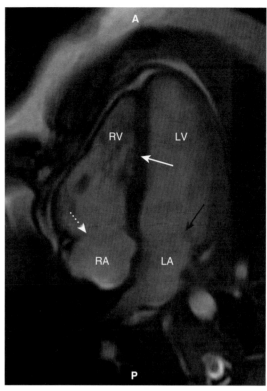

Figure 9-30 Cardiac MRI, horizontal long axis view. This is another standard view of the heart using MRI called the **horizontal long axis** or **four-chamber view**. The right (*RV*) and left ventricles (*LV*) are separated by the interventricular septum (*solid white arrow*). Posterior to each of them are the right atrium (*RA*) and left atrium (*LA*) separated by the regions of the tricuspid (*dotted white arrow*) and mitral valves (*solid black arrow*), respectively. (*A* is anterior and *P* is posterior.)

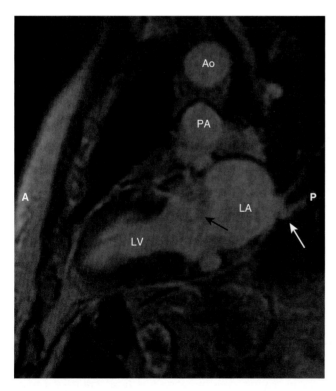

Figure 9-31 Cardiac MRI, vertical long axis view. The **vertical long axis** or **two-chamber view** demonstrates the left ventricle (*LV*) separated from the more posterior left atrium (*LA*) by the mitral valve area (*solid black arrow*). Pulmonary veins drain into the left atrium (*solid white arrow*). The aorta (*Ao*) sits atop the pulmonary artery (*PA*). (*A* is anterior and *P* is posterior.)

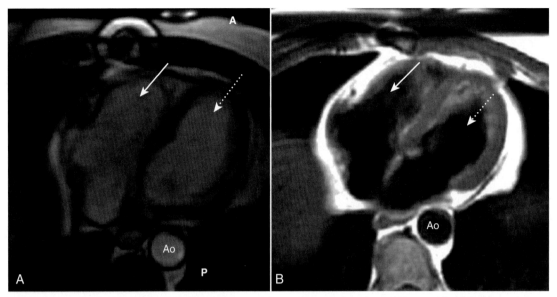

Figure 9-32 Cardiac MRI, *bright blood* and *black blood* images. Using different imaging algorithms, MRI is capable of displaying the same tissues with differing appearances. **(A)** and **(B)** are both axial sections through the heart, showing the right ventricle (*solid white arrows*), the left ventricle (*dotted white arrows*) and the aorta (*Ao*). The **bright blood** technique **(A)** is utilized to assess cardiac function while the **black blood** technique **(B)** is usually better at depicting cardiac morphology. (*A* is anterior and *P* is posterior.)

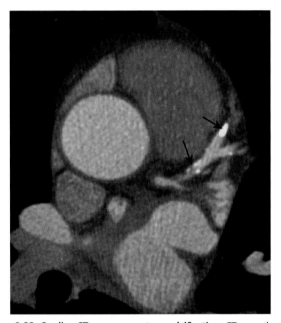

Figure 9-33 Cardiac CT, coronary artery calcification. CT scan through the heart without intravenous contrast demonstrates calcified plaque in the left anterior descending coronary artery (*solid black arrows*). The amount of calcium detected on a cardiac CT scan and calculated by computer can be a helpful prognostic tool for coronary artery disease.

- Nuclear medicine studies can also estimate left ventricular function.

WEBLINK

Registered users may obtain more information on Recognizing Adult Heart Disease on StudentConsult.com.

TAKE-HOME POINTS

Recognizing Adult Heart Disease

In adults, a quick assessment of heart size can be made using the *cardiothoracic ratio*, which is the ratio of the widest transverse diameter of the heart compared to the widest internal diameter of the rib cage. In normal adults, the cardiothoracic ratio is usually <50%.

There are extracardiac causes which can make the heart appear to be enlarged, even if it is actually normal, including AP portable studies, factors which inhibit a deep inspiration, abnormalities of the bony thorax, and the presence of a pericardial effusion.

The heart will appear slightly larger on an AP projection than a PA projection of the chest because the heart is closer to the imaging surface on a PA exposure.

On the lateral projection, the heart usually does not extend posteriorly to overlap the spine unless it is enlarged or there is a pericardial effusion.

In an infant, the heart may normally be up to 65% of the cardiothoracic ratio; other factors should be assessed in an infant with apparent cardiomegaly such as the pulmonary vasculature and the clinical signs and symptoms.

The thymus gland is usually seen in infants superimposed on the upper portion of the cardiac silhouette and could mimic cardiac enlargement.

The normal contours of the heart and the normal appearance of the pulmonary vasculature are reviewed.

Two major patterns of congestive heart failure are pulmonary interstitial and pulmonary alveolar edema.

The four key findings of **pulmonary interstitial edema** are thickening of the interlobular septa, peribronchial cuffing, fluid in the fissures, and pleural effusions.

The key findings in **pulmonary alveolar edema** are fluffy, indistinct, patchy airspace densities; bat-wing or butterfly configuration frequently sparing the outer third of lungs; and pleural effusions, especially with cardiogenic pulmonary edema.

Causes of pulmonary edema can be divided into two major categories: cardiogenic and noncardiogenic causes.

Cardiogenic pulmonary edema is more likely to have pleural effusions and Kerley B lines, cardiomegaly, and an elevated pulmonary capillary wedge pressure than noncardiogenic pulmonary edema.

The noncardiogenic causes of pulmonary edema are a diverse group of diseases, including uremia, disseminated intravascular coagulopathy, smoke inhalation, near-drowning, volume overload, and lymphangitic spread of malignancy.

Adult respiratory distress syndrome (ARDS) can be considered a subset of noncardiogenic pulmonary edema in which the clinical picture is one of severe hypoxia, cyanosis, tachypnea, and dyspnea.

Essential hypertension is a common disease that can lead to congestive heart failure and coronary artery disease as well as secondary hypertrophic cardiomyopathy.

Mitral stenosis has become less common with antibiotic treatment of rheumatic fever but can lead to left and then right heart failure through chronic elevation of the pulmonary venous and arterial pressures with increased pulmonary vascular resistance.

Pulmonary arterial hypertension may either be idiopathic (primary) or secondary to emphysema or recurrent thromboembolic disease. It produces *pruning* of the pulmonary vasculature and might be suspected when the main pulmonary artery achieves a diameter of 3 cm or more on CT or MRI.

Aortic stenosis in the elderly is most often secondary to degeneration of a tricuspid aortic valve and can lead to angina, syncope, or congestive heart failure. The ascending aorta may be prominent from *post-stenotic dilatation*.

Cardiomyopathies are divided into dilated, hypertrophic, and restrictive forms. Restrictive cardiomyopathy must be differentiated from constrictive pericarditis with which it shares its clinical findings.

Aortic aneurysms can be saccular or fusiform or can dissect. Most thoracic aortic dissections begin in the ascending aorta (Stanford type A) and are treated surgically.

Coronary artery disease is the leading cause of death worldwide. It or its sequelae can be imaged using a variety of techniques, including CT, MRI, and single photon emission computed tomography (SPECT).

Chapter 10

Recognizing the Correct Placement of Lines and Tubes: Critical Care Radiology

- Patients in the critical or intensive care units (ICU) are monitored on a frequent basis with portable chest radiography both to check on the position of their multiple assistive devices and to assess their cardiopulmonary status.
  - Diseases commonly seen in critically ill patients are discussed in other chapters (Table 10-1).
- In this chapter, you'll get practical advice for evaluating the successful (or not so successful) insertion and ultimate position of multiple tubes, lines, catheters, and other supportive apparatus used in the ICU.
- Most times, a conventional radiograph is obtained after the insertion or attempted insertion of one of these devices to check on its position and to rule out any unintended complications.
- Therefore, **for each tube or device, you'll learn**:
  - **Why they are used.**
  - **Where they belong** when properly placed.
  - Where such devices can be **malpositioned** and what **complications** may occur from the device.

ENDOTRACHEAL AND TRACHEOSTOMY TUBES

Endotracheal Tubes (ETT)

- **Why they are used**
  - Assist ventilation
  - Isolate the trachea to permit control of the airway
  - Prevent gastric distension
  - Provide a direct route for suctioning
  - Administer medications
- **Correct placement of an ETT** (Box 10-1)
  - Endotracheal tubes are usually **wide-bore tubes** (about 1 cm) with a **radioopaque marker stripe** and **no side holes**. The tip is **frequently diagonally shaped**.
  - With the patient's head in the neutral position (i.e., bottom of mandible is at the level of C5-C6), the **tip of ETT should be 3-5 cm from the carina.**
    - This is roughly **half the distance between the medial ends of clavicles and the carina** (Fig. 10-1).
    - Ideally the **diameter of the ETT should be one half to two thirds the width of the trachea.**
      - An inflated cuff (balloon), if present, may fill—but shouldn't distend—the lumen of the trachea (Fig. 10-2).

  ➡️ How to find the carina on a frontal chest radiograph

  - Follow the right or left main bronchus backward until it meets the opposite main bronchus. The carina projects over the T5, T6, or T7 vertebral bodies in 95% of people.

- Movement of tip with flexion and extension
  - Neck **flexion** may cause **2 cm of descent** of the tube tip. This is why the tip should be 3-5 cm from the carina.
  - Neck **extension** from neutral may cause **2 cm of ascent** of the tip.
- **Incorrect placement and complications of an ETT**
  - **Most common malposition**: because of the shallower angle and wider diameter of the **right main bronchus** or bronchus intermedius, the tip of the ETT will tend to slide **into the right-sided bronchial tree** preferentially to the left.
    - This can lead to **atelectasis** (especially of the non-aerated right upper lobe and left lung) (see Fig. 5-13).
    - Intubation of the right main bronchus could also lead to a **right-sided tension pneumothorax.**
  - Inadvertent **esophageal intubation** will produce a grossly dilated stomach.
  - The tip of the tube should not be positioned in the larynx or pharynx—the tip should be at least 3 cm distal to level of vocal cords; otherwise, **the tube can damage the vocal cords or lead to aspiration** (Fig. 10-3).

Tracheostomy Tubes

- Why they are used
  - In patients with airway obstruction at or above level of larynx
  - In respiratory failure requiring long-term intubation (>21 days)
  - For airway obstruction during sleep apnea
  - When paralysis of the muscles affects swallowing or respiration
- **Correct placement of a tracheostomy tube** (Box 10-2)
  - The tip **should be about halfway between the stoma in which the tracheostomy tube was inserted and the carina.** This is usually around the **level of T3** (Fig. 10-4).
  - Unlike an ETT, the placement of the tip of a tracheostomy tube is not affected by flexion and extension of the head.
  - **The width of the tracheostomy tube should be about two thirds the width of trachea.**
- **Incorrect placement and complications of a tracheostomy tube**
  - Immediately after insertion, **look for signs** of inadvertent **perforation of the trachea,** such as:
    - Pneumomediastinum
    - Pneumothorax
    - Subcutaneous emphysema

TABLE 10-1 COMMON DISEASES IN CRITICALLY ILL PATIENTS

Finding or Disease	Discussed in
Adult respiratory distress syndrome	Chapter 9
Aspiration	Chapter 7
Atelectasis	Chapter 5
Congestive heart failure (pulmonary edema)	Chapter 9
Pleural effusion	Chapter 6
Pneumomediastinum	Chapter 8
Pneumonia	Chapter 7
Pneumothorax	Chapter 8
Pulmonary thromboembolic disease	Chapter 12

Box 10-1 Endotracheal Tubes

The tip should be about 3-5 cm above the carina.

The inflated cuff should not distend the lumen of the trachea.

They are most commonly malpositioned in the right main or right lower lobe bronchi.

If positioned with their tip in the neck, damage to vocal cords can occur.

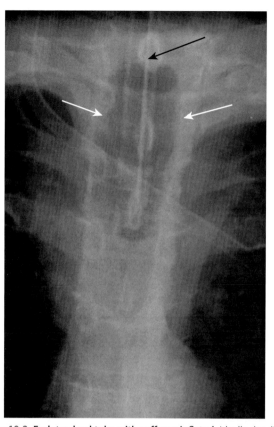

Figure 10-2 Endotracheal tube with cuff overinflated. Ideally the diameter of the endotracheal tube (*solid black arrow*) should be one third to one half the width of trachea. An inflated cuff (balloon), if present, may fill—but shouldn't distend—the lumen of the trachea. Here the inflated balloon (*solid white arrows*) is wider than the diameter of the trachea and was subsequently deflated. Prolonged compression on the tracheal wall by an overinflated cuff can result in necrosis of the wall and tracheal stenosis.

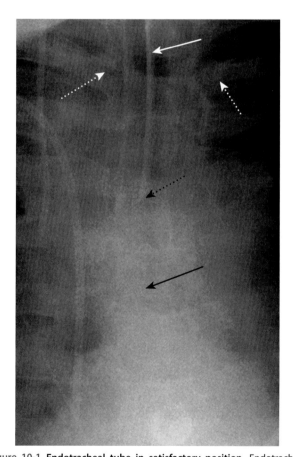

Figure 10-1 Endotracheal tube in satisfactory position. Endotracheal tubes are usually wide-bore tubes (about 1 cm) with a radioopaque marker stripe (*solid white arrow*) and no side holes. The tip is frequently diagonally angled (*dotted black arrow*). With the patient's head in the neutral position, the tip of ETT should be 3-5 cm from the carina (*solid black arrow*), which is roughly half the distance between the medial ends of clavicles (*dotted white arrows*) and the carina.

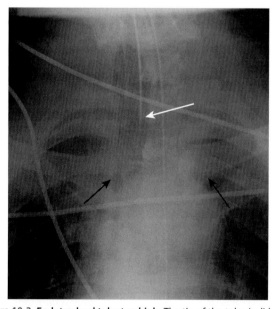

Figure 10-3 Endotracheal tube too high. The tip of the tube (*solid white arrow*) should not be positioned in the larynx or pharynx. The tip should be at least 3 cm distal to the level of the vocal cords so that damage to the vocal cords and aspiration do not occur. The medial ends of the clavicles are marked by the *solid black arrows*.

INTRAVASCULAR CATHETERS

Central Venous Catheters (CVC)

- **Why they are used**
  - For venous access to instill chemotherapeutic and hyperosmolar agents not suitable for peripheral venous administration
  - Measurement of central venous pressure
  - To maintain and monitor intravascular blood volume
- **Correct placement of CVCs** (Box 10-3)
  - **CVCs are small** (3 mm) and **uniformly opaque without a marker stripe**.
  - They are usually inserted either by the **subclavian** or **internal jugular** route. The internal jugular veins join the subclavian veins to form the brachiocephalic (innominate) veins, which, in turn, drain into the superior vena cava. The junctions of the subclavian and brachiocephalic veins generally occur posterior to the **medial ends** of the clavicles.
  - A CVC should reach the **medial end of clavicle before descending**, and its **tip** should **lie medial** to the **anterior** end of the 1st rib.
  - The catheter should **descend lateral to the spine, and the tip should lie in the superior vena cava** (Fig. 10-5).
    - You should be able to recognize the indentation of the cardiac contour that marks the junction between the superior vena cava and the right atrium (see Fig. 2-1).
  - **All bends in the catheter should be smooth curves**, not sharp kinks.
- **Incorrect placement and complications of CVCs**
  - CVCs, more frequently those placed by the subclavian route, can be malpositioned.
  - They are **most often malpositioned with their tips in the right atrium or internal jugular vein** (if inserted via the subclavian vein) (Fig. 10-6).
    - In the **right atrium**, they can **produce cardiac arrhythmias**.
    - When CVCs are malpositioned, they may provide **inaccurate central venous pressure readings**.
  - **Pneumothorax** can occur in up to 5% of CVC insertions, more often with the subclavian approach than the internal jugular route.
  - **Occasionally CVCs may perforate the vein** and lie outside of the blood vessel. Look for sharp bends in the catheter as a clue to a possible perforation.
  - Sometimes, they may be **inadvertently inserted in the subclavian artery** rather than the subclavian vein.
    - Suspect **arterial placement** if the **flow is pulsatile** and the course of the catheter **parallels the aortic arch** or **fails to descend to the right of the spine** (Fig. 10-7).

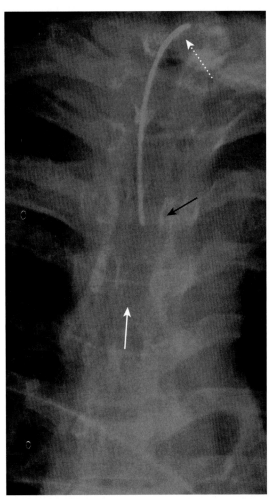

Figure 10-4 Tracheostomy tube in correct position. The tip (*solid black arrow*) should be about halfway between the stoma in which the tracheostomy tube was inserted (*dotted white arrow*) and the carina (*solid white arrow*). This is usually around the level of T3. Unlike the tip of an endotracheal tube, the placement of the tip of a tracheostomy tube is not affected by flexion and extension of the neck.

- If the tracheostomy tube is equipped with a **cuff, the cuff should generally be inflated to a diameter that fills but does not distend the normal tracheal contour.**
- **Long-term complication of tracheostomies:**
  - **Tracheal stenosis is the most common late-occurring complication** of a tracheostomy tube and can occur at the entrance stoma, level of the cuff, or at the tip of tube, but is **most common at the stoma.**

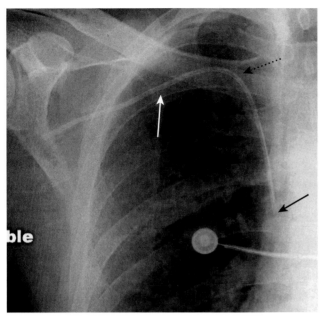

Figure 10-5 Subclavian central venous catheter in correct position. Central venous catheters are small (3 mm) and uniformly opaque without a marker stripe (*solid white arrow*). The subclavian vein joins the brachio-cephalic vein behind the medial end of the clavicle. A central venous catheter should reach the medial end of the clavicle (*dotted black arrow*) before descending. The catheter should descend to the right of the tho-racic spine, and the tip should be in the superior vena cava (*solid black arrow*).

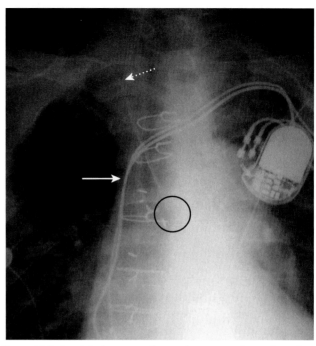

Figure 10-7 Arterial placement of central venous catheter. Sometimes central lines may be inadvertently inserted in the subclavian artery rather than the subclavian vein. This catheter does not reach the medial end of the clavicle (*dotted white arrow*) before descending, and its tip (*black circle*) is oriented over the spine, directed away from the superior vena cava (*solid white arrow*). Suspect arterial placement if the flow is pulsatile.

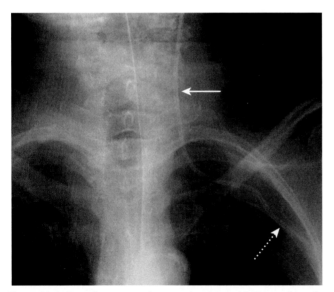

Figure 10-6 Central venous catheter malpositioned in internal jugular vein. Central venous catheters, especially those placed by the subclavian route (*dotted white arrow*), are often malpositioned. They are most often malpositioned with their tips in the right atrium or internal jugular vein (*solid white arrow*). In the right atrium, they can produce cardiac arrhyth-mias. When central venous catheters are malpositioned, they may provide inaccurate central venous pressure measurements.

 Two or more attempts at inserting a CVC

- A frontal chest radiograph is obtained following place-ment of a CVC.
- **Should initial placement fail,** you should **obtain a chest radiograph before trying insertion on the**

Box 10-4 PICC Lines

The tip should lie in the superior vena cava or axillary vein.
They may be difficult to visualize because of their small size.
Thrombosis of the line may occur over time.

---

other side to avoid the possibility of producing bilat-eral pneumothoraces.

Peripherally Inserted Central Catheters: "PICC Lines"

- **Why they are used**
  - For long-term venous access (months)
  - To administer medications such as chemotherapy or antibiotics
  - For frequent blood sampling
  - Because of their small size, they can be inserted into an antecubital vein.
- **Correct placement of PICC lines** (Box 10-4)
  - **Tip** should lie **within** the **superior vena cava** but may be placed in an axillary vein. Because the lines are so small, they may be difficult to visualize (Fig. 10-8).
- **Incorrect placement and complications of PICC lines**
  - Tips may become malpositioned over time.
  - Thrombosis of the line may occur because of its small lumen size.

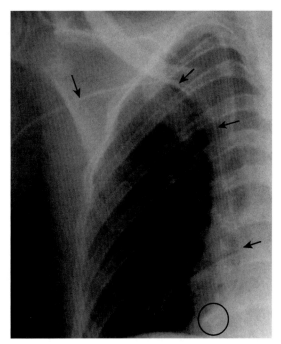

Figure 10-8 Peripherally inserted central catheter (PICC line) in right atrium. A PICC line (*solid black arrows*) can be used for long-term venous access. Because the lines are so small, they may be difficult to visualize. The tip should lie within the superior vena cava but may be placed in an axillary vein. In this case, the tip extends to the region of the right atrium (*black circle*).

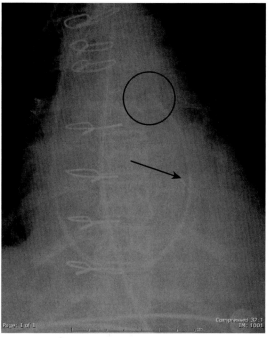

Figure 10-9 Swan-Ganz catheter in correct position. Swan-Ganz catheters have the same appearance as central venous lines but are longer (*solid black arrow*). They are inserted via the subclavian vein or internal jugular vein, and their tips (*black circle*) are floated out into the proximal right or proximal left pulmonary artery. The tip should be no more than 2 cm from the hilar shadow.

> **Box 10-5 Pulmonary Artery Catheters (Swan-Ganz Catheters)**
>
> Tip should be about 2 cm from the hilum in either the right or left pulmonary artery.
>
> Balloon should be inflated only when pressure measurements are performed.
>
> The tip of the catheter should not lie within a peripheral pulmonary artery.

Pulmonary Artery Catheters: Swan-Ganz Catheters

- **Why they are used**
  - Monitor hemodynamic status of critically ill patients
  - Help in differentiating cardiac from noncardiac pulmonary edema
- **Correct placement of Swan-Ganz catheters (also known as *pulmonary capillary wedge pressure catheters*) (Box 10-5)**
  - Swan-Ganz catheters have the **same appearance as central venous lines but are longer**.
  - Inserted via the subclavian vein or internal jugular vein, their tips are floated out into the **proximal right or proximal left pulmonary artery**.
    - The **tip of the Swan-Ganz catheter should be no more than about 2 cm from the hila** (Fig. 10-9).
  - The catheter's balloon is temporarily inflated only when pressure measurements are made and should then be deflated.
- **Incorrect placement and complications of Swan-Ganz catheters**
  - **Serious complications are uncommon**.

- The most common significant complication is **pulmonary infarction** from occlusion of a pulmonary artery by the catheter or from emboli arising from the catheter.
- Peripherally placed catheters may produce a localized, confined perforation or ***pseudoaneurysm***, which can be recognized by consolidation or a mass that forms at the site of the catheter tip in a critical-care patient who also develops hemoptysis.
- **Make sure the catheter tip does not lie in a distal branch of a pulmonary artery,** as this increases the risk of complication (Fig. 10-10).

Double Lumen Catheters: "Quinton Catheters," Hemodialysis Catheters

- **Why they are used**
  - Hemodialysis
  - Simultaneous ports for administration of medication and blood sampling
- **Correct placement of double lumen catheters for hemodialysis (Box 10-6)**
  - These are **large-bore catheters** that are **typically marked with a central stripe**.
  - Designs vary among different commercial brands, but all have at least two lumens arranged coaxially inside a single catheter with the goal to minimize the amount of recirculation that occurs between the two ports.
    - The **"arterial" port** from which blood is **withdrawn from the patient is proximal** to the "venous" port through which blood is **returned to the patient** to minimize recirculation of blood.

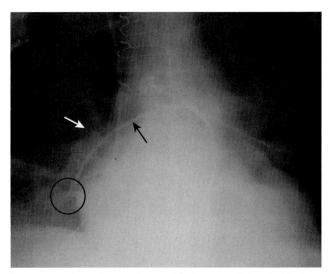

Figure 10-10 **Swan-Ganz catheter with tip too peripheral.** This Swan-Ganz catheter is directed toward the right pulmonary artery (*solid black arrow*). The tip of a Swan-Ganz catheter should lie within 2 cm of the hilar shadow (*solid white arrow*). The tip of this catheter (*black circle*) lies in a peripheral branch of the right descending pulmonary artery. This increases the risk of complication, such as pulmonary infarction or pseudoaneurysm formation.

Box 10-6 Double Lumen Catheters

The tip should either be in the superior vena cava or right atrium; some catheters are designed with separate lumens so that one tip is in the superior vena cava and the other is in the right atrium.

The right internal jugular vein has the lowest incidence of clotting so it is the preferred access route.

Complications include pneumothorax, thrombosis, and infection.

- Some catheters are designed as two separate single-lumen catheters with one catheter tip in the superior vena cava and the other catheter tip in the right atrium (Fig. 10-11).
- The **right internal jugular route is most often used for access.**
- Those that are used temporarily (2-3 weeks) usually have their tips in the superior vena cava, while the tips of the more permanent catheters may be in the right atrium.
- **Incorrect placement and complications of double lumen catheters**
  - **Immediate complications** can include **pneumothorax** or **malposition** or **perforation** of the tip.
  - **Long-term complications** include **infection** and **thrombosis** of the vein containing the catheter or **occlusion** of the catheter itself.

PLEURAL DRAINAGE TUBES (CHEST TUBES, THORACOTOMY TUBES)

- **Why they are used**
  - To remove either air or abnormal collections of fluid from the pleural space
- **Correct placement of pleural drainage tubes** (Box 10-7)

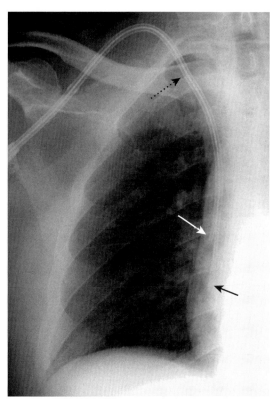

Figure 10-11 **Double lumen catheter in correct position.** These large-bore catheters are typically marked with a central stripe (*dotted black arrow*). All have at least two lumens arranged coaxially inside a single catheter with the tip for blood withdrawal (*solid white arrow*) farther from the heart than the tip for blood return to the patient (*solid black arrow*) in order to minimize recirculation. The right internal jugular route is most often used for access. Some catheters, such as this one, are designed as two, separate single-lumen catheters with one tip in the superior vena cava and the other in the right atrium.

Box 10-7 Pleural Drainage Tubes (Chest Tubes)

In general, chest tubes work well no matter where they are positioned, but malpositioning can result in inadequate drainage.

For pleural effusions, they work best with their tip placed posteriorly and inferiorly.

For pneumothorax, they work best with their tip placed anteriorly and superiorly.

Rapid drainage of a large pleural effusion or large pneumothorax can produce reexpansion pulmonary edema in the underlying lung.

- Chest tubes are **wide-bore tubes with a radioopaque stripe** used as a marker. The **stripe "breaks" at the site of a side hole.**
- Ideal position is **anterosuperior for evacuating a pneumothorax and posteroinferior for draining an effusion,** but chest tubes usually work well no matter where positioned (Fig. 10-12).
- **None of the side holes should lie outside of the thoracic wall** (Fig. 10-13).
- **Incorrect placement and complications of pleural drainage tubes**
  - Most malpositions lead to **inadequate drainage** rather than serious complication.
  - This includes malpositions in which the tube is inadvertently placed in the major fissure (Fig. 10-14).

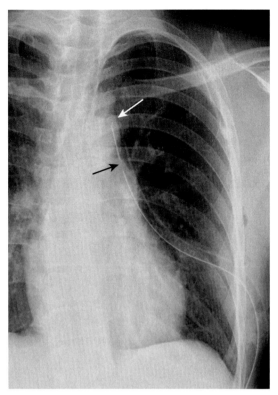

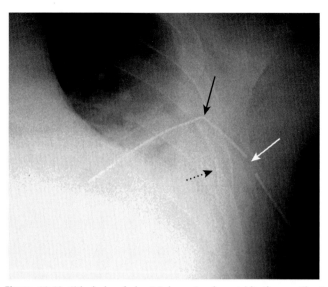

Figure 10-13 Side hole of chest tube extends outside thorax. Chest tubes typically have one or more side holes marked by a discontinuity in the marker stripe. None of the side holes (*solid white arrow*) should lie outside the thoracic wall (*dotted black arrow*) as it does in this patient. An air leak can develop leading to persistence of the underlying problem, in this case a pleural effusion. This tube is also kinked as it enters the chest (*solid black arrow*), which may further reduce its efficiency.

Figure 10-12 Chest tube in correct position. Chest tubes are wide-bore tubes with a radioopaque stripe used as a marker. The stripe "breaks" at the site of the side hole (*solid black arrow*). The ideal position is anterosuperior (*solid white arrow*), such as in this patient, for evacuating a pneumothorax and posteroinferior for draining an effusion. Chest tubes usually work well no matter where positioned.

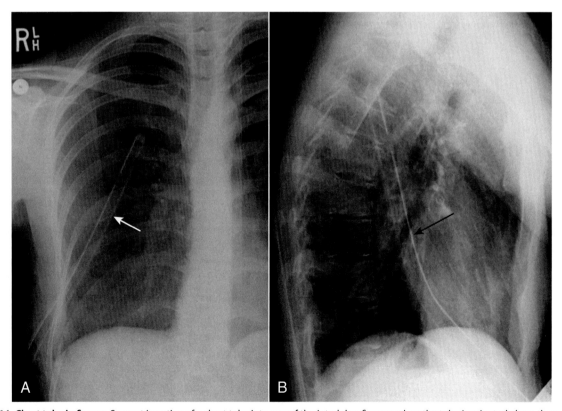

Figure 10-14 Chest tube in fissure. Suspect insertion of a chest tube into one of the interlobar fissures when the tube is oriented along the course of the fissure (*solid white arrow* on the frontal view **[A]** and *solid black arrow* on the lateral view **[B]**). This tube lies within the right major fissure. Malpositions like this can lead to inadequate drainage rather than a serious complication.

- **If the side hole extends outside of the chest wall**, this can lead to an *air leak* causing both inadequate drainage and subcutaneous emphysema.
- **Serious complications are uncommon:**
  - Bleeding secondary to laceration of intercostal artery
  - Laceration of liver or spleen on insertion
  - Rapid reexpansion of a collapsed lung, caused either by a large pneumothorax or a large pleural effusion, may lead to unilateral *reexpansion pulmonary edema* (see Fig. 9-18).

CARDIAC DEVICES

Pacemakers

- **Why they are used**
  - Used for cardiac conduction abnormalities
  - Certain conditions refractory to medical treatment (e.g., congestive heart failure)
- **Correct placement of cardiac pacemakers** (Box 10-8)
  - All **pacemakers consist of a pulse generator** usually implanted subcutaneously in the left anterior chest wall and **at least one lead (electrode)** inserted percutaneously most often into the subclavian vein.
  - **The tip of one lead is almost always located in the apex of the right ventricle.**

Remember that in the frontal projection, the apex of the right ventricle lies to the left of the spine and on the lateral film the apex of the right ventricle is located anteriorly (Fig. 10-15).

- Some pacemakers have two leads (usually their tips are in the right atrium and right ventricle) while others may have three leads (with their tips usually in the right atrium, right ventricle, and coronary sinus).
- **All leads should have gentle curves.** The electrodes should have no sharp kinks.
- **Incorrect placement and complications of cardiac pacemakers**
  - **Pneumothoraces** are infrequent complications of either pacemaker or AICD insertion.
  - **Fracture of the leads** may occur at any of three places: the pacer itself, the tip of the lead, or the site of venous access. Breaks in the lead can be **recognized by discontinuity in the wire lead itself** (Fig. 10-16).
  - **Leads can perforate the heart** producing cardiac tamponade. **Look for sharp bends** in leads secondary to perforation of a blood vessel.
  - **Leads may retract from normal contact with the ventricular wall** because the patient twists or twiddles the pacemaker generator under the skin, unknowingly winding the leads around the pacer causing retraction of

---

Box 10-8 Pacemakers

The generator is usually placed in the left anterior chest wall with at least one lead in the right ventricular apex.

Remember that the right ventricle projects to the left of the spine on the frontal view and anteriorly on the lateral view of the chest.

Complications are infrequent but include fractures in the lead wires and pneumothorax.

Ectopically placed leads may result in failure of the pacemaker to function properly.

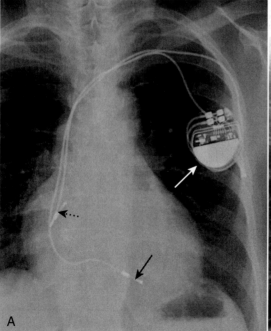 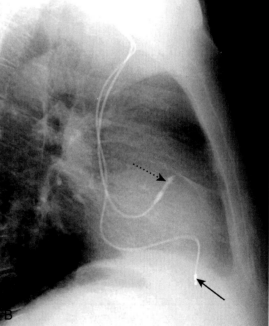

Figure 10-15 Dual-lead pacemaker in correct position. Pacemakers consist of a pulse generator (*solid white arrow*) usually implanted in the left chest wall and one or more electrode leads usually inserted into the subclavian vein. This patient has a dual-lead pacemaker. One of the leads is in the apex of the right ventricle (*solid black arrow* in **[A]** and **[B]**) while the other lead is in the right atrium (*dotted black arrow* in **[A]** and **[B]**). Notice that the right ventricular lead (*solid black arrows*) projects to the left of the midline **(A)** and anteriorly **(B),** and the right atrial lead typically curls upward.

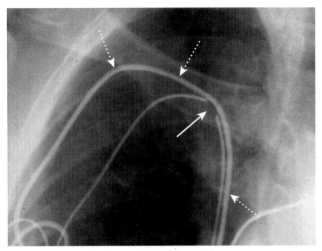

Figure 10-16 Fractured pacemaker lead. Fractures of pacemaker or automatic implantable cardiac defibrillator (AICD) leads may occur at any of three places: the generator itself, the tip of the lead, or the site of venous access. Breaks in the lead can be recognized by discontinuity in the wire lead itself (*solid white arrow*) which, in this patient, occurred at the site of venous access to the subclavian vein. The broken lead had been discovered earlier and a second, intact lead is already in place (*dotted white arrows*).

the tips (*Twiddler syndrome*) (Fig. 10-17) or from subcutaneous migration of the pacer.
- Leads may be ectopically placed, e.g., hepatic vein.

Automatic Implantable Cardiac Defibrillators (AICDs)

- **Why they are used**
  - To prevent sudden death, usually from tachyarrhythmias like ventricular fibrillation or ventricular tachycardia.
- **Correct placement of automatic implantable cardiac defibrillators** (Box 10-9)
  - AICDs can usually be **differentiated from pacemakers by the wider and more opaque segment of at least one of the electrodes** (Fig. 10-18). One electrode is usually placed in the superior vena cava or brachiocephalic vein. If present, the other electrode tip is placed in the apex of the right ventricle.
  - **All bends in the leads should be smooth curves,** not sharp kinks.
- **Incorrect placement and complications of automatic implantable cardiac defibrillators**
  - Leads may migrate and become dislodged.
  - Leads may fracture.

Intraaortic Counterpulsation Balloon Pump (IACB or IABP)

- **Why they are used**
  - Used to improve cardiac output and improve perfusion of the coronary arteries following surgery or in patients with cardiogenic shock or refractory ventricular failure. Placed in the proximal descending thoracic aorta, **the balloon is inflated in diastole and deflated in systole.**
- **Correct placement of intraaortic balloon pumps** (Box 10-10)

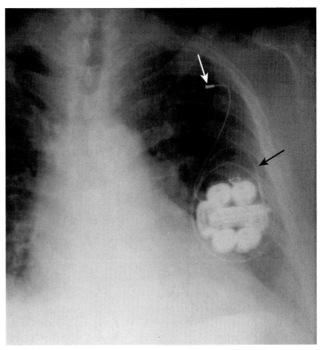

Figure 10-17 Twiddler syndrome. Some patients inadvertently "twiddle" with their subcutaneous pulse generator and, if the subcutaneous tissue allows, may rotate the generator many times on its own axis, curling the lead(s) around the device (*solid black arrow*). This can retract the tip of the electrode from the inner wall of the right ventricle, rendering the pacemaker useless. This lead has retracted to the left subclavian vein (*solid white arrow*).

Box 10-9 Automatic Implantable Cardiac Defibrillator

Can be differentiated from pacemakers by the presence of a thicker electrode on at least one lead.

May have one (right ventricle), two (right atrium and right ventricle), or three leads (right atrium, right ventricle, and coronary sinus).

Bends in the leads should be smooth curves, not sharp kinks.

Visible complications can include lead breakage and dislodgement.

- **Tip can be identified by a small, linear metallic marker** (Fig. 10-19).
  - **The tip should lie distal to origin of the left subclavian artery** so as not to occlude it.
  - Metallic **marker may point slightly toward the right** in region of aortic arch.
- When inflated, the sausage-shaped balloon may be visualized as an air-containing structure in the descending thoracic aorta.
- **Incorrect placement and complications of intraaortic balloon pumps**
  - If catheter is **too proximal, the balloon may occlude the great vessels** leading to stroke.
  - If the balloon is **too distal, the device has decreased effectiveness.**
  - Aortic dissection and arterial perforation may occur infrequently.

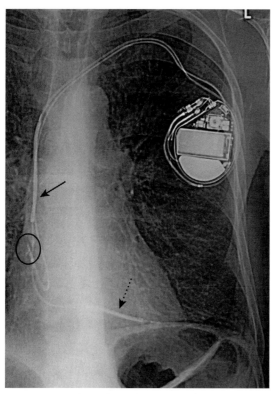

Figure 10-18 Automatic implantable cardiac defibrillator (AICD). AICDs can usually can be differentiated from pacemakers by the wider and more opaque segment of at least one of the electrodes (*solid and dotted black arrows*). One electrode is usually placed in the superior vena cava (*solid black arrow*) or brachiocephalic vein with its tip in the right atrium (*black circle*), and the other electrode tip is placed in the apex of the right ventricle (*dotted black arrow*). All bends in the leads should be smooth curves, not sharp kinks.

Box 10-10 Intraaortic Balloon Pumps
The tip has a metallic marker which should lie distal to the origin of the left subclavian artery.
When inflated, the balloon will be visible as an air-containing "sausage" in thoracic aorta.
Catheters placed too proximally may occlude the great vessels.
Catheters placed too distally may be ineffective.

GASTROINTESTINAL TUBES AND LINES

Nasogastric Tubes (NGTs)

- **Why they are used**
  - Short-term feeding
  - Gastric sampling and decompression through suction
  - Administering medication
- **Correct placement of nasogastric tubes** (Box 10-11)
  - **Nasogastric tubes** are **wide tubes** (about 1 cm) marked with a **radioopaque stripe** that "breaks" at a **side hole**, usually about **10 cm from the tip.**
  - **The tip and all side holes** of the tube should **extend about 10 cm into the stomach beyond the esophagogastric (EG) junction** to prevent aspiration from administration of a feeding into esophagus. If the NGT is to be used only for suction, the position of the side holes is less important.

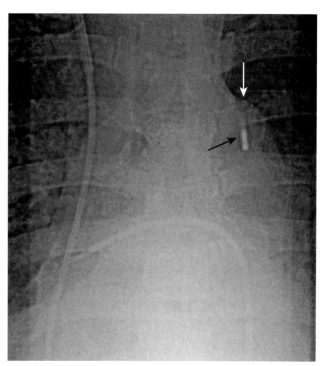

Figure 10-19 Intraaortic counterpulsation balloon pump (IABP). The tip of this assistive device can be identified by a small, linear metallic marker in the region of the descending thoracic aorta (*solid black arrow*). The tip should lie distal to origin of the left subclavian artery so as not to occlude it. In this case, the tip is about 1 cm from the top of the aortic knob (*solid white arrow*). The metallic marker may sometimes point slightly toward the right in the region of the arch.

Box 10-11 Nasogastric Tube (Levin Tube)
The tip of a nasogastric tube should extend into the stomach about 10 cm past the EG junction.
NG tubes are the most commonly malpositioned of all tubes; always check their positioning with a radiograph.
When malpositioned, they most frequently coil in the esophagus.
If inserted in the trachea, they can extend into a bronchus to periphery of lung, more often on the right side.

 How to recognize the location of the EG junction

- The **EG junction** is usually **located at the junction of the left hemidiaphragm and the left side of the thoracic spine** (this is called the *left cardiophrenic angle*) (Fig. 10-20).
- **Incorrect placement and complications of nasogastric tubes**
  - **The nasogastric tube is the most commonly malpositioned of all tubes and lines.**
    - **Coiling of the NG tube in the esophagus is the most common malposition.**
    - **May be inadvertently inserted into the trachea** and enter a bronchus (Fig. 10-21).
    - **Perforation caused by an NG tube is rare**, but when it occurs, it is usually in the cervical esophagus.
    - Long-term indwelling NG tube **can lead to gastroesophageal reflux**, which may, in turn, produce **esophagitis** and **stricture.**

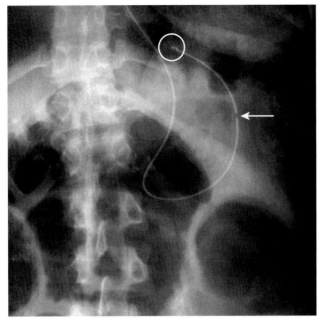

Figure 10-20 Nasogastric tube in stomach. Nasogastric tubes are wide-bore tubes marked with a radiopaque stripe that "breaks" in the position of the side hole, usually about 10 cm from the tip (*solid white arrow*). The tip and all side holes of the tube should extend about 10 cm into the stomach beyond the esophagogastric (EG) junction to prevent aspiration from administration of the feeding into esophagus. This tube is coiled back upon itself, and the tip (*white circle*) is too near the EG junction.

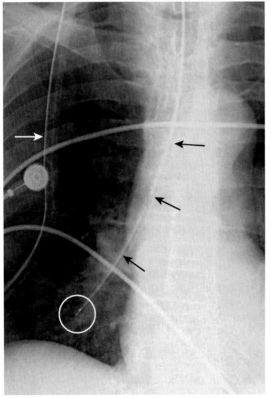

Figure 10-21 Nasogastric tube in right lower lobe bronchus. Nasogastric tubes are the most commonly malpositioned of all tubes and lines. Coiling of the NG tube in the esophagus is the most common malposition. In this patient, the nasogastric tube (*solid black arrows*) entered the trachea instead of the esophagus, and its tip extends to the right lower lobe (*white circle*). It is important to obtain a radiograph to confirm positioning of an NG tube before using it for feeding. A portion of the NG tube that lies outside the patient is superimposed on the chest (*solid white arrow*), as are several heart monitor leads.

> **Box 10-12 Feeding Tubes (Dobbhoff Tubes)**
>
> The tip should ideally be in the duodenum, although most lie in the stomach.
>
> The tip is recognizable by a metallic marker.
>
> If inadvertently inserted into the trachea, the tip may extend into the lung.
>
> Always obtain a confirmatory radiograph before using the tube for feedings.

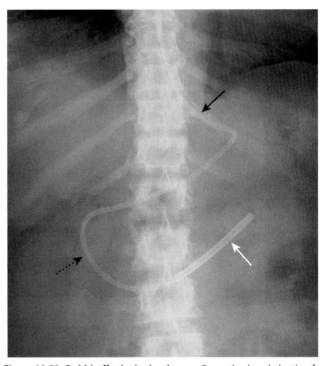

Figure 10-22 Dobbhoff tube in duodenum. Correctly placed, the tip of a Dobbhoff feeding tube should be in the duodenum to reduce risk of aspiration after feeding. The tip is recognizable by a weighted, metallic end (*solid white arrow*). This Dobbhoff tube enters the stomach (*solid black arrow*), courses around the duodenal sweep (*dotted black arrow*), and ends at the junction between the fourth portion of the duodenum and the jejunum. Placement in the stomach rather than the duodenum is very common. Note that the EG junction is usually located at the junction of the left hemidiaphragm and the left side of the thoracic spine (the left cardiophrenic angle) (*solid black arrow*).

- Always obtain a confirmatory radiograph before feeding the patient or administering any medication through the tube.

Feeding Tubes (Dobbhoff Tubes, DHTs)

- **Why they are used**
  - For nutrition
- **Correct placement of feeding tubes** (Box 10-12)
  - The ideal position of the **tip of the feeding tube is considered to be postpyloric, i.e., in the duodenum or jejunum,** the rationale being to reduce risk of aspiration after feeding (Fig. 10-22). In fact, placement in the stomach is very common.
  - The tip of a Dobbhoff tube is recognizable by a weighted, metallic, linear density.

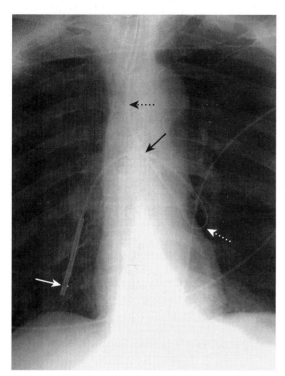

Figure 10-23 Dobbhoff tube in left and right lower lobe bronchi. In this case, the Dobbhoff tube inadvertently entered the trachea (*dotted black arrow*), entered the left lower lobe bronchus (*dotted white arrow*), then coiled back on itself (*solid black arrow*) to cross the midline and end in the right lower lobe bronchus (*solid white arrow*). It is important to obtain a confirmatory radiograph prior to using the tube for feedings.

- Did you know that the Dobbhoff tube was not named after a person called "Dobbhoff"? The tube is named after two physicians, Drs. Dobbie and Hoffmeister.
- **Incorrect placement and complications of feeding tubes**
  - **Placement in the trachea** rather than the esophagus may lead to the tip entering the lung. Always obtain a confirmatory radiograph before feeding the patient (Fig. 10-23).
  - **Perforation of the esophagus by the guide wire** is an uncommon complication.
    - Once the guide wire is removed, it is not reinserted.

WEBLINK

Registered users may obtain more information on Recognizing the Correct Placement of Lines and Tubes: Critical Care Radiology on StudentConsult.com.

TAKE-HOME POINTS

Recognizing the Correct Placement of Lines and Tubes: Critical Care Radiology

Tube or Line	Desired Position
Endotracheal tube (ETT)	Tip 3-5 cm from carina
Tracheostomy tube tip	Halfway between stoma and carina
Central venous catheter (CVC)	Tip in superior vena cava
Peripherally inserted central catheters (PICC)	Tip in superior vena cava
Swan-Ganz catheter	Tip in proximal right or left pulmonary artery, within 2 cm from hilum
Double-lumen (Quinton) catheters	Tips in either superior vena cava or right atrium (or both) depending on type of catheter
Pleural drainage tube	Anterosuperior for pneumothorax; posteroinferior for pleural effusion
Pacemaker	Tip at apex of right ventricle; other lead(s) in right atrium and/or coronary sinus
Automatic implantable cardiac defibrillator (AICD)	One lead in superior vena cava; other lead(s) in right ventricle and/or coronary sinus
Intraaortic balloon pump (IABP)	Tip about 2 cm from top of aortic arch in descending thoracic aorta
Nasogastric (Levin) tube (NGT)	Tip in stomach 10 cm from esophagogastric junction
Feeding (Dobbhoff) tube (DHT)	Tip ideally in the duodenum but more frequently in stomach

Chapter 11

Computed Tomography: Understanding the Basics and Recognizing Normal Anatomy

INTRODUCTION TO CT

- A computed tomographic (CT) image is composed of a matrix of thousands of tiny squares called *pixels*, each of which is computer-assigned a *CT number* from –1000 to +1000 measured in something called *Hounsfield units (HU)*, after Sir Godfrey Hounsfield, the man credited with developing the first CT scanner (for which he won the Nobel prize in Medicine in 1979 along with Allan Cormack).
  - A *tomogram* is a **slice** through the body measured in **millimeters** that allows for the accurate localization of objects in that section, unlike conventional radiographs that superimpose all of the structures within a given field of view.
  - **A CT scanner uses x-rays** transmitted to multiple *detectors* connected to a **computer**, which processes the data though various **algorithms** to produce **images** of diagnostic quality.
- The CT number will **vary according to the density of the tissue** scanned and is a **measure of how much of the x-ray beam is absorbed** by the tissues at each point in the scan. By convention, **air is assigned a Hounsfield number of –1000 HU** and **bone is about 400 to 600 HU (fat is –40 to –100, water is 0, and soft tissue 20 to 100).**
- CT images are displayed or viewed using a range of Hounsfield numbers preselected to best demonstrate the tissues being studied (for example, from –100 to +300) and anything within that range of CT numbers is displayed over the levels of density in the available gray scale.
- This range of densities is called the *window* or *window-width* setting, and the number within that range that is arbitrarily chosen to be the center of the gray scale is called the *center* or the *window level*.

> **Denser substances** that absorb more x-rays have **high CT numbers**, are said to demonstrate *increased attenuation*, and are displayed as **whiter densities** on CT scans.

- On conventional radiographs, these substances (like **metal** and **calcium**) would also appear whiter and be said to have *increased density* or be *more opaque*.
- **Less dense substances** that absorb fewer x-rays have **low CT numbers**, are said to demonstrate *decreased attenuation,* and are displayed as **blacker densities** on CT scans.
  - On conventional radiographs, these substances (like air and fat) would also appear as blacker densities and be said to have *decreased density* (or *increased lucency*).
- **High-resolution computed tomography (HRCT)**, or thin-slice CT, is now a potential part of every chest CT, making these studies particularly useful for the imaging and characterization of diffuse parenchymal lung diseases.
- **Spiral CT** (helical CT) uses a continuously rotating x-ray source and detector array combined with constant table movement to permit data acquisition through the chest or abdomen so quickly it can be done while the patient holds a single breath.
  - This results in an extremely **rapid acquisition** of data that has **no "gaps"** between slices, which, in turn, allows for seamless reconstruction (also called *reformatting*) of those images in almost any plane. As importantly, the resolution of the reconstructions is equivalent to the clarity of the original scan with most modern scanners.
  - Traditionally, CT images were viewed mostly in the axial plane. With volumetric data acquisition and seamless reconstruction, CT scans now provide **diagnostically useful images** in the **coronal** and **sagittal planes** as well as **three-dimensional reconstructions** that can be viewed at any angle.

> **Multislice CT** (also called *multidetector CT*) makes use of multiple rows of detectors that allow for images to be reconstructed in a range of **slice thicknesses after the scan is completed** without reimaging the patient.

- Because of increasingly sophisticated arrays of detectors and acquisition of many as 256 slices simultaneously, **multislice CT scanners permit very fast imaging** (head to toe in less than 30 seconds) that has allowed for development of new applications for CT, such as *virtual colonoscopy* (see Chapter 18) and *virtual bronchoscopy, cardiac calcium scoring,* and *CT coronary angiography* (see Chapter 9).
- Such examinations can contain a thousand or more images so that the older convention of filming each image for study on a view box is impractical and such examinations are almost always viewed on computer workstations.
- So, you might ask, why not scan everyone at the thinnest possible slice thickness from head to toe?
  - The reason is that doing so might expose a patient to an **unnecessarily high dose of radiation**. The radiation dose delivered by CT studies is dependent on many factors, including the type of equipment, the energy of the x-rays used to produce the images, and the size of the patient. The economic and personal costs of evaluating unexpected and often inconsequential findings may also outweigh any potential benefit from whole-body screening.
  - Dose-reducing measures are being employed, including the use of optimized CT settings, reduction in the x-ray

Box 11-1 **Contrast Reactions and Renal Failure**

Intravenous contrast materials available today are nonionic, low-osmolar solutions containing a high concentration of iodine that circulate through the bloodstream, opacify those tissues and organs with high blood flow, are absorbed by x-ray (and therefore appear "whiter" on images), and are finally excreted in the urine by the kidneys.

In some patients (e.g., those with diabetes, dehydration, multiple myeloma) who have compromised renal function evidenced by creatinine > 1.5, iodinated contrast can produce a nephrotoxic effect resulting in acute tubular necrosis. Though usually reversible, in a small number of patients with underlying renal insufficiency, renal dysfunction may permanently worsen. This effect is dose related.

Iodinated contrast agents can sometimes produce mild side effects, including a feeling of warmth, nausea, vomiting, local irritation at the site of injection, itching, and hives; these side effects usually require no treatment. Occasional idiosyncratic, allergic-like reactions include itching, hives, and laryngeal irritation.

Asthmatics and those with a history of severe allergies or prior reactions to IV contrast have a higher likelihood of contrast reactions (but still very low overall) and may benefit from steroids, benadryl, and cimetidine administered prior and/or after injection. Prior shellfish allergy bears absolutely NO relationship to iodinated contrast reactions.

In about 0.01 to 0.04% of all patients, severe and idiosyncratic reactions to contrast can occur that can produce intense bronchospasm, laryngeal edema, circulatory collapse, and very rarely death (1 in 200,000 to 300,000).

TABLE 11-1 CT SCANS: WHEN CONTRAST IS USED

IV Contrast Used	IV Contrast Usually Not Used
Chest	
CT-pulmonary angiogram (CT-PA) for pulmonary embolism	Evaluation of diffuse infiltrative lung diseases using HRCT
Evaluation of the mediastinum or hila for mass or adenopathy	Confirmation of the presence of a nodule suspected from conventional radiographs
Detect aortic aneurysm or dissection	Detect pneumothorax/ pneumomediastinum
Evaluate blunt or penetrating trauma	Calcium scoring for the coronary arteries
Characterize pleural disease (metastases, empyema)	Known allergies to contrast or renal failure
CT densitometry of pulmonary masses	
Evaluate the coronary arteries	
Abdomen and Pelvis	
Evaluate for the presence of and/or to characterize a mass and to stage or follow up malignancies	Virtual colonoscopy
Trauma	Search for a ureteral calculus
Abdominal pain (e.g., appendicitis)	
Detect aortic aneurysm or dissection	
When Oral Contrast Is Used	
Most cases of nontraumatic abdominal pain	
Inflammatory bowel disease	
Abdominal or pelvic abscess	
Locate the site of bowel perforation, including fistulae	

energy used, limiting the number of repeat scans, and assuring—through appropriate consultation—that the benefits derived from obtaining the study outweigh any potential risks of the radiation exposure.

INTRAVENOUS CONTRAST IN CT SCANNING

- CT scans **can be performed with or without the intravenous administration of iodinated contrast** material but, in general, **they yield more diagnostic information** that is more easily recognizable **when intravenous contrast can be used**.
  - All radiographic contrast agents, in general, are **administered to increase the differences in density between two tissues**. CT scans done **with intravenous contrast** are called *contrast-enhanced* or simply *enhanced*. Most of the time, the radiologist will choose the scanning parameters to optimize the CT study for the patient's clinical issues. For example, different rates of contrast administration and timing of the scan will allow diagnostic enhancement of hepatic vessels versus the liver parenchyma.
  - While it might sound like a wonderful idea to give everyone contrast for all CT studies, keep in mind that **iodinated contrast** can have **adverse effects** and produce **serious reactions** in **susceptible individuals** (Box 11-1).

ORAL CONTRAST IN CT SCANNING

- For abdominal and pelvic CT imaging, **oral contrast** may also be administered to define the bowel, although its

use has diminished as the quality of CT images has improved. Oral contrast is usually not employed in chest CT scanning unless there is a question concerning the esophagus.

- Orally administered contrast, frequently given in temporally divided doses to allow earlier contrast to reach the colon while later contrast opacifies the stomach, is utilized for most abdominal CT scans except those performed for **trauma**, the **stone search study**, and studies specifically directed towards evaluating vascular structures like the **aorta**.
- One of two different types of oral contrast may be used. The most widely used is a dilute solution of **barium sulfate**, the same contrast agent employed in upper gastrointestinal studies and barium enemas. If there is concern for bowel perforation and the possibility that contrast may exit from the lumen of the bowel, an iodine-based, water-soluble contrast is sometimes used (**Gastrografin**). Contrast may also be introduced rectally to opacify the colon more quickly than it would take for orally administered contrast to reach the large bowel or through a Foley catheter to quickly opacify the urinary bladder.
- You will probably not be required to make the decision of when or if to use contrast because **the radiologist will usually tailor the examination to best answer the clinical question being asked**, so it is always important to provide as much clinical information as possible when requesting a study.
- Table 11-1 summarizes **when intravenous and oral contrasts are utilized** for particular problems.

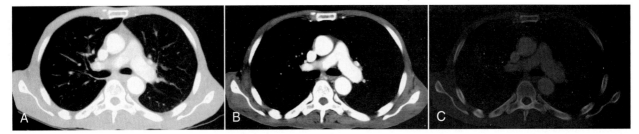

Figure 11-1 Windowing the thorax. Chest CT scans are usually "windowed" and displayed in several formats in order to optimize anatomic definition. Lung windows **(A)** are chosen to maximize our ability to image abnormalities of the lung parenchyma and to identify normal and abnormal bronchial anatomy. Mediastinal windows **(B)** are chosen to display the mediastinal, hilar, and pleural structures to best advantage. Bone windows **(C)** are utilized as a third way of displaying the data, visualizing the bony structures to their best advantage. It is important to recognize that the displays of these different windows are manipulations of the data obtained during the original scan and do not require rescanning the patient.

- By convention, **CT scans**, like most other radiologic studies, **are viewed** with the **patient's right on your left and the patient's left on your right**.
  - If the patient is scanned in the supine position, as most usually are, the **top** of each image is **anterior** and the **bottom** of each image is **posterior**.

NORMAL CHEST CT ANATOMY

Chest CT scans are usually "windowed" and **displayed in** at least **two formats** designed to be viewed as parts of the same study in order to optimize anatomic definition.

- *Lung windows* are chosen to maximize our ability to image abnormalities of the **lung parenchyma**, identify unusual collections of air such as **pneumothorax**, and to identify **normal and abnormal bronchial anatomy**. The mediastinal structures usually appear as a homogenous white density on lung windows.
- *Mediastinal windows* are chosen to display the **mediastinal, hilar, and pleural structures** to best advantage. The lungs usually appear completely black when viewed with mediastinal windows.
- *Bone windows* are also utilized quite often as a third way of displaying the data, demonstrating the bony structures to their best advantage.
- It is important to know that the displays of these different windows are **manipulations of the data** obtained during the **original scan** and **do not require rescanning the patient** (Fig. 11-1).
- We will cover only a few of the major anatomic landmarks demonstrable on chest CT. All of the scans utilized will be *contrast-enhanced*, i.e., the patient will have received intravenous contrast to opacify the blood vessels.
- It is best to read the text in conjunction with its associated photograph. Any references to "right" or "left" mean the patient's right or left side, not yours.
- We will start at the top of the chest and progress inferiorly, highlighting the major structures visible at **six key levels**. This is a good way to systematically study every CT study of the chest.

Five-Vessel Level

- At this level, you should be able to identify the **lungs, the trachea, and the esophagus** (Fig. 11-2).

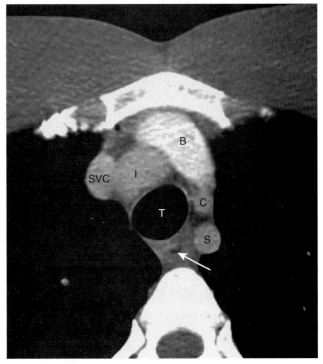

Figure 11-2 Five vessel level. At this level, you should be able to identify the lungs, the trachea (*T*), and the esophagus (*solid white arrow*). Depending on the exact level of the image, several of the great vessels will be visible. The venous structures tend to be more anterior than the arterial. The superior vena cava is the large vessel to the right of the trachea (*SVC*). The brachiocephalic vein (*B*) lies just posterior to the sternum. From the patient's right to the patient's left, the arteries you see may include the innominate artery (*I*), left common carotid (*C*), and left subclavian artery (*S*).

- The **trachea** is black because it contains air and is usually oval in shape and about 2 cm in diameter.
- The **esophagus** lies posterior to the trachea, either to its left or right. It is usually collapsed but may contain swallowed air.
- Depending on the exact level of the image, several of the great vessels will be visible.
  - The venous structures tend to be more anterior than the arterial.
- The **brachiocephalic veins** lie just posterior to the sternum.
  - From the patient's **right** to the patient's **left**, the visible arteries may include the **innominate artery**, **left common carotid**, and **left subclavian arteries**.

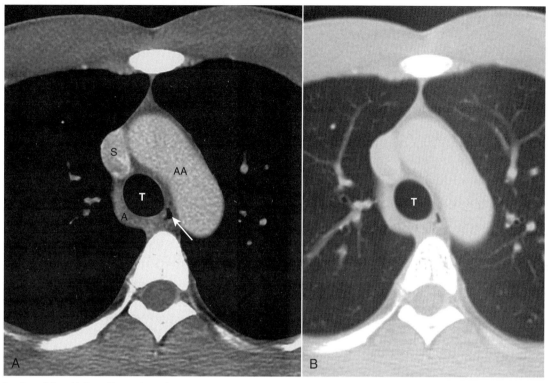

Figure 11-3 Aortic arch level (A) mediastinal window and (B) lung window. A, At this level, you should be able to identify the aortic arch (*AA*), superior vena cava (*S*) and azygous vein (*A*). The aortic arch is an upside-down U-shaped tube. If the scan skims the top of the arch, it will appear as a comma-shaped tubular structure with roughly the same diameter anteriorly as posteriorly, as is seen here. The *solid white arrow* points to air in the esophagus. **B** is the same image as **A** but windowed to best visualize lung anatomy. Lung windows are chosen to maximize our ability to image abnormalities of the lung parenchyma and to identify normal and abnormal bronchial anatomy (*T* = trachea).

Aortic Arch Level

- At this level, you should be able to identify the **aortic arch, superior vena cava, and azygous vein** (Fig. 11-3).
- The *aortic arch* is an upside-down U-shaped tube. If the scan skims the very top of the arch, it will appear as a comma-shaped tubular structure with roughly the same diameter anteriorly as posteriorly.
- To the right of the trachea will be the *superior vena cava* into which the *azygous vein* enters.

Aortopulmonary Window Level

- At this level you should be able to identify the **ascending and descending aorta, superior vena cava,** and possibly the **uppermost aspect of the left pulmonary artery** (Fig. 11-4).
- As we scan lower through the opening of the upside-down "U" shaped aortic arch, the **ascending aorta** will appear as a rounded density anteriorly while the **descending aorta** will appear as a rounded density **posteriorly** and **to the left** of the spine.
  - The **ascending aorta** usually measures **2.5 to 3.5 cm** in diameter; the **descending** thoracic aorta is slightly **smaller at 2 to 3 cm**.
- In most people, there is a space visible just underneath the arch of the aorta but above the pulmonary artery called the *aortopulmonary window*. The aortopulmonary window is an important landmark because it is a favorite location for **enlarged lymph nodes to appear**.

- At or slightly below this level, the trachea bifurcates at the **carina** into the **right and left main bronchi.**

Main Pulmonary Artery Level

- At these levels (it may require more than one image to see all of these structures), you should be able to identify the **main, right, and left pulmonary arteries,** the **right and left main bronchi,** and the **bronchus intermedius** (Fig. 11-5).
- The **left pulmonary artery** is higher than the right and appears as if it were a continuation of the main pulmonary artery.
- The **right pulmonary artery** originates at a 90° angle to the main pulmonary artery and crosses to the right side.
- The **right main bronchus** will appear as a circular, air-containing structure, which will then become tubular as the **right upper lobe bronchus** comes into view.
  - There should be nothing but lung tissue posterior to the bronchus intermedius.
- The **left main bronchus** will appear as an air-containing circular structure on the left.

High Cardiac Level

- At this level, you should be able to identify the **left atrium, right atrium, aortic root, and right ventricular outflow tract** (Fig. 11-6).
  - The **left atrium** occupies the posterior and central portion of the heart. One or more **pulmonary veins** may be seen to enter the left atrium.

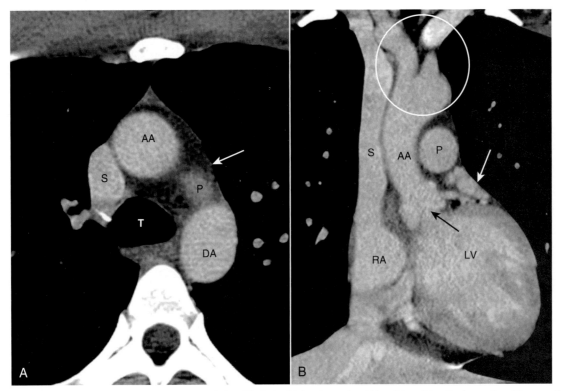

Figure 11-4 Aortopulmonary window level (A) and coronal view (B). A, At this level you should be able to identify the trachea (*T*), ascending (*AA*) and descending aorta (*DA*), superior vena cava (*S*), and possibly the uppermost aspect of the left pulmonary artery (*P*). In most people, there is a space visible just under the arch of the aorta and above the pulmonary artery called the aortopulmonary window (*solid white arrow*). **B,** Coronal reformatted CT enables us to also see the right atrium (*RA*), left ventricle (*LV*), aortic valve (*solid black arrow*), left atrial appendage (*solid white arrow*), and origin of the great vessels (*white circle*).

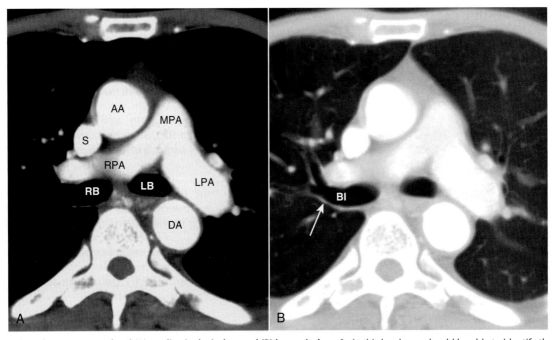

Figure 11-5 Main pulmonary artery level (A) mediastinal window and (B) lung window. A, At this level, you should be able to identify the main (*MPA*), right (*RPA*), and left pulmonary arteries (*LPA*), and the right (*RB*) and left main bronchi (*LB*). The left pulmonary artery is higher than the right and appears as if it were a continuation of the main pulmonary artery. The right pulmonary artery originates at a 90° angle to the main pulmonary artery and crosses to the right side. **B,** Distal to the takeoff of the right upper lobe bronchus is the bronchus intermedius (*BI*). The posterior wall of the right upper lobe bronchus is 2-3 mm in thickness with only lung posterior to it (*solid white arrow*). (*AA* = ascending aorta; *DA* = descending aorta; *S* = superior vena cava.)

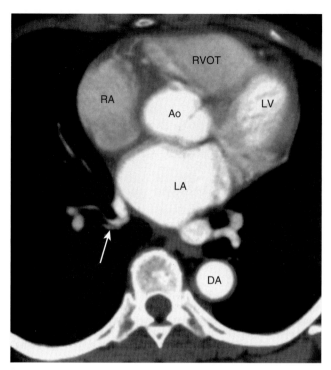

Figure 11-6 High cardiac level. At this level, you should be able to identify the left atrium, right atrium, aortic root, and right ventricular outflow tract. The left atrium (*LA*) occupies the posterior and central portion of the heart. One or more pulmonary veins may be seen to enter the left atrium (*solid white arrow*). The right atrium (*RA*) produces the right heart border and lies anteriorly and to the right of the left atrium. The right ventricular outflow tract (*RVOT*) lies anterior, lateral and superior to the root of the aorta (*Ao*). (*DA* = descending thoracic aorta; *LV* = left ventricle.)

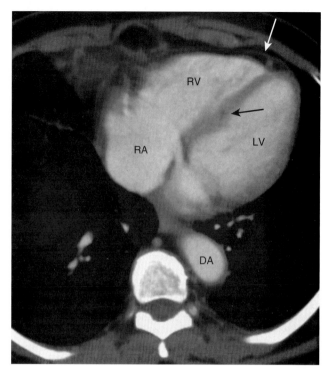

Figure 11-7 Low cardiac level. At this level, you should be able to identify the right atrium, right ventricle, left ventricle, pericardium, and interventricular septum. The right atrium (*RA*) continues to form the right heart border. The right ventricle (*RV*) is anteriorly located, just behind the sternum. The left ventricle (*LV*) produces the left heart border. The interventricular septum is visible between the right and left ventricles (*solid black arrow*). The normal pericardium is about 2 mm thick and is usually outlined by mediastinal fat (outside the pericardium) and epicardial fat (on its inner surface) (*solid white arrow*). (*DA* = descending thoracic aorta.)

- The **right atrium** forms the right heart border and lies immediately to the right of and slightly anterior to the left atrium.
- The **right ventricular outflow tract** lies anterior, lateral and superior to the root of the aorta.
  - The normal relationship between the pulmonic and aortic valves can be remembered by the acronym "**PALS.**" The Pulmonic valve lies Anterior, Lateral, and Superior to the aortic valve.

Low Cardiac Level

- At this level, you should be able to identify **the right atrium, right ventricle, left ventricle, pericardium, and interventricular septum** (Fig. 11-7).
  - The **right atrium** continues to form the right heart border.
  - The **right ventricle** is anteriorly located, just behind the sternum.
  - The **left ventricle** produces the left heart border and normally has a thicker wall than the right ventricle.
  - With IV contrast, you should be able to see the **interventricular septum** between the right and left ventricles.
  - The **normal pericardium** is about **2 mm thick** and usually outlined by **mediastinal fat** (outside the pericardium) and **epicardial fat** (on its inner surface).

The Fissures

- Depending on slice thickness and the plane of the image, the **major fissures** will be visible either as thin white lines or by an avascular band about 2 cm thick, which they produce as they travel obliquely through the lungs **from posterosuperior to anteroinferior.**
- The **minor fissure** travels in the same plane as an axial CT image so that it is normally not visible. Its **location can be inferred by an avascular zone** between the right upper and middle lobes (Fig. 11-8).
- The fissures will also be visible on coronal and sagittal reformatted images of the lungs (Fig. 11-9).

CARDIAC CT

- Faster multislice CT scanners and ECG-gated acquisition to reduce degradation of the image by cardiac motion, along with powerful computer algorithms, now allow for the imaging and three-dimensional reconstruction of the coronary arteries and quantitative measurement of the amount of **coronary artery calcium.** The administration of intravenous contrast allows evaluation of **vessel patency** with identification of **thrombus** in the lumen or **plaque** in the vessel wall.
- By reconstructing multiple phases of the cardiac cycle, it is also possible to analyze wall motion and evaluate ejection fraction and myocardial perfusion.

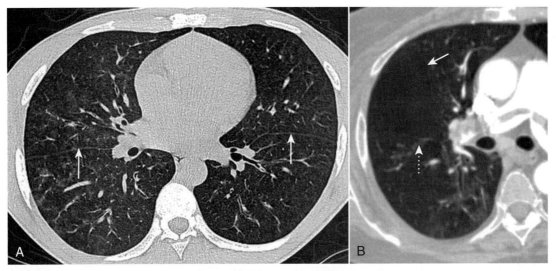

Figure 11-8 Minor fissure and major fissures. A, The major fissures will be visible either as thin white lines (*solid white arrows*) or by the avascular band about 2 cm thick that they produce as they travel obliquely through the lungs from posterosuperior to anteroinferior. **B,** The minor fissure travels in the same plane as the axial CT scan so that it is normally not visible. Like the major fissures, though, the location of the minor fissure can be inferred by an avascular zone between the right upper and middle lobes (*solid white arrow*). The major fissure is also visible (*dotted white arrow*).

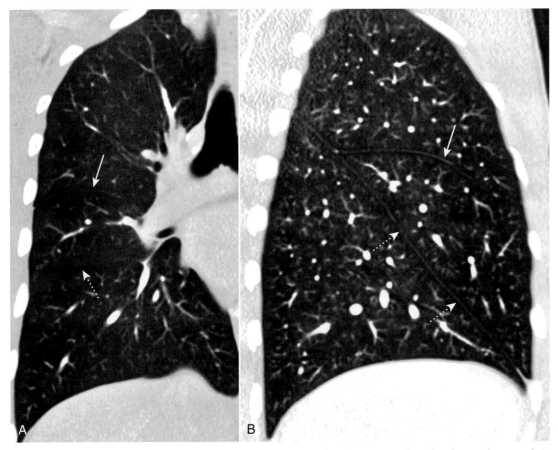

Figure 11-9 Fissures seen on coronal and sagittal reformatted views. A, The minor fissure is seen as a thin white line on the coronal view of the right lung (*solid white arrow*), while the major fissure, traveling obliquely in the plane of the image, is seen as an avascular zone (*dotted white arrow*). **B,** Sagittal reformatted image of right lung shows the minor fissure (*solid white arrow*) and major fissure (*dotted white arrows*) each as thin white lines.

- **Calcium scoring** is based on the premise that the amount of calcium in the coronary arteries is related to the degree of atherosclerosis and that quantifying the amount of calcium may help predict future cardiac events related to coronary artery disease.
  - The scoring is done by calculations that include the amount of calcium visualized in the coronary arteries (Fig. 11-10).
  - The **absence** of coronary artery calcification has a high negative predictive value for significant luminal narrowing.
- It is possible to perform an ultrafast CT scan in the emergency department that will allow for the simultaneous evaluation of **coronary artery disease, aortic dissection,** and **pulmonary thromboembolic disease**—the so-called *triple scan* for patients who present with **acute chest pain**.

ABDOMINAL CT

General Considerations

- Conventional radiography, ultrasonography, CT, and MRI are all utilized in the imaging evaluation of abdominal abnormalities.
- Each has advantages and disadvantages inherent to its own particular technology and the choice of modality is frequently based on the patient's clinical condition (Table 11-2).
- History and physical examination continue to be an essential part of evaluating abdominal abnormalities, not only to suggest an etiology but also to help determine which, if any,

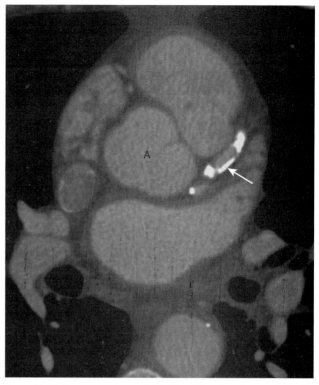

Figure 11-10 Coronary artery calcification. There is a dense calcification (*solid white arrow*) seen in the left anterior descending coronary artery arising from the aorta (*A*). It is now possible to image the coronary arteries and measure the amount of coronary artery calcium, evaluate for vessel patency and identify the presence of thrombus in the lumen or plaque in the vessel wall following the administration of intravenous contrast.

TABLE 11-2 IMAGING OF THE ABDOMEN AND PELVIS: MODALITIES COMPARED

Uses	Advantages	Disadvantages
Conventional Radiography		
Primarily used for screening in abdominal pain	Availability Cost Patients tolerate procedure well	Lower sensitivity Ionizing radiation
Ultrasonography		
Primary imaging mode for gallbladder and biliary tree Screening for aortic aneurysm Identification of vascular abnormalities and flow Detection of ascites Primary imaging mode for the female pelvis	Availability Cost No ionizing radiation Patients tolerate procedure well Portable	Operator dependent More difficult to interpret
CT		
Diagnostic modality of choice for most abdominal abnormalities, including trauma	Availability Cost High spatial resolution and image reconstruction Evaluates multiple organ systems simultaneously	Ionizing radiation Contrast reactions Inability to use IV contrast in renal insufficiency Patient weight and size may exclude scanning
MRI		
Problem solving for difficult diagnoses Extension of known disease into surrounding soft tissues (staging) Vascular anatomy	Soft tissue contrast No ionizing radiation No iodinated contrast Image reconstruction	Cost Availability Longer scan times Claustrophobia Monitoring issues in acutely ill patients Patient weight and size may degrade or exclude scanning Incompatible with aneurysm clips, pacemakers, etc.

imaging study will provide the best yield in establishing the correct diagnosis.

Liver

- The liver receives its blood **supply** from both **hepatic arteries** and **portal veins** and **drains** to the inferior vena cava via the **hepatic veins.**
- For practical purposes, the **vascular distribution of the liver defines its anatomy** because the vascular anatomy directs the surgical approach to liver lesions.
- The liver is divided into **right, left, and caudate lobes** by its vessels.
  - The **right lobe** is subdivided into **two segments:** the **anterior** and **posterior.** The **left lobe** is subdivided into **two segments:** the **medial** and **lateral.**
  - A prominent, fat-filled fissure that contains the **falciform ligament** and **ligamentum teres** (formerly the umbilical vein) separates the **medial and lateral segments** of the **left lobe** of the liver (Fig. 11-11).

Spleen

- **The liver should always be denser than or equal to the density of the spleen on noncontrast scans.**

⚠ On early contrast-enhanced scans, the spleen may be inhomogeneous in its attenuation, a finding that should disappear over the course of the next several minutes.

- The spleen is usually **about 12 cm long, does not project** substantially below the margin of the **12th rib**, and is about the **same size as the left kidney.**

Pancreas

- The pancreas is a retroperitoneal organ oriented obliquely so that the entire organ is not seen on any one axial image of the upper abdomen.
  - The **tail** is usually **most superior,** lying in the hilum of the spleen.

- Proceeding inferiorly, the **body of the pancreas** crosses the midline and rests anterior to the **superior mesenteric artery.** The **head of the pancreas** is nestled in the duodenal loop (Fig. 11-12). The **uncinate process** is part of the head and curves around the **superior mesenteric vein.**
- The **splenic vein** courses along the posterior border of the pancreas to the **superior mesenteric vein,** and the **splenic artery** runs along the superior border of the pancreas from the **celiac axis** to the spleen. The main pancreatic duct empties into the duodenum as the **duct of Wirsung** and sometimes through an **accessory duct of Santorini.**

Kidneys

- The kidneys are retroperitoneal organs, encircled by varying amounts of fat and enclosed within a fibrous capsule.
  - They are surrounded by the *perirenal space,* which, in turn, is delineated by the **anterior and posterior renal**

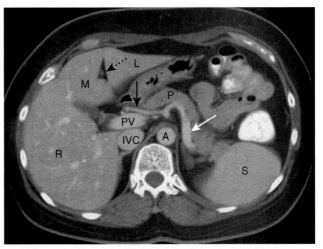

Figure 11-11 Normal liver anatomy. The ligamentum teres (*dotted black arrow*) divides the left lobe of the liver into a medial (*M*) and lateral segment (*L*) with the larger right lobe (*R*) lying more posterior. The portal vein (*PV*) lies just posterior to the hepatic artery (*solid black arrow*). The splenic artery (*solid white arrow*) follows the path of the pancreas (*P*) toward the spleen (*S*). The inferior vena cava (*IVC*) lies to the right of the aorta (*A*).

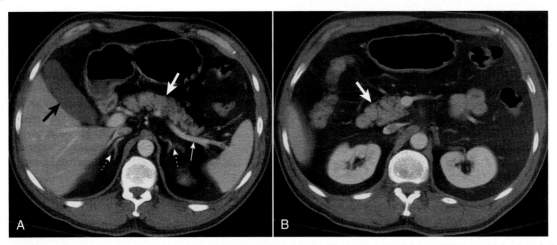

Figure 11-12 Normal pancreas. A, Body of pancreas (*thick white arrow*). Splenic artery (*thin white arrow*). Also well seen are both adrenal glands (*dotted white arrows*) and gallbladder (*black arrow*). **B,** Normal head (*thick white arrow*). The pancreas is a retroperitoneal organ oriented obliquely so that the entire organ is not seen on any one axial image of the upper abdomen. The tail is most superior, and the body and then head are usually visualized on successively more inferior slices.

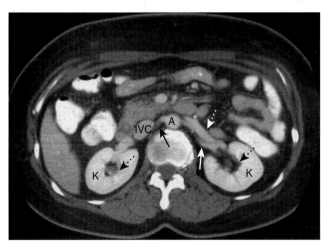

Figure 11-13 Normal kidneys. The kidneys (*K*) lie in the renal fossae bilaterally. The normal renal pelvis, containing fat, occupies the central portion of the kidneys (*dotted black arrows*). The right renal artery (*solid black arrow*) runs posterior to the inferior vena cava (*IVC*). The left renal vein (*dotted white arrow*) lies anterior to the left renal artery (*solid white arrow*). (*A* = abdominal aorta.)

fasciae. Certain fascial attachments, muscles, and other organs define a series of spaces that produce predictable patterns of abnormality when those spaces are filled with fluid, pus, blood, or air.

- In adults, the left kidney is minimally larger than the right, each kidney being about **11 cm in size** or about the same size as the spleen.

■ So long as they are functioning properly, the **kidneys are the major route** for excretion of iodinated **contrast** material. They should therefore enhance whenever intravenous contrast is administered. Over time, the urine will become more opacified, increasing significantly from its normal water density, sometimes requiring delayed imaging of the urinary tract (Fig. 11-13).

- If the kidneys are not functioning properly, contrast is excreted though alternative pathways (bile, bowel), a process called *vicarious excretion* of contrast.

Small and Large Bowel

■ Opacification and distension of the bowel lumen is helpful for proper evaluation of the bowel wall regardless of the modality used to evaluate it. Wall thickness may artificially seem increased in collapsed bowel.

■ The **small bowel** is usually **2.5 cm or less in diameter** with a **wall thickness usually less than 3 mm**. Adjacent loops of small bowel are usually in contact with each other, depending in part on the amount of intraperitoneal fat present.

■ The **colonic wall** is usually **less than 3 mm thick** with the colon distended and less than 5 mm with the colon collapsed. The cecum is recognizable by the presence of the terminal ileum. The position of the transverse and sigmoid segments of the colon is variable, depending upon the degree of redundancy (Fig. 11-14).

Urinary Bladder

■ The bladder is an **extraperitoneal organ**, the extraperitoneal space being continuous with the retroperitoneum. The

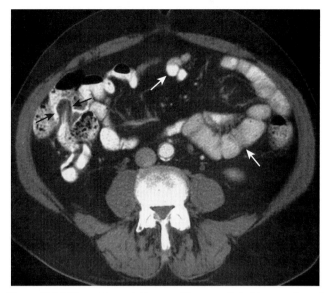

Figure 11-14 Normal bowel. Contrast fills a nondilated lumen of small bowel (less than 2.5 cm). The small bowel wall is so thin that it normally is almost invisible (*white arrows*). The terminal ileum can be recognized by the fat-containing "lips" of the ileocecal valve outlined with contrast (*black arrows*).

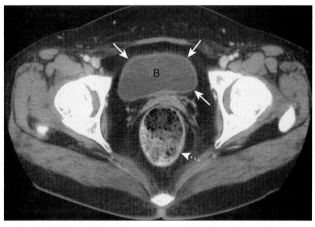

Figure 11-15 Normal bladder. The urinary bladder (*B*) contains unopacified urine in this early image of a contrast-enhanced CT scan of the pelvis. The bladder wall (*solid white arrows*) is thin and of equal thickness around the circumference of the bladder. The rectum lies posterior to the bladder (*dotted white arrow*).

dome of the bladder is covered by the **inferior reflection of the peritoneum**.

■ The **bladder wall measures 5 mm or less with the bladder distended**.

■ The bladder is **best evaluated when distended** with either urine or urine-containing contrast, but the **bladder wall is usually visible** whether or not intravenous contrast has been administered (Fig. 11-15).

WEBLINK

Registered users may obtain more information on Computed Tomography: Understanding the Basics and Recognizing Normal Anatomy on StudentConsult.com.

TAKE-HOME POINTS

Computed Tomography: Understanding the Basics and Recognizing Normal Anatomy

CT scanners produce a computer-generated representation of human anatomy based on measurements of the density of the tissue scanned, which is determined by the amount the x-ray beam is absorbed or transmitted by the tissues at each point in the scan.

Spiral CT scanners use a continuously rotating x-ray detector combined with constant table movement to permit rapid and "gapless" data acquisition that can be obtained in a single breath-hold by the patient. This allows for diagnostically useful images in the coronal and sagittal planes and 3D reconstructions that can be viewed at any angle.

CT scans can be performed with or without intravenous contrast and displayed in any number of *windows* that allow the original data acquired to be viewed with optimum density settings for the lungs, mediastinum, or bone without the need for rescanning the patient.

Iodinated contrast agents may produce occasional side effects such as warmth, nausea, and vomiting and rare idiosyncratic, allergic-like reactions leading to anaphylaxis and death.

Oral and/or rectal contrast may be used to define the bowel and help in differentiating the bowel from adjacent lymph nodes or pathologic, fluid-containing lesions.

There are a number of clinical settings in which either iodinated or oral contrast (or both) improve the diagnostic accuracy of CT scanning. The radiologist usually tailors imaging studies based on the clinical problem.

Normal anatomy of the major structures is described at six levels in the chest from top to bottom: five-vessel view, aortic arch, aortopulmonary window, main pulmonary artery, upper cardiac, and lower cardiac levels.

The normal anatomy of the liver, spleen, pancreas, kidneys, bowel, and bladder is described.

Chapter 12

Recognizing Diseases of the Chest

In this chapter, you'll learn how to recognize mediastinal masses, benign and malignant pulmonary neoplasms, pulmonary thromboembolic disease, and selected airway diseases.

- Several chest abnormalities are discussed in other chapters (Table 12-1).
- A complete discussion of all of the abnormalities visible in the chest is beyond the scope of this text. We'll begin here with mediastinal masses and work our way outward to the lungs.

MEDIASTINAL MASSES

- The mediastinum is an area whose **lateral margins are defined by the medial borders of each lung,** whose **anterior margin is the sternum and anterior chest wall,** and whose **posterior margin is the spine,** usually including the paravertebral gutters.
- The mediastinum can be arbitrarily subdivided into three compartments: the *anterior, middle,* and *posterior* compartments—and each contains its favorite set of diseases (Fig. 12-1).
  - The *superior mediastinum*, roughly the area above the plane of the aortic arch, is a division that is now usually combined with one of the other three compartments mentioned above.

⚠️ **Pitfall:** Since these compartments have no true anatomic boundaries, **diseases from one compartment may extend into another compartment.** When a mediastinal abnormality becomes extensive or a mediastinal mass becomes quite large, it is often impossible to determine which compartment was its site of origin.

- **Differentiating a mediastinal from a parenchymal lung mass on frontal and lateral chest radiographs:**
  - **Mediastinal masses will originate in the mediastinum** (makes sense, doesn't it?), although large masses may be difficult to place.
  - If a **mass is surrounded by lung tissue in both the frontal and lateral projections, it lies within the lung;** if a **mass is surrounded by lung tissue in one but not both projections, it may be in either the lung or the mediastinum.**
    - Unfortunately, masses may not be surrounded by lung tissue in either projection and still originate within the lung.
  - In general (note that this is a generalization), **the margin of a mediastinal mass is sharper** than a mass originating in the lung.

- Mediastinal masses frequently **displace, compress,** or **obstruct** other mediastinal structures.
- Ultimately, CT scans of the chest are more accurate than conventional radiographs in determining the location and nature of a mediastinal mass.

ANTERIOR MEDIASTINUM

- The **anterior mediastinum** is the compartment that extends from the **back of the sternum** to the **anterior border of the heart and great vessels.**
- The **differential diagnosis for anterior mediastinal masses** most often includes:
  - Substernal **thyroid masses**
  - **Lymphoma**
  - **Thymoma**
  - **Teratoma**
  - Lymphoma is sometimes called "terrible lymphoma" so that all of the diseases in this list start with the letter "T" (Table 12-2).

Thyroid Masses

- In **everyday practice, enlarged substernal thyroid masses** are the **most frequently encountered anterior mediastinal mass.** The vast majority of these masses are **multinodular goiters,** and the mass is called a *substernal goiter* or *substernal thyroid* or *substernal thyroid goiter.*
- On occasion, the isthmus or lower pole of either lobe of the thyroid may enlarge but project **downward** into the upper thorax rather than **anteriorly** into the neck.
  - About 3 out of 4 thyroid masses extend anterior to the trachea; the remaining (almost all of which are right-sided) descend posterior to the trachea.
- **Substernal goiters characteristically displace the trachea** either to the left or right **above the level of the aortic arch,** a tendency the other anterior mediastinal masses do not typically demonstrate. Classically, **substernal goiters do not extend below the top of the aortic arch** (Fig. 12-2).

➡️ Therefore, you should **think of an enlarged substernal thyroid** whenever you see **an anterior mediastinal mass that displaces the trachea.**

- Radioisotope **thyroid scans are the study of choice** in **confirming** the diagnosis of a substernal thyroid because virtually all goiters will display some uptake of the radioactive tracer that can be imaged and recorded with a special camera.

TABLE 12-1 CHEST ABNORMALITIES DISCUSSED ELSEWHERE IN THIS TEXT

Topic	Appears in
Atelectasis	Chapter 5
Pleural effusion	Chapter 6
Pneumonia	Chapter 7
Pneumothorax, pneumomediastinum, and pneumopericardium	Chapter 8
Cardiac and thoracic aortic abnormalities	Chapter 9
Chest trauma	Chapter 17

TABLE 12-2 ANTERIOR MEDIASTINAL MASSES ("3 Ts and an L")

Mass	What to Look For
Thyroid goiter	The only anterior mediastinal mass that routinely deviates the trachea
Lymphoma (lymphadenopathy)	Lobulated, polycyclic mass, frequently asymmetrical, that may occur in any compartment of the mediastinum
Thymoma	Look for a well-marginated mass that may be associated with myasthenia gravis
Teratoma	Well-marginated mass that may contain fat and calcium on CT scans

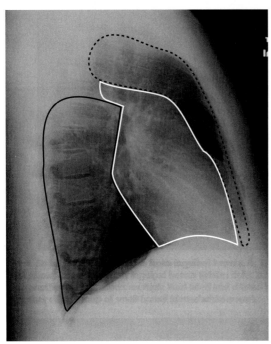

Figure 12-1 The mediastinum. The mediastinum can be arbitrarily subdivided into three compartments: anterior, middle, and posterior, with each containing its favorite set of diseases. The anterior mediastinum is the compartment that extends from the back of the sternum to the anterior border of the heart and great vessels (*dotted black outline*). The middle mediastinum is the compartment that extends from the anterior border of the heart and aorta to the posterior border of the heart and origins of the great vessels (*solid white outline*). The posterior mediastinum is the compartment that extends from the posterior border of the heart to the anterior border of the vertebral column (*solid black outline*). For practical purposes, however, it is considered to extend into the paravertebral gutters.

- **On CT scans,** substernal thyroid masses are **contiguous with the thyroid gland, frequently contain calcification,** and **avidly take up intravenous contrast** but with a **mottled, inhomogeneous appearance** (Fig. 12-3).

Lymphoma

- **Lymphadenopathy,** whether from lymphoma, metastatic carcinoma, sarcoid, or tuberculosis, is the most common cause of a mediastinal mass overall.
- **Anterior mediastinal lymphadenopathy is most common in Hodgkin disease, especially the nodular sclerosing variety.**
- Hodgkin disease is a malignancy of the lymph nodes, more common in females, which most often presents with painless, enlarged lymph nodes in the neck.

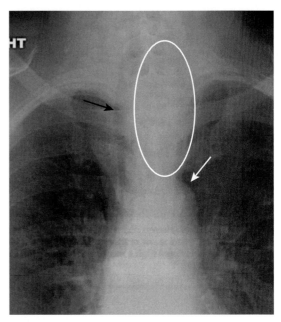

Figure 12-2 Substernal thyroid mass. The lower pole of the thyroid may enlarge but project downward into the upper thorax (*white oval*) rather than anteriorly into the neck. Classically, substernal thyroid goiters produce mediastinal masses that do not extend below the top of the aortic arch (*solid white arrow*). Substernal goiters characteristically displace the trachea (*solid black arrow*) either to the left or right above the aortic knob, a tendency the other anterior mediastinal masses do not typically demonstrate. Therefore, you should think of an enlarged substernal thyroid goiter whenever you see an anterior mediastinal mass that displaces the trachea.

- Unlike teratomas and thymomas, which are presumed to expand outward from a single abnormal cell, lymphomatous masses are frequently composed of several contiguously enlarged lymph nodes. As such, **lymphadenopathy frequently presents with a border that is lobulated or polycyclic in contour** owing to the conglomeration of enlarged nodes that make up the mass.

➤ On chest radiographs, this finding **may help differentiate lymphadenopathy from other mediastinal masses.**

- **Mediastinal lymphadenopathy** in Hodgkin disease is usually **bilateral and asymmetrical** (Fig. 12-4). In addition, **asymmetrical hilar adenopathy** is associated with mediastinal adenopathy in many patients with Hodgkin disease.

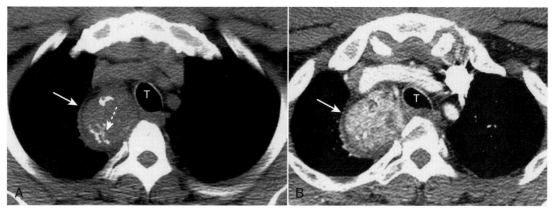

Figure 12-3 CT of a substernal thyroid goiter without and with contrast enhancement. These are two images at the same level in a patient who was scanned both before **(A)** and then after intravenous contrast administration **(B). A,** On CT scans, substernal thyroid masses (*solid white arrow*) are contiguous with the thyroid gland, frequently contain calcification (*dotted white arrow*) and **(B)** avidly take up intravenous contrast but with a mottled, inhomogeneous appearance (*solid white arrow*). This mass is displacing the trachea (*T*) slightly to the left.

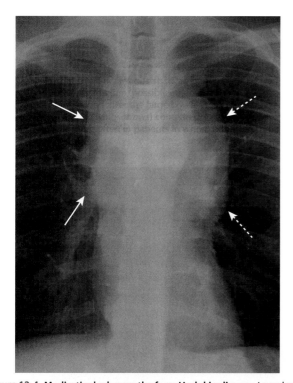

Figure 12-4 Mediastinal adenopathy from Hodgkin disease. Lymphadenopathy frequently presents with a lobulated or polycyclic border due to the conglomeration of enlarged nodes that produce the mass (*solid white arrows*). This finding may help differentiate lymphadenopathy from other mediastinal masses. Mediastinal lymphadenopathy in Hodgkin disease is usually bilateral (*dotted white arrows*) and frequently asymmetric.

- In general, **mediastinal lymph nodes that exceed 1 cm** measured along their **short axis** on CT scans of the chest are **considered to be enlarged.**
- Lymphoma will **produce multiple, lobulated soft-tissue masses** or **one large soft-tissue mass** from lymph node aggregation.
- The **mass is usually homogeneous** in density on CT but **may be heterogeneous** when it achieves a sufficient size to undergo **necrosis (areas of lower attenuation, i.e., blacker)** or hemorrhage (**areas of higher attenuation, i.e., whiter)** (Fig. 12-5).

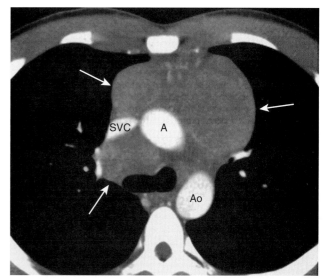

Figure 12-5 CT of anterior mediastinal adenopathy in Hodgkin disease. On CT, lymphomas will produce multiple, lobulated soft-tissue masses or a large soft-tissue mass from lymph node aggregation (*solid white arrows*). The mass is usually homogeneous in density, as in this case, but may be heterogeneous when the nodes achieve a sufficient size to undergo necrosis (areas of low attenuation, i.e., blacker) or hemorrhage (areas of high attenuation, i.e., whiter). The superior vena cava (*SVC*) is compressed by the nodes while the ascending (*A*) and descending aorta (*Ao*) are typically less so.

- Some findings of lymphoma may mimic those of sarcoid since both produce thoracic adenopathy. Table 12-3 helps to differentiate them.

Thymic Masses

- **Normal thymic tissue can be visible on CT throughout life,** although the gland begins to **involute after age 20.**
- **Thymomas** are **neoplasms of thymic epithelium and lymphocytes.** They occur most often in **middle-aged adults,** generally at an **older** age than those with **teratomas.** Most thymomas are **benign.**

 Thymomas are **associated with myasthenia gravis about 35% of the time** they are present. Conversely, about **15% of patients with** clinical **myasthenia gravis will** be found to **have a thymoma.** The importance of identifying a thymoma in patients with myasthenia gravis lies in the **favorable prognosis** for patients with myasthenia **after thymectomy.**

- **On CT scans, thymomas** classically present as a **smooth or lobulated mass** that arises near the **junction of the heart and great vessels,** which, like a teratoma, **may contain calcification** (Fig. 12-6).
- Other lesions that can produce enlargement of the thymus include thymic cysts, thymic hyperplasia, thymic lymphoma, carcinoma, or lipoma.

Teratoma

- Teratomas are **germinal tumors** that typically **contain all three germ layers** (ectoderm, mesoderm, and endoderm). Most teratomas are benign and occur earlier in life than thymomas. Usually asymptomatic and discovered serendipitously, about 30% of mediastinal teratomas are malignant and have a poor prognosis.
- The most common variety of teratoma is **cystic;** it produces a **well-marginated** mass near the origin of the great vessels that **characteristically contains fat, cartilage, and possibly bone on CT examination** (Fig. 12-7).

TABLE 12-3 SARCOIDOSIS VS. LYMPHOMA

Sarcoid	Lymphoma
Bilateral hilar and right paratracheal adenopathy classic combination	More often mediastinal adenopathy, associated with asymmetrical hilar enlargement
Bronchopulmonary nodes more peripheral	Hilar nodes more central
Pleural effusion in about 5%	Pleural effusion more common—in 30%
Anterior mediastinal adenopathy is uncommon	Anterior mediastinal adenopathy is common

MIDDLE MEDIASTINUM

- The **middle mediastinum** is the compartment that extends from the **anterior border of the heart and aorta** to the **posterior border of the heart and contains the heart, the origins of the great vessels, trachea,** and **main bronchi** along with **lymph nodes** (see Fig. 12-1).
- **Lymphadenopathy produces the most common mass in this compartment.** While Hodgkin disease is the most likely cause of mediastinal adenopathy, other malignancies and several benign diseases can produce such findings.
  - Other malignancies that produce mediastinal lymphadenopathy include **small cell lung carcinoma** and **metastatic disease** such as from primary **breast carcinoma** (Fig. 12-8).
  - Benign causes of mediastinal lymphadenopathy include **infectious mononucleosis** and **tuberculosis, the latter usually producing unilateral mediastinal adenopathy.**

POSTERIOR MEDIASTINUM

- The **posterior mediastinum** is the compartment that extends from the **posterior border of the heart** to the **anterior border of the vertebral column.** For practical purposes, however, it is **considered to extend to either side of the spine into the paravertebral gutters** (see Fig. 12-1).
- It contains the **descending aorta, esophagus, and lymph nodes** and is the site of masses representing **extramedullary hematopoiesis.** Most importantly, it is the home of **tumors of neural origin.**

Neurogenic Tumors

- Although neurogenic tumors produce the largest percentage of posterior mediastinal masses, none of these lesions is particularly common. Neurogenic tumors include such

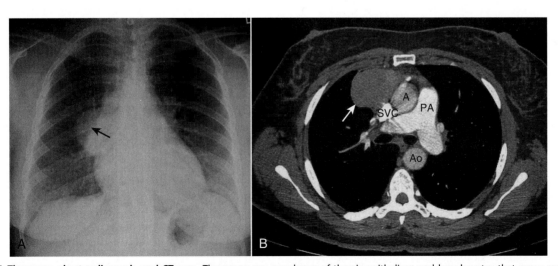

Figure 12-6 Thymoma, chest radiograph, and CT scan. Thymomas are neoplasms of thymic epithelium and lymphocytes that occur most often in middle-aged adults, generally at an older age than those with teratomas. **A,** The chest radiograph shows a smoothly marginated anterior mediastinal mass (*solid black arrow*). **B,** Contrast-enhanced CT scan confirms the anterior mediastinal location and homogeneous density of the mass (*solid white arrow*). The patient had myasthenia gravis and improved following resection of the thymoma. (*A* = ascending aorta; *Ao* = descending aorta; *PA* = main pulmonary artery; *SVC* = superior vena cava.)

entities as **neurofibroma, schwannoma (neurilemmoma), ganglioneuroma,** and **neuroblastoma.**

- **Nerve sheath tumors** (Schwannoma or neurilemmoma) are the **most common** and are almost always **benign.** They usually affect persons 20-50 years of age. These slow-growing tumors may produce no symptoms until late in their course.
- Neoplasms that arise from nerve elements **other than the sheath,** such as ganglioneuromas and neuroblastoma, are usually **malignant.**

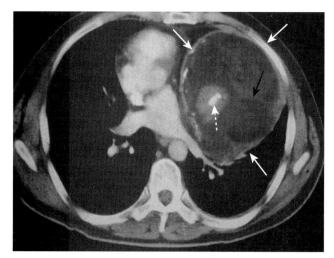

Figure 12-7 Mediastinal teratoma. Teratomas are germinal tumors that typically contain all three germ layers. They tend to be discovered at a younger age than thymomas. The most common variety of teratoma is cystic, as in this case (*solid white arrows*). As shown here, they usually produce a well-marginated mass near the origin of the great vessels. On CT, they characteristically contain fat (*solid black arrow*), cartilage, and sometimes bone (*dotted white arrow*).

- **Neurogenic tumors** will produce a soft tissue **mass, usually sharply marginated,** in the paravertebral gutter (Fig. 12-9). Both benign and malignant tumors **may erode ribs** (Fig. 12-10A). They may **enlarge the neural foramina** producing **dumbbell-shaped** lesions that arise from the spinal canal but project through the neural foramen into the mediastinum (Fig. 12-10B).
- **Neurofibromas** can occur as an **isolated tumor** arising from the Schwann cell of the nerve sheath **or as part of a syndrome** called *neurofibromatosis.* As part of the latter, they are a component of a neurocutaneous bone dysplasia that can cause numerous abnormalities, including **subcutaneous nodules, erosion of adjacent bone** (*rib notching*), **scalloping** of the posterior aspect of the vertebral bodies (Fig. 12-11), **absence** of the **sphenoid wings, pseudarthroses,** and **sharp-angled kyphoscoliosis** at the thoracolumbar junction.

SOLITARY NODULE/MASS IN THE LUNG

- **The difference between a *nodule* and a *mass* is size:** under 3 cm, it is usually called a *nodule*; over 3 cm a *mass.*
- Much has been written about the workup of a patient in whom a single nodular density is discovered in the lung on imaging of the thorax, i.e., the *solitary pulmonary nodule.* It is estimated that as many as 50% of smokers have a nodule discovered by chest CT, but fewer than 1% of the nodules < 5 mm in size show any malignant tendencies (growth or metastases) when followed for 2 years.
- In evaluating a solitary pulmonary nodule, the **critical question** to be answered is **whether the nodule is most likely benign or malignant.**

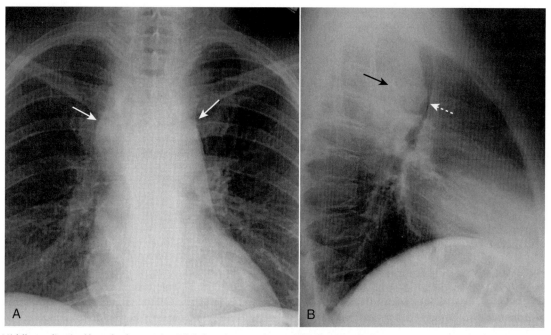

Figure 12-8 Middle mediastinal lymphadenopathy. While lymphoma is the most likely cause of adenopathy in the middle mediastinum, other malignancies, such as small cell lung carcinoma and metastatic disease, as well as several benign diseases, can produce these findings. This patient has a mediastinal mass demonstrated on both the frontal **(A)** (*solid white arrows*) and lateral **(B)** views (*solid black arrow*). The mass is pushing the trachea forward (*dotted white arrow*) on the lateral view. The biopsied lymph nodes in this patient demonstrated small cell carcinoma of the lung.

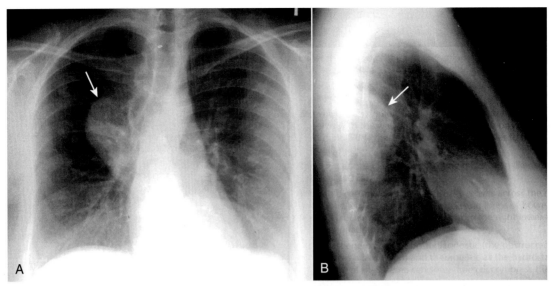

Figure 12-9 Neurofibromatosis. Neurofibromas can occur as an isolated tumor arising from the Schwann cell of the nerve sheath or as part of the syndrome *neurofibromatosis*, as in this case. There is a large, posterior mediastinal neurofibroma (*solid white arrows*) seen in the right, paravertebral gutter on the frontal **(A)** and lateral **(B)** views.

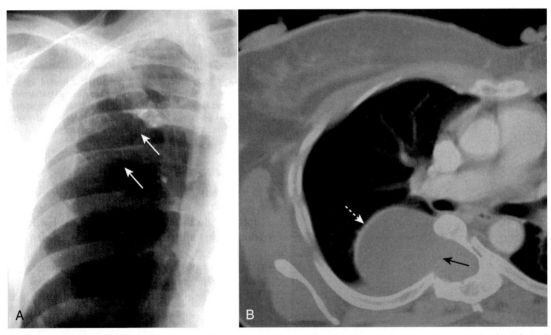

Figure 12-10 Rib-notching and a dumbbell-shaped neurofibroma. A, Plexiform neurofibromas can produce erosions along the inferior borders of the ribs (where the intercostal nerves are located) and produce either notching or a wavy appearance called **ribbon ribs** (*solid white arrows*). **B,** Another patient demonstrates a large neurofibroma that is enlarging the neural foramen, eroding half of the vertebral body (*solid black arrow*) and producing a dumbbell-shaped lesion that arises from the spinal canal but projects through the foramen into the mediastinum (*dotted white arrow*).

- If most likely benign, it can be watched. If most likely malignant, it will almost certainly be treated aggressively with therapies that carry some degree of morbidity and mortality.
- The answer to the question of benign versus malignant will depend on many factors, including the availability of **prior imaging studies** which **can help greatly in establishing stability of a lesion over time.**
- In 2005, an international society of chest radiologists (Fleischner Society) approved a set of evidence-based criteria setting guidelines for the follow-up of noncalcified nodules found incidentally during chest CT (Table 12-4).

Signs of a Benign Versus Malignant Solitary Pulmonary Nodule

- **Size of the lesion.** Nodules less than 4 mm rarely show malignant behavior. Masses **larger than 5 cm have a 95% chance of malignancy** (Fig. 12-12).
- **Calcification.** The presence of calcification is usually determined by CT. **Lesions containing central, laminar, or diffuse patterns of calcification are invariably benign.**
- **Margin.** Lobulation, spiculation, and shagginess all suggest malignancy (Fig. 12-13).
- **Change in size over time.** This requires a previous study or sufficient confidence so that a follow-up study will

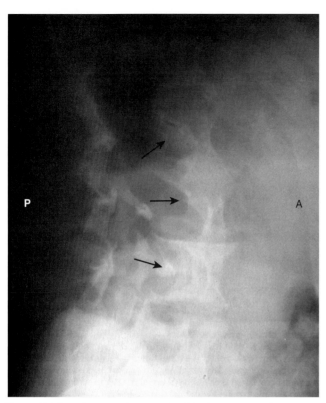

Figure 12-11 Scalloping of the vertebral bodies in neurofibromatosis. Neurofibromatosis is a neurocutaneous disorder associated with a skeletal dysplasia. There may be numerous skeletal abnormalities associated with the disease, including scalloping of posterior vertebral bodies (*solid black arrows*), especially in the thoracic or lumbar spine (as shown here). This is produced by diverticula of the thecal sac caused by dysplasia of the meninges that leads to erosion of adjacent bone through the pulsations transmitted via the spinal fluid. (*A* is anterior and *P* is posterior.)

TABLE 12-4 FLEISCHNER SOCIETY CRITERIA FOR FOLLOW-UP OF INCIDENTAL, NONCALCIFIED SOLITARY PULMONARY NODULES

Nodule Size (mm)	Low-Risk Patients*	High-Risk Patients**
≤ 4	No follow-up needed	Follow-up at 12 months; if no change, no further imaging needed
> 4-6	Follow-up at 12 months; if no change, no further imaging needed	Initial follow-up CT at 6-12 months and then at 18-24 months if no change
> 6-8	Initial follow-up CT at 6-12 months and then at 18-24 months if no change	Initial follow-up CT at 3-6 months and then at 9-12 and 24 months if no change
> 8	Follow-up CTs at around 3, 9, and 24 months; dynamic contrast-enhanced CT, PET, and/or biopsy	Same as for low-risk patients

*__Low-risk patients:__ Minimal or absent history of smoking and of other known risk factors (e.g., radon exposure).
**__High-risk patients:__ History of smoking or of other known risk factors.

provide a basis of comparison of size over time. **Malignancies** tend to **increase in size at a rate that is not so brief as to suggest an inflammatory etiology** (changes in weeks) **nor so prolonged as to suggest benignity** (no change over a year or more).
- **Large cell carcinomas,** as a cell type, **grow the most rapidly.**
- **Squamous cell carcinomas** and small cell carcinomas tend to grow slightly **less rapidly.**
- **Adenocarcinomas** grow the **most slowly.**
- When clinical signs or symptoms are present, the chance of malignancy rises. Solitary pulmonary nodules that are surgically removed (clinical signs or symptoms and imaging findings suggested malignancy) are **malignant 50% of the time in men over the age of 50.**

Benign Causes of Solitary Pulmonary Nodules

- **Granulomas.** Tuberculosis and histoplasmosis usually produce calcified nodules < 1 cm in size, although tuberculomas and histoplasmomas can reach up to 4 cm.
  - **When calcified, they are clearly benign. Tuberculous granulomas are usually homogeneously calcified. Histoplasmomas** may contain a **central** or **"target" calcification** or may have a **laminated calcification,** which is diagnostic (Fig. 12-14).
  - If the nodule is large enough, **CT densitometry** can be used to help differentiate between a calcified and a

noncalcified pulmonary nodule by detecting occult calcification within nodules using calculations based on numerical density measurements of the lesion.
- **Positron emission tomographic** scans (PET scans) can also help in differentiating benign from malignant nodules and provide insight into the site of any metastatic disease. Using a glucose analog (FDG), the test is based on the enhanced glucose metabolism and uptake of lung cancer cells. Usually, the nodules must be > 1 cm in size for accurate characterization as being "PET-avid" (i.e., most likely malignant).
- **Hamartomas.** Peripherally located lung tumors of **disorganized lung tissue** that characteristically **contain fat and calcification** on CT scan. The **classical calcification** of a hamartoma is called *popcorn calcification* (Fig. 12-15).
- Other uncommon benign lesions that can produce solitary pulmonary nodules include rheumatoid nodules, fungal diseases such as nocardiosis, arteriovenous malformations, and granulomatous vasculitis (Wegener granulomatosis).
- Round atelectasis may mimic a solitary pulmonary nodule and is discussed in Chapter 5, *Recognizing Atelectasis.*

BRONCHOGENIC CARCINOMA

- In the United States, **lung cancer is the most common fatal malignancy in men** and the **second most common in women** (next to breast cancer).
- The **number** of nodules in the lung can help direct the further work-up. **Primary lung cancer** usually presents as a **solitary nodule,** while **metastatic disease** to the lung from another organ characteristically produces **multiple nodules.**
- Table 12-5 summarizes the classical manifestations and growth tendencies of the four types of bronchogenic carcinoma by cell type.

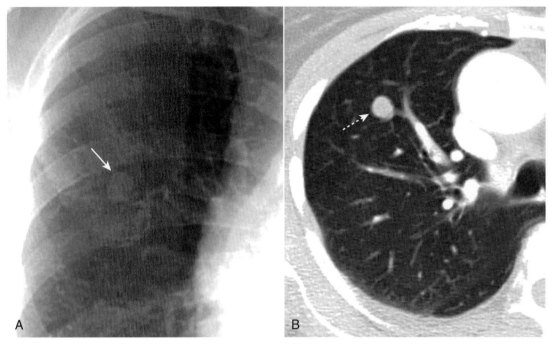

Figure 12-12 Solitary pulmonary nodule, conventional radiograph (A) and CT (B). A 1.8 cm nodule is seen in the right upper lobe (*solid and dotted white arrows*) in this 53-year-old male with an episode of hemoptysis. The critical question to be answered in evaluating any solitary pulmonary nodule is whether the lesion is benign or malignant. The answer to the question will depend on many factors, including the lesion's size and availability of prior imaging studies, which can help greatly in establishing growth of a lesion over time. A PET scan in a lesion of this size might help in indicating if the nodule is benign or not. This patient had a biopsy that revealed an adenocarcinoma of the lung.

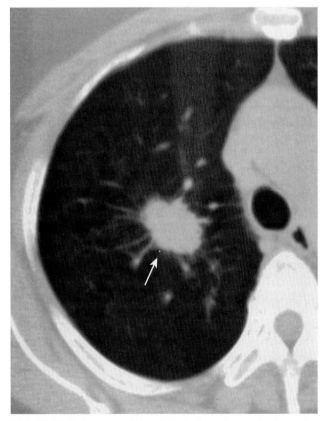

Figure 12-13 Right upper lobe bronchogenic carcinoma. A 3.2 cm spiculated mass is demonstrated in the right upper lobe (*solid white arrow*). The relatively large size and irregular margins of this mass point toward a malignant process. A percutaneous biopsy revealed an adenocarcinoma of the lung.

- **Recognizing bronchogenic carcinomas**
  - They may be recognized by visualization of the **tumor itself**: i.e., a **nodule/mass in the lung.**
  - They may be suspected by recognizing the **effects of bronchial obstruction**: i.e., **pneumonitis** and/or **atelectasis.**
  - They may be suspected by recognizing the results of either their **direct extension or metastatic spread** to the lung or to other organs.

Bronchogenic Carcinomas Presenting as a Nodule/Mass in the Lung

- These are most often **adenocarcinomas.**
- The nodule may have **irregular** and **spiculated margins** (see Fig. 12-13).
- It **may cavitate**, more often if it is of squamous cell origin (although cavitation also occurs with adenocarcinoma), producing a **relatively thick-walled** cavity with a **nodular and irregular inner margin** (Fig. 12-16).

Bronchogenic Carcinoma Presenting with Bronchial Obstruction

- **Bronchial obstruction is most often caused by a squamous cell carcinoma.** Endobronchial lesions produce varying degrees of bronchial obstruction, which can lead to pneumonitis or atelectasis.
- **Obstructive pneumonitis and atelectasis.**
  - *Pneumonitis* is the term used because the obstructed lung is consolidated but frequently not infected (though it can be).

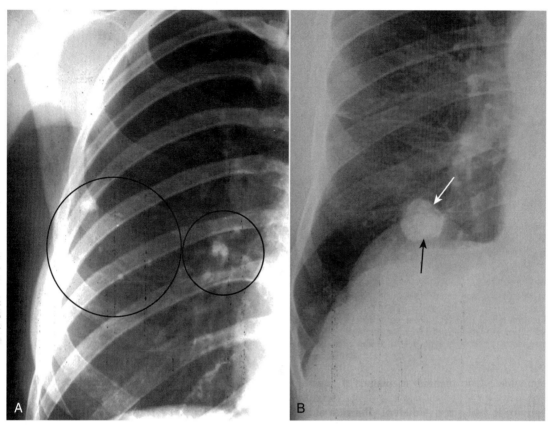

Figure 12-14 Calcified tuberculous granulomas and histoplasmoma. When a pulmonary nodule is heavily calcified, it is almost always benign. **A,** Tuberculous granulomas are common sequelae of prior, usually subclinical, tuberculous infection and are usually homogeneously calcified (*black circles*). **B,** Histoplasmomas (*solid white arrow*) may contain a central or "target" calcification (*solid black arrow*) or may have a laminated calcification, which is diagnostic. CT can be used to differentiate between a calcified and a noncalcified pulmonary nodule with greater sensitivity than conventional radiographs.

- **Atelectasis** secondary to an endobronchial obstructing lesion features the usual shifts of the fissures or mobile mediastinal structures toward the side of the atelectasis (see Chapter 5) in addition to visualization of the obstructing mass (see Fig. 5-11).

Bronchogenic Carcinoma Presenting with Direct Extension or Metastatic Lesions

- **Rib destruction by direct extension.** *Pancoast tumor* is the eponym for a tumor arising from the superior sulcus of the lung, frequently producing destruction of one or more of the first three ribs on the affected side (Box 12-1; Fig. 12-17).
- **Hilar adenopathy.** Usually unilateral on the same side as the tumor (Fig. 12-18).
- **Mediastinal adenopathy.** May be the sole manifestation of a small cell carcinoma, the peripheral lung nodule being invisible (see Fig. 12-8).
- **Other nodules in the lung.** One of the manifestations of diffuse bronchoalveolar cell carcinoma may be multiple nodules throughout both lungs and, as such, may mimic metastatic disease.
- **Pleural effusion.** Frequently, there is associated lymphangitic spread of tumor when there is a pleural effusion.
- **Metastases to bones.** These tend to be mixed osteolytic and osteoblastic.

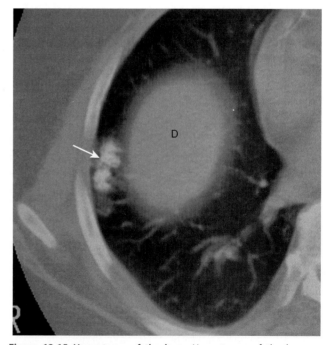

Figure 12-15 Hamartoma of the lung. Hamartomas of the lung are peripherally located tumors of disorganized lung tissue that classically contain fat and calcification on CT scans. The classical calcification of a hamartoma is called **popcorn calcification** (*solid white arrow*). The small island of soft tissue in the middle of the right lung (*D*) is the uppermost part of the right hemidiaphragm.

TABLE 12-5 CARCINOMA OF THE LUNG: CELL TYPES

Cell Type	Graphic Representation	Classical Manifestations
Squamous cell carcinoma		Primarily central in location Arise in segmental or lobar bronchi Invariably produce bronchial obstruction leading to obstructive pneumonitis or atelectasis Tend to grow rapidly
Adenocarcinoma, including bronchoalveolar cell carcinoma		Primarily peripheral in location Usually solitary except in the case of diffuse bronchoalveolar cell carcinoma, which can present as multiple nodules Slowest growing
Small cell, including oat cell carcinoma		Primarily central in location May contain neurosecretory granules that lead to an association of small cell carcinoma with paraneoplastic syndromes such as Cushing syndrome, inappropriate secretion of antidiuretic hormone
Large cell carcinoma		Diagnosis of exclusion for lesions that are nonsmall cell and not squamous or adenocarcinoma Larger peripheral lesions Grow extremely rapidly

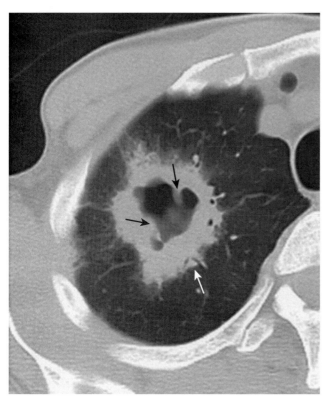

Figure 12-16 Cavitary bronchogenic carcinoma. A large, cavitating neoplasm with a thick wall (*solid white arrow*) is present in the right upper lobe. The outer margin of the lesion is spiculated. The internal contour of the cavity is nodular (*solid black arrows*). These features point toward a cavitating malignancy. This was a squamous cell carcinoma.

Box 12-1 Pancoast Tumor: Apical Lung Cancer
Manifests as a soft tissue mass in the apex of the lung
Most often squamous cell carcinoma or adenocarcinoma
Frequently produces adjacent rib destruction
May invade brachial plexus or cause Horner syndrome on affected side
On the right side, it may produce superior vena caval obstruction

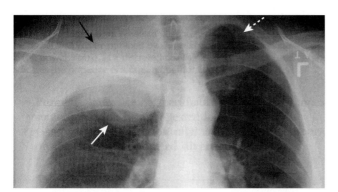

Figure 12-17 Pancoast tumor, right upper lobe. A large, soft tissue mass is seen in the apex of the right lung (*solid white arrow*). It is associated with rib destruction (*solid black arrow*). On the normal left side, the ribs are intact (*dotted white arrow*). The finding of an apical soft tissue mass with associated rib destruction is classical for a Pancoast or superior sulcus tumor.

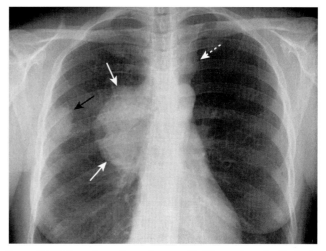

Figure 12-18 Bronchogenic carcinoma with hilar and mediastinal adenopathy. A peripheral lung mass (*solid black arrow*) shows evidence of ipsilateral hilar and mediastinal adenopathy (*solid white arrows*) and contralateral mediastinal adenopathy (*dotted white arrow*). Bronchogenic carcinoma may present with metastatic lesions that can manifest in distant organs or in the thorax itself. This was an adenocarcinoma of the lung.

METASTATIC NEOPLASMS IN THE LUNG

Multiple Nodules

- Multiple nodules in the lung are most often metastatic lesions that have traveled through the bloodstream from a distant primary (*hematogenous spread*). Multiple metastatic nodules are **usually of slightly differing sizes** indicating tumor embolization that occurred at different times.
- They are **frequently sharply marginated,** varying in size from **micronodular** to **"cannonball" masses** (see Fig. 3-15A).
- For all practical purposes it is **impossible to determine the primary site** by the **appearance of the metastatic nodules,** i.e., all metastatic nodules appear similar.
- Tissue sampling, whether by bronchoscopic or percutaneous biopsy, is the best means of determining the organ of origin of the metastatic nodule.
- Table 12-6 summarizes the primary malignancies most likely to metastasize to the lung hematogenously.

Lymphangitic Spread of Carcinoma

- In lymphangitic spread of carcinoma, a tumor grows in and obstructs lymphatics in the lung, producing a pattern that is **radiologically similar to pulmonary interstitial edema** from heart failure **including Kerley B lines, thickening of the fissures,** and **pleural effusions.**

 The findings **may be unilateral or may involve only one lobe,** which should alert you to suspect the possibility of lymphangitic spread rather than congestive heart failure, which is usually bilateral (Fig. 12-19).

- The **most common primary malignancies to produce lymphangitic spread** to the lung are those that arise around the thorax: **breast, lung, and pancreatic carcinoma.**

TABLE 12-6 SOME COMMON PRIMARY SITES OF METASTATIC LUNG NODULES

Males	Females
Colorectal carcinoma	Breast cancer
Renal cell carcinoma	Colorectal carcinoma
Head and neck tumors	Renal cell carcinoma
Testicular and bladder carcinoma	Cervical or endometrial carcinoma
Malignant melanoma	Malignant melanoma
Sarcomas	Sarcomas

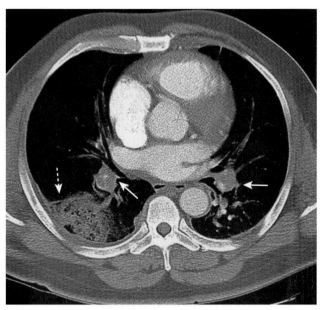

Figure 12-20 Hampton hump. There is a wedge-shaped, peripheral air-space density present (*dotted white arrow*) associated with filling defects in both the left and right pulmonary arteries (*solid white arrows*). The wedge-shaped infarct is called a **Hampton hump**. Without the associated emboli present, the pleural-based airspace disease could have a differential diagnosis that includes pneumonia, lung contusion, or aspiration.

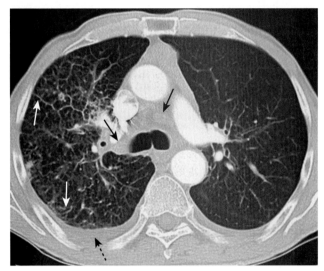

Figure 12-19 Bronchogenic carcinoma with lymphangitic spread of tumor. In lymphangitic spread of carcinoma, a tumor grows in and obstructs lymphatics in the lung producing a pattern that is radiologically similar to pulmonary interstitial edema from heart failure. The findings may be unilateral, as in this case, which should alert you to the possibility of lymphangitic spread rather than congestive heart failure. There is extensive hilar and mediastinal adenopathy (*solid black arrows*) from a carcinoma of the lung. The interstitial markings are prominent in the right lung compared to the left, and there are thickened septal lines (Kerley B lines) present (*solid white arrows*) along with a right pleural effusion (*dotted black arrow*).

PULMONARY THROMBOEMBOLIC DISEASE

- **Over 90% of pulmonary emboli develop from thrombi in the deep veins of the leg,** especially above the level of the popliteal veins. They are usually a **complication of surgery** or **prolonged bed rest** or **cancer.** Because of the **dual** circulation of the lungs (pulmonary and bronchial), **most pulmonary emboli do not result in infarction.**

- Although conventional chest radiographs are frequently abnormal in patients with pulmonary embolus (PE), they demonstrate nonspecific findings, such as **subsegmental atelectasis, small pleural effusions,** or elevation of the hemidiaphragm. Conventional chest radiography has a **high false-negative rate** in detecting PE.

- Chest radiographs infrequently manifest one of the "classic" findings for PE, which can include:
  - Wedge-shaped peripheral air-space disease (*Hampton hump*) (Fig. 12-20).
  - Focal oligemia (*Westermark sign*)
  - A prominent central pulmonary artery (*knuckle sign*)

- If the chest radiograph is normal, a nuclear medicine ventilation-perfusion scan (V/Q scan) may be diagnostic. If, however, the chest radiograph is abnormal, CT is usually performed.

- **CT pulmonary angiography (CT-PA)** is made possible by the **fast data acquisition** of **spiral CT** scanners (one breath hold) combined with **thin slices** and **rapid bolus intravenous injection of iodinated contrast** that produce maximal opacification of the pulmonary arteries with little or no motion artifact.

- Another benefit of CT-PA studies is the ability to acquire images of the veins of the pelvis and legs by obtaining slightly delayed images following the pulmonary arterial phase of the study. In this way, a deep venous thrombus may be detected even if the pulmonary portion of the angiogram is nondiagnostic.

- CT-PA has a **sensitivity in excess of 90%** and has replaced the use of V/Q scans in patients with **chronic obstructive pulmonary disease** or a **positive chest radiograph** in whom a V/Q scan is known to be less sensitive.

- On CT-PA, acute **pulmonary emboli** appear as **partial- or complete-filling defects centrally located** within the **contrast-enhanced** lumina of the **pulmonary arteries** (Fig. 12-21).

- CT-PA has the **additional benefit** of **demonstrating other diseases** that may be present, such as pneumonia, even if the study is negative for PE.

CHRONIC OBSTRUCTIVE PULMONARY DISEASE

- Chronic obstructive lung disease (COPD) is defined as a disease of **airflow obstruction due to chronic bronchitis or emphysema.**

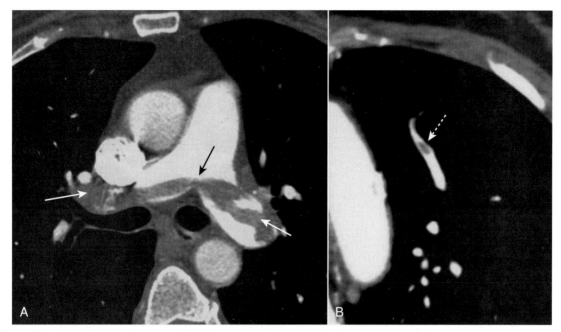

Figure 12-21 Saddle and peripheral pulmonary emboli. Acute pulmonary emboli appear as partial or complete filling defects centrally located within the contrast-enhanced lumina of the pulmonary arteries. **A,** A large pulmonary embolus almost completely fills both the left and right pulmonary arteries (*solid white and black arrows*). This is a **saddle embolus. B,** A small, central filling defect is seen in a more peripheral pulmonary artery (*dotted white arrow*). This pulmonary artery seems to be floating disconnected in the lung because the plane of this particular image does not display its connection to the left pulmonary artery.

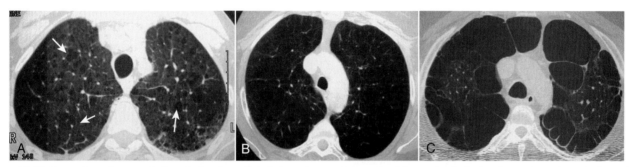

Figure 12-22 Types of emphysema. A, *Centriacinar (centrilobular) emphysema* features focal destruction limited to the respiratory bronchioles and the central portions of the acinus (*solid white arrows*). It is associated with cigarette smoking and is most severe in the upper lobes. **B,** *Panacinar (panlobular) emphysema* involves the entire alveolus distal to the terminal bronchiole, is most severe in the lower lung zones, and generally develops in patients with homozygous alpha1-antitrypsin deficiency. **C,** *Paraseptal emphysema* is the least common form, involves distal airway structures, alveolar ducts, and sacs, tends to be subpleural, and may cause pneumothorax.

- **Chronic bronchitis** is defined **clinically** by **productive cough,** whereas **emphysema** is defined **pathologically** by the presence of **permanent and abnormal enlargement and destruction of the air spaces distal to the terminal bronchioles**.
- **Emphysema has three pathologic patterns:**
  - **Centriacinar (centrilobular) emphysema** features focal destruction limited to the respiratory bronchioles and the central portions of acinus. It is **associated with cigarette smoking** and is most severe in the **upper lobes** (Fig. 12-22A).
  - **Panacinar emphysema** involves the entire alveolus distal to the terminal bronchiole. It is most severe in the **lower lung zones** and generally develops in patients with homozygous **alpha 1-antitrypsin deficiency** (Fig. 12-22B).
  - **Paraseptal emphysema** is the **least common** form. It involves distal airway structures, alveolar ducts, and

sacs. Localized to fibrous septa or to the pleura, it can lead to formation of bullae, which **may cause pneumothorax**. It is not associated with airflow obstruction (Fig. 12-22C).
- On conventional radiographs, the **most reliable finding of COPD is hyperinflation,** including **flattening of the diaphragm,** especially on the **lateral** exposure (Fig. 12-23). Other findings may include an **increase** in the **retrosternal clear space, hyperlucency** of the lungs with fewer than normal vascular markings visible, and **prominence of the pulmonary arteries** from pulmonary arterial hypertension.
- With CT, findings of COPD may include **focal areas of low density** in which the cystic areas lack visible walls except where bounded by interlobular septa. CT is helpful in evaluating the extent of emphysematous disease and in planning for surgical procedures designed to remove bullae to reduce lung volume.

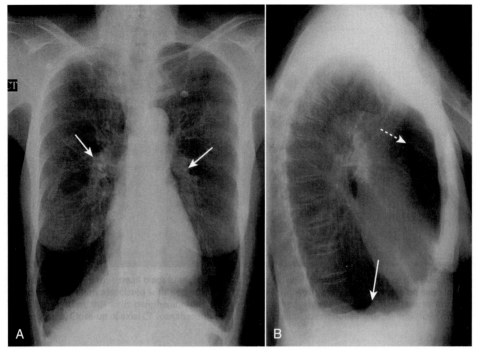

Figure 12-23 Emphysema. On conventional radiographs, the imaging findings of COPD are hyperinflation, including flattening of the diaphragm, especially on the lateral exposure (*solid white arrow* in **B**), increase in the retrosternal clear space (*dotted white arrow*), hyperlucency of the lungs with fewer than normal vascular markings, and prominence of the pulmonary arteries secondary to pulmonary arterial hypertension (*solid white arrows* in **A**).

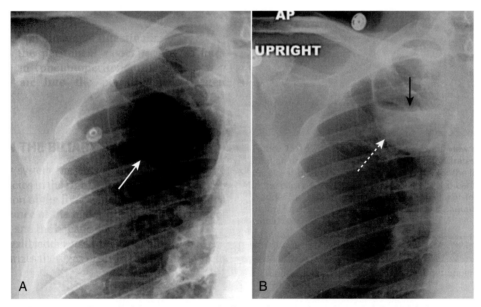

Figure 12-24 Infected bulla. A, Several thin-walled, but air-containing, bullae are shown in the right upper lobe (*solid white arrow*). **B,** Several weeks later, one of the bullae (*dotted white arrow*) contains both fluid and air (*solid black arrow*). Bullae normally contain air but can become partially or completely fluid-filled from infection or hemorrhage.

BLEBS AND BULLAE, CYSTS AND CAVITIES

- Blebs, bullae (singular: bulla), cysts, and cavities are all **air-containing lesions in the lung** of differing **size, location,** and **wall composition**.
- Almost any of these lesions can contain **fluid** instead of, or in addition to, air.
  - Fluid usually develops as a result of **infection, hemorrhage,** or **liquefaction necrosis**.

- When these lesions are **completely filled with fluid,** they **will appear solid** on conventional radiographs and CT scans, but they will typically demonstrate a **low CT number** that will differentiate them from a solid tumor.
- When they contain some fluid and some air, they will manifest an **air-fluid level** on a conventional radiograph (exposed with a horizontal x-ray beam) or on CT scans (Fig. 12-24).

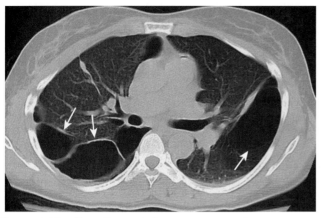

Figure 12-25 Bullous disease. Bullae measure more than 1 cm in size. They have a very thin wall that is often only partially visible on conventional radiography. CT demonstrates them more easily (*solid white arrows*). Characteristically, they contain no blood vessels but septae may appear to traverse the bulla. On conventional radiographs their presence is often inferred by a localized paucity of lung markings (see Fig. 12-24A).

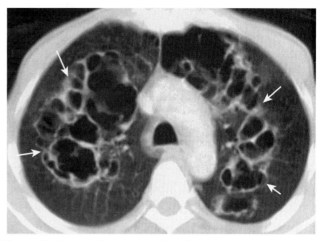

Figure 12-26 Cysts (pneumatocoeles) in *Pneumocystis* pneumonia (PCP). Cysts are visible on chest radiographs in 10% of patients with PCP and far more frequently with CT scans (up to 1 in 3 patients). Cysts may occur in the acute or in the postinfective phase of the disease. They have a predilection for the upper lobes and are commonly multiple (*solid white arrows*). Their etiology is unclear.

Blebs

- Blebs are **very small, blisterlike lesions that form in the visceral pleura**, usually at the **apex** of the lung. They are **very thin-walled** and, while they may be seen by CT, they are too small to be visible on chest radiographs. They are thought to be associated with spontaneous pneumothoraces.

Bullae

- Bullae measure **more than 1 cm** in size. They are usually **associated with emphysema.** They occur in the **lung parenchyma** and have a **very thin wall** (<1 mm) that is frequently **only partially visible** on conventional radiography but well seen on CT (Fig. 12-25).
  - On **conventional radiographs** their **presence is often inferred** by a localized paucity of lung markings.
- They can **grow to fill the entire hemithorax** and compress the lung to such an extent on the affected side that it seems to disappear (*vanishing lung syndrome*).
- Bullae can develop an **air-fluid level** through infection or hemorrhage.

Cysts

- Cysts are either congenital or acquired. They can occur in either the **lung parenchyma** or the **mediastinum.** They have a **thin wall** that is usually thicker than that of a bulla (<3 mm).
  - *Pneumatocoeles* represent **thin-walled cysts** that usually develop after a lung infection caused by such organisms as *Staphylococcus* or *Pneumocystis* (Fig. 12-26).

Cavities

- Cavities can **vary in size** from a few millimeters to many centimeters. They occur in the **lung parenchyma** and usually **result from a process** that produces necrosis of the central portion of the lesion.

TABLE 12-7 DIFFERENTIATING THREE CAVITATING LUNG LESIONS

Lesion	Thickness of the Cavity Wall	Inner Margin of Cavity
Bronchogenic carcinoma (Fig. 12-27A)	Thick*	Nodular
Tuberculosis (Fig. 12-27B)	Thin	Smooth
Lung abscess (Fig. 12-27C)	Thick	Smooth

*Thick = more than 5 mm; thin = less than 5 mm.

- Cavities usually have the **thickest wall** of any of these four air-containing lesions with a **wall thickness from 3 mm to several cm** (see Fig. 12-16).
- Differentiation between three of the most frequent causes of cavities (carcinoma, pyogenic abscess, and tuberculosis) is summarized in Table 12-7 (Fig. 12-27).

BRONCHIECTASIS

- Bronchiectasis is defined as **localized irreversible dilatation of part of the bronchial tree.** Although it can be associated with many other diseases, it is **usually caused by necrotizing bacterial infections,** like those of *Staphylococcus* and *Klebsiella,* and it usually affects the lower lobes.
  - Bronchiectasis may also occur with cystic fibrosis, primary ciliary dyskinesia (*Kartagener syndrome*), allergic bronchopulmonary aspergillosis, and *Swyer-James syndrome* (unilateral hyperlucent lung).
- Clinically, **chronic productive cough** and associated **hemoptysis** are the major symptoms.
- **Conventional radiographs** may demonstrate findings suggestive of the disease but are **usually not specific.**
  - Findings include parallel-line opacities (*tram-tracks*) due to thickened, dilated bronchial walls, **cystic lesions**

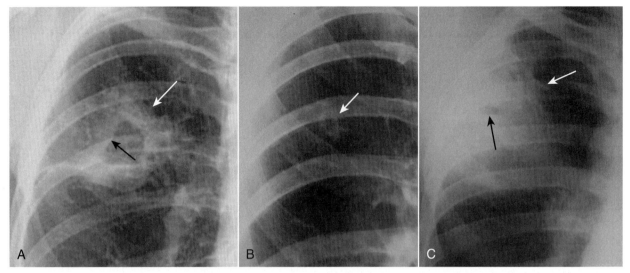

Figure 12-27 Cavitary lesions of the lung. Three of the most common cavitary lesions of the lung can frequently be differentiated from each other by noting the thickness of the wall of the cavity and the smoothness or nodularity of its inner margin. **A,** Squamous cell bronchogenic carcinoma produces a cavity with a thick wall (*solid white arrow*) and a nodular interior margin (*solid black arrow*). **B,** Tuberculosis usually produces a relatively thin-walled, upper lobe cavity with a smooth inner margin (*solid white arrow*). **C,** A staphylococcal lung abscess demonstrates a characteristically thickened wall (*solid white arrow*), which in this case has a very small cavity with a smooth inner margin (*solid black arrow*).

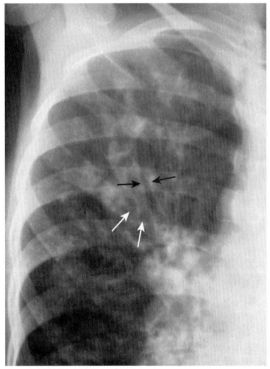

Figure 12-28 Bronchiectasis in cystic fibrosis. Conventional radiographs may demonstrate parallel line opacities called *tram tracks* due to thickened walls of dilated bronchi (*solid black arrows*) and cystic lesions as large as 2 cm in diameter due to cystic bronchiectasis (*solid white arrows*). Bilateral upper lobe bronchiectasis in children is highly suggestive of cystic fibrosis.

as large as 2 cm in diameter due to cystic bronchiectasis, and **tubular densities** from fluid-filled bronchi (Fig. 12-28). **CT is the study of choice in diagnosing bronchiectasis.**

- The hallmark lesion on CT is the *signet-ring sign* in which the **bronchus**, frequently with a thickened wall, **becomes larger than its associated pulmonary artery;** this is the opposite of the normal relationship between the two. The bronchus may also show a failure to taper normally (Fig. 12-29).

WEBLINK

Registered users may obtain more information on Recognizing Diseases of the Chest on StudentConsult.com.

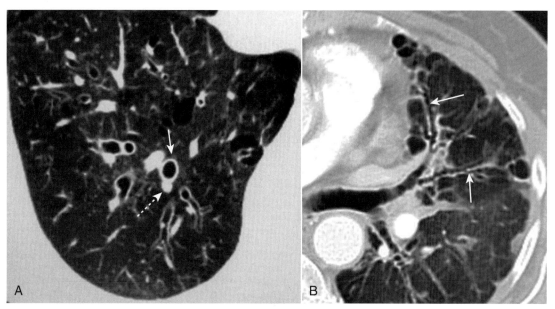

Figure 12-29 Bronchiectasis. CT is the study of choice in diagnosing bronchiectasis. **A,** The hallmark lesion is the *signet-ring sign* in which the bronchus with a thickened wall (*solid white arrow*) becomes larger than its associated pulmonary artery (*dotted white arrow*); this is the opposite of the normal relationship between the two. **B,** The bronchus may also show *tram-tracking*, thickened walls, and a failure to taper normally (*solid white arrows*).

TAKE-HOME POINTS

Recognizing Diseases of the Chest

The **mediastinum** lies in the central portion of the thorax between the two lungs and is arbitrarily divided into anterior, middle, and posterior compartments.

Masses in the **anterior mediastinum** include substernal thyroid goiters, lymphoma, thymoma, and teratoma.

The **middle mediastinum** is home primarily to lymphadenopathy from lymphoma and metastatic disease, such as from small cell carcinoma of the lung.

The **posterior mediastinum** is the location of neurogenic tumors, which originate either from the nerve sheath (mostly benign) or tissues other than the sheath (mostly malignant).

Incidental **solitary pulmonary nodules (SPNs)** less than 4 mm in size are rarely malignant; when clinical or imaging findings suggest malignancy, 50% of SPNs in men over the age of 50 are malignant. The key question is to determine whether a nodule is most likely benign or most likely malignant in any given individual.

Criteria on which an evaluation of benignity can be made include absolute size of the nodule upon discovery, presence of calcification within it, the margin of the nodule, and the change in the size of the nodule over time.

Bronchogenic carcinomas present in one of three ways: visualizing the tumor itself; recognizing the effects of bronchial obstruction such as pneumonitis and/or atelectasis; or recognizing the results of either their direct extension or metastatic spread to the chest or to distant organs.

Bronchogenic carcinomas presenting as a solitary nodule/mass in the lung are most often adenocarcinomas; bronchoalveolar cell carcinoma is a subset of adenocarcinoma that may present with multiple nodules, mimicking metastatic disease.

Bronchogenic carcinoma presenting with bronchial obstruction is most often due to squamous cell carcinoma; squamous cell carcinomas are most likely to cavitate.

Small cell carcinomas are highly aggressive, centrally located, peribronchial tumors, the majority of which have already metastasized at the time of initial presentation; they can be associated with paraneoplastic syndromes such as inappropriate secretion of antidiuretic hormone and Cushing syndrome.

Multiple nodules in the lung are most often **metastatic lesions** that have traveled through the bloodstream from a distant primary (*hematogenous spread*); common sites of primaries for such metastases include colorectal, breast, renal cell, head and neck, bladder, uterine and cervical, soft tissue sarcomas, and melanoma.

In **lymphangitic spread** of carcinoma, a tumor grows in and obstructs lymphatics in the lung producing a pattern that is radiologically similar to pulmonary interstitial edema; primaries that metastasize to the lung in this fashion include breast, lung, and pancreatic cancer.

Conventional radiography has a high false negative rate in **pulmonary thromboembolic disease** because demonstration of "classic" findings such as Hampton hump, Westermark sign, and the knuckle sign is infrequent.

CT-pulmonary angiography (CT-PA) is now widely used for the diagnosis of pulmonary embolism producing images of the pulmonary arteries with little or no motion artifact.

Chronic obstructive pulmonary disease (COPD) consists of emphysema and chronic bronchitis; of the two, chronic bronchitis is a clinical diagnosis while emphysema is defined pathologically and has findings that can be seen on both conventional radiographs and CT scans.

Blebs, bullae, cysts, and cavities are all air-containing lesions in the lung that differ in size, location, and wall composition; bullae, cysts, and cavities are seen on CT and may also be seen on conventional radiographs.

Although **bronchiectasis** may be seen on conventional radiographs, CT is the study of choice demonstrating tram-tracks, cystic lesions, or tubular densities.

Chapter 13

Recognizing the Normal Abdomen: Conventional Radiographs

- While imaging of the abdomen is now largely performed utilizing CT, ultrasound, or MRI, many patients have "plain films" of the abdomen as a first step before other imaging studies are performed or as a method of following up on findings demonstrated by other modalities.
  - As always, the principles that guide the interpretation of conventional radiographs apply to the modalities of CT, MRI, and ultrasound.
- In order to recognize *abnormal* findings on conventional radiographs of the abdomen, you first must familiarize yourself with the appearance of normal.

WHAT TO LOOK FOR

 First, look at the **overall gas pattern** (Box 13-1).

- You are looking for the overall pattern, so don't spend too much time trying to identify every bubble of bowel gas you see.
- **Second,** check for **extraluminal air** (see Chapter 15).
- **Third,** look for **abnormal abdominal calcifications**.
- **Fourth,** look for any **soft tissue masses**.

NORMAL BOWEL GAS PATTERN

- Virtually all gas in the bowel comes from swallowed air. Only a fraction comes from the bacterial fermentation of food.
- In the abdomen, the terms *gas* and *air* are used interchangeably to refer to the contents of the bowel.
- Loops of bowel that contain a sufficient amount of air to fill the lumen completely are said to be *distended*. *Distension* of bowel is **normal**.
- Loops of bowel that are filled beyond their normal size are said to be *dilated*. *Dilatation* of the bowel is **abnormal**.
- Stomach
  - There is almost **always air in the stomach,** unless
    - The patient has recently vomited, or
    - There is a nasogastric tube in the stomach and the tube is attached to suction.
- Small bowel
  - There is usually a small amount of **air in about two or three loops of nondilated small bowel** (Fig. 13-1).

- The **normal diameter of small bowel is less than 2.5 cm,** which is about 1 inch or the diameter of one U.S. quarter.
- Large bowel
  - **There is almost always air in the rectum or sigmoid.** There may be **varying amounts of gas** in the remainder of the **colon** (Fig. 13-2).
  - Use this rule to decide if the large bowel is dilated or not:
    - **The large bowel can normally distend to about the same size as it does on a barium enema examination.** To give you an idea of how large that is, look at Figure 13-3.
    - Stool is recognizable by the **multiple, small bubbles of gas** present within a semisolid-appearing mass. Recognizing the appearance of stool will help in localizing the large bowel (Fig. 13-4).

Individuals who swallow large quantities of air may develop *aerophagia*, characterized by numerous polygonal-shaped, air-containing loops of bowel, none of which is dilated (Fig. 13-5).

NORMAL FLUID LEVELS

- Stomach
  - Fluid is almost always seen in the stomach, so **an air-fluid level is almost always demonstrated in the stomach** on an upright abdominal or upright chest radiograph or if the patient is in the decubitus position.
    - **To see an air-fluid level, the x-ray beam must be directed horizontally**—parallel to the floor (see Chapter 1, *Recognizing Anything*).
- Small bowel
  - **Two or three air-fluid levels** in the small bowel may be seen normally on an upright or decubitus view of the abdomen.
- Large bowel
  - The large bowel functions, in part, to remove fluid, so there are **no** or **very few air-fluid levels in the colon** (Fig. 13-6).

Many air-fluid levels may be present in the colon if the patient has had a **recent enema** or if the patient is **taking medication with a strong anticholinergic, antiperistaltic effect.**

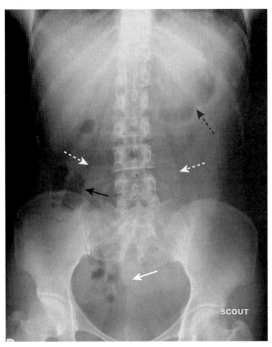

Figure 13-1 Normal supine abdomen. This is the "scout" film of the abdomen, the one that gives a general idea of the bowel gas pattern and allows you to search for radiopaque calculi and detect organomegaly. There is usually a small amount of air in about two to three loops of non-dilated small bowel (*solid black arrow*). There will almost always be air in the stomach (*dotted black arrow*) and in the rectosigmoid (*solid white arrow*). Depending on the amount of fat around the visceral organs, their outlines may be partially visible on conventional radiographs. The psoas muscles are outlined by fat (*dotted white arrows*) making them visible on this image.

- The normal distribution of bowel gas and fluid is summarized in Table 13-1.

DIFFERENTIATING LARGE FROM SMALL BOWEL

- **Recognizing large bowel**
  - **Large bowel is peripherally placed** around the perimeter of the abdominal cavity except for the right upper quadrant, which is occupied by the liver (Fig. 13-7).
  - **Haustral markings usually do not extend completely across the large bowel** from one wall to the other. If they do connect one wall with another, **haustral markings are spaced more widely apart** than the valvulae conniventes of the small bowel (Fig. 13-8).
- **Recognizing small bowel**
  - **Small bowel is centrally placed** in the abdomen. Valvulae markings typically extend across the lumen of

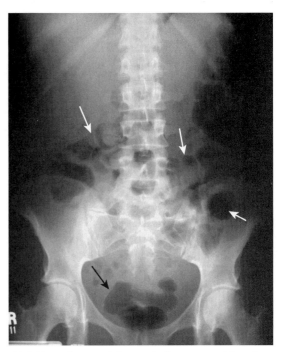

Figure 13-2 Normal prone abdomen. In the prone position, the ascending and descending colon and the rectosigmoid—all posterior structures—are the highest parts of the large bowel and thus most likely to fill with air. There is air seen in the S-shaped rectosigmoid (*solid black arrow*) and throughout the remainder of the colon (*solid white arrows*).

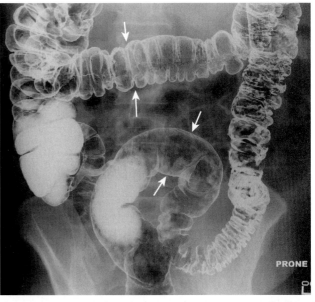

Figure 13-3 Normal colonic distension. The colon can normally distend to the size of the diameter of the colon as seen on a barium enema (*solid white arrows*). Beyond this size, the colon would be considered dilated. This patient has had a double-contrast barium enema examination in which both air and barium are instilled as contrast agents. The combination allows for excellent visualization of the mucosal surface of the colon.

small bowel from one wall to the other. The **valvulae are spaced much closer together** than the haustra of the large bowel (Fig. 13-9).
- Small bowel can achieve a maximum diameter, even when dilated, of about 5 cm. Large bowel can dilate to many times that size.

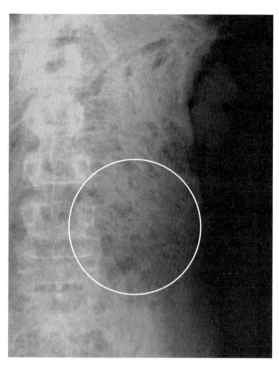

Figure 13-4 Appearance of stool. Stool is recognizable by the multiple, small bubbles of gas present within a semisolid-appearing soft tissue density (*white circle*). Stool marks the location of the large bowel and can help in identification of individual loops of bowel on conventional radiographs. This patient has a markedly dilated sigmoid colon from chronic constipation.

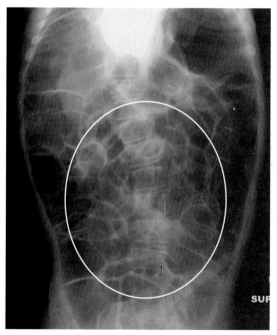

Figure 13-5 Aerophagia. Virtually all bowel gas comes from swallowed air. Swallowing large quantities of air may produce a picture called **aerophagia**, characterized by numerous polygonal-shaped, air-containing loops of bowel, none of which is dilated (*white circle*).

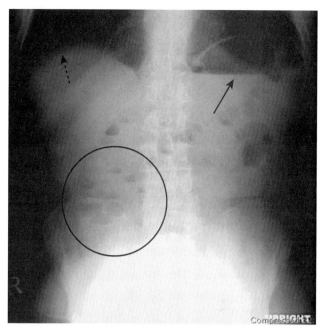

Figure 13-6 Normal upright abdomen. There for two things to look for on an upright view of the abdomen: air-fluid levels and free intraperitoneal air. Normally, there is an air-fluid level in the stomach (*solid black arrow*). There may be short, air-fluid levels present in a few nondilated loops of small bowel (*black circle*). There are usually very few or no air-fluid levels seen in the colon. Free air, if present, should be visible just below the hemidiaphragm (*dotted black arrow*) and would be easier to recognize on the right than on the left.

TABLE 13-1 NORMAL DISTRIBUTION OF GAS AND FLUID IN THE ABDOMEN

Organ	Normally Contains Gas	Normally Has Air-Fluid Levels
Stomach	Yes	Yes
Small bowel	Yes—2-3 loops	Yes
Large bowel	Yes, especially rectosigmoid	No

ACUTE ABDOMINAL SERIES: THE VIEWS AND WHAT THEY SHOW

- Almost every Department of Radiology has a series of radiographic images (a protocol) that is routinely obtained in patients who have acute abdominal pain.
  - These series are sometimes called "obstructions series," "complete abdominal series," "acute abdominal series," or something similar. For the purposes of this book, we'll call such series "acute abdominal series."
- **Acute abdominal series: what it may contain**
  - **Supine view** of the abdomen. This view is almost always obtained.
  - **Prone or lateral rectum view.** The inclusion of these views is the most variable in different hospitals' acute abdominal series.
  - **Upright or left-side down (left lateral) decubitus view.** One or the other is almost always included.
  - **Chest—upright or supine view.** Inclusion of a chest radiograph depends upon hospital practices.
- Table 13-2 summarizes what to look for on each of the views of an acute abdominal series.

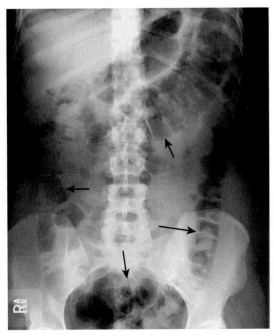

Figure 13-7 Location of large bowel. The large bowel usually occupies the periphery of the abdomen. The small bowel is located more centrally. Here, the large bowel (*solid black arrows*) contains a normal amount of air. The liver occupies the right upper quadrant and normally displaces all bowel from this area.

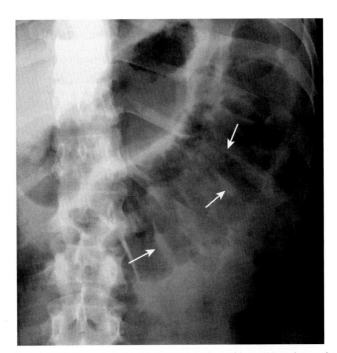

Figure 13-8 Normal large bowel haustral markings. Most haustral markings in the colon do not traverse the entire lumen to extend from one wall to the opposite wall (*solid white arrows*). This is unlike the appearance of the valvulae conniventes in the small bowel. The haustral markings are also spaced more widely apart than the valvulae of the small bowel (see Fig. 13-9).

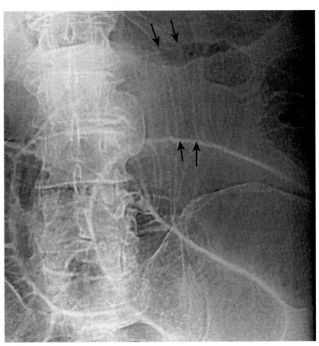

Figure 13-9 Normal small bowel valvulae. Markings representing the valvulae typically do extend across the lumen of the small bowel to extend from one wall to the other. In addition, the valvulae are spaced much closer together than the haustra of the large bowel, even when the small bowel is dilated. The *solid black arrows* point to two valvulae that traverse the entire lumen in this enhanced close-up of dilated small bowel in this patient with a small bowel obstruction.

Acute Abdominal Series: Supine View ("Scout Film")

- **What it's good for**
  - **Overall appearance of the gas pattern**
    - The **overall appearance of the bowel gas pattern**, including how much air and fluid there are and their most likely location, is **more important** than identifying every small bubble of air on the radiograph.
  - Identifying the **presence or absence of calcifications.**
  - Identifying the **presence of soft tissue masses** (see Fig. 13-1).
- **How it's obtained**
  - The patient lies on his or her back on the x-ray table or stretcher and the x-ray beam is directed vertically downward (Fig. 13-10).
- **Substitute view**
  - There is really no other view that substitutes for a supine view of the abdomen. Virtually all patients, regardless of their condition, can tolerate this part of the examination.

Acute Abdominal Series: Prone View

- **What it's good for**
  - **Identifying gas in the rectum and/or sigmoid**
    - Since the rectum and sigmoid are the **highest points of the large bowel** with the person lying prone on the x-ray table, air will rise into the rectosigmoid.
    - By the way, almost no air is introduced into the rectosigmoid during the course of a routine rectal examination.

TABLE 13-2 ACUTE ABDOMINAL SERIES: THE VIEWS AND WHAT TO LOOK FOR

View	Look for
Supine abdomen	Bowel gas pattern, calcifications, masses
Prone abdomen	Gas in the rectosigmoid
Upright abdomen	Free air, air-fluid levels in the bowel
Upright chest	Free air, pneumonia, pleural effusions

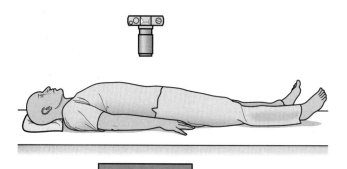

Figure 13-10 Positioning for supine view of the abdomen. The patient lies on his or her back on the x-ray table or stretcher and the x-ray beam is directed vertically downward. The camera icon represents the x-ray tube, which would actually be positioned about 40 inches above the cassette, represented by the thick line.

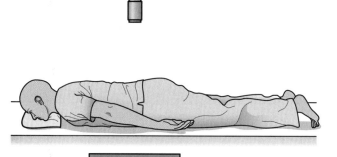

Figure 13-11 Positioning for prone view of the abdomen. The patient lies on his or her abdomen on the x-ray table or stretcher and the x-ray beam is directed vertically downward. The camera icon represents the x-ray tube, which would actually be positioned about 40 inches above the cassette, represented by the thick line.

- • **Identifying gas in ascending and descending colon**
  - • Since these two parts of the large bowel, besides the rectosigmoid, are also posteriorly positioned, air will collect in them when the patient is lying prone (see Fig. 13-2).
- ■ **How it's obtained**
  - • The patient lies on his or her abdomen on the x-ray table or stretcher, and the x-ray beam is directed vertically downward (Fig. 13-11).
- ■ **Substitute view**
  - • Frequently, patients are **unable to lie prone** because of their physical condition (e.g., recent surgery, severe abdominal pain).
  - • These patients can turn on their **left side** and have a **lateral view of the rectum** exposed with a **vertical beam** to substitute for the prone radiograph (Fig. 13-12).

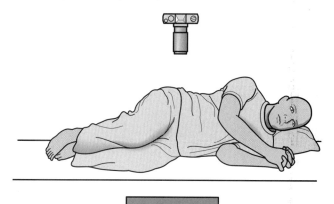

Figure 13-12 Positioning for the lateral rectum view. Patients who cannot lie prone can turn on their left side and have a lateral view of the rectum exposed with a vertical beam to substitute for the prone radiograph. The camera icon represents the x-ray tube, which would actually be positioned about 40 inches above the cassette, represented by the thick line.

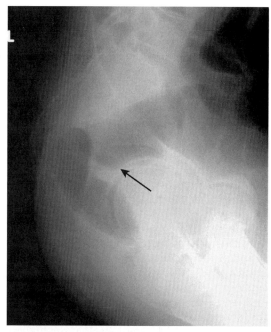

Figure 13-13 Normal lateral view of the rectum. Frequently, patients are unable to lie prone because of their physical condition (e.g., recent surgery, severe abdominal pain). These patients can turn on their left side and have a lateral view of the rectum exposed with a vertical beam to substitute for the prone radiograph. The lateral view of the rectum will usually demonstrate the presence or absence of air in the rectum and sigmoid (*solid black arrow*).

- • The lateral view of the rectum will usually demonstrate the presence or absence of air in the rectum and sigmoid (Fig. 13-13).

Acute Abdominal Series: Upright View of Abdomen

- ■ **What it's good for**
  - • Seeing **free air in the peritoneal cavity** (i.e., extraluminal air)

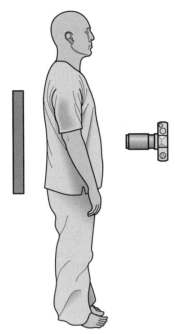

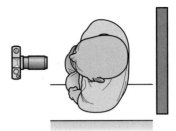

Figure 13-15 Positioning of the patient for a left lateral decubitus view of the abdomen. Patients who cannot tolerate an upright view of their abdomen usually have a left lateral decubitus view as a substitute. The patient lies on his or her left side on the examining table, the x-ray tube is usually positioned anteriorly (camera icon) and the cassette (thick line) is placed in back of the patient. The x-ray beam is directed horizontally, parallel to the floor at a distance of about 40 inches from the patient.

Figure 13-14 Positioning of patient for an upright view of the abdomen. The patient stands or sits up and the x-ray beam is directed horizontally, parallel to the plane of the floor. The camera icon represents the x-ray tube, which would actually be positioned about 40 inches from the cassette, represented by the thick line.

- Seeing **air-fluid levels within the bowel lumen** (see Fig. 13-6)
■ **How it's obtained**
- The patient stands or sits up and the exposure is made with the **x-ray beam directed horizontally**, parallel to the plane of the floor (Fig. 13-14).
■ **Substitute view**
- Frequently, patients with the signs and symptoms of an acute abdomen cannot tolerate standing or sitting up for an upright view of their abdomen.
- In such cases, a **left lateral decubitus view** of the abdomen is substituted for the upright radiograph. For a left lateral decubitus view, the **patient lies on his or her left side on the x-ray table.** This is done so that any "free air" will distribute itself at the highest part of the abdominal cavity which will be the patient's **right** side (Fig. 13-15).
  - **Free air should be easily visible** over the **outside edge of the liver** where no bowel gas normally is present (Fig. 13-16).
  - If a right lateral decubitus view were obtained, any free air would rise to the left side of the abdomen. The left side of the abdomen is the normal location of the stomach bubble as well as gas in the splenic flexure of the colon, either of which could be mistaken for free air.
- In order **to see free air, the x-ray beam must be directed horizontally**, parallel to the floor, when a decubitus view is obtained.

 Box 13-2 summarizes what is needed to visualize air-fluid levels in the abdomen.

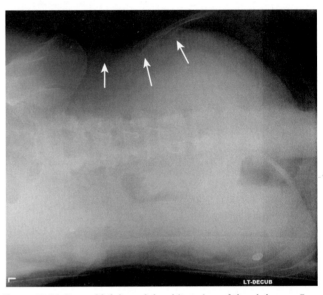

Figure 13-16 Normal left lateral decubitus view of the abdomen. For a left lateral decubitus view, the patient lies on his or her left side on the examining table and an exposure is made with a horizontal x-ray beam (parallel to the floor). This is done so that any "free air" will distribute itself at the highest part of the abdominal cavity which will be the patient's right side. Free air, if present, should be easily visible as a black crescent over the outside edge of the liver (*solid white arrows*), a location in which no bowel gas is normally present.

Box 13-2 To See an Air-Fluid Level on Conventional Radiographs, You Must Have:
Air
Fluid
A horizontal x-ray beam (parallel to the plane of the floor)
Air-fluid interfaces cannot be visualized on conventional radiographs taken with a vertical x-ray beam.

Acute Abdominal Series: Upright View of Chest

■ **What it's good for**
- Seeing **free air beneath the diaphragm**
- Finding **pneumonia at the lung bases**, which might mimic the symptoms of an acute abdomen
- Finding **pleural effusions**, which could be secondary to an intraabdominal process and help identify its presence

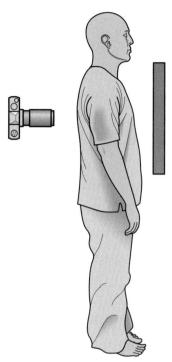

Figure 13-17 Positioning of patient for an upright chest radiograph. The patient sits upright or stands with the anterior chest wall closest to the cassette. The camera icon represents the x-ray tube, which is actually about 72 inches from the cassette, represented by the thick line.

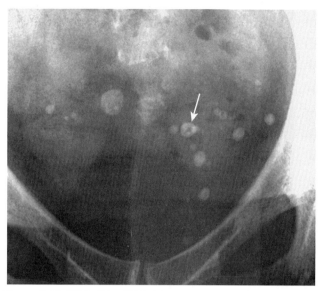

Figure 13-18 Phleboliths. Phleboliths are small, rounded calcifications that represent calcified venous thrombi that occur with increasing age, most often in the pelvic veins of women. They classically have a lucent center (*solid white arrow*). In the pelvic veins, they are considered incidental and nonpathologic calcifications, but they can be confused with ureteral calculi.

- **Pancreatitis,** for example, may be **associated with a left pleural effusion.**
- Some **ovarian tumors** may occasionally be associated **with right-sided or bilateral pleural effusions.**
- An abscess beneath the right hemidiaphragm (**subphrenic abscess**) **may be associated with a right pleural effusion.**
- See Chapter 6 for more on the laterality of pleural effusions.
- **How it's obtained**
  - The **patient stands or sits up** and an exposure of the thorax is made using a **horizontal x-ray beam** (Fig. 13-17).
- **Substitute view for an upright chest x-ray**
  - Frequently, patients with the signs and symptoms of an acute abdomen cannot tolerate standing for an upright view of their chest. In those cases, **a supine view of the chest may be obtained** with the patient lying on the stretcher or x-ray table.
  - In a supine view, the x-ray beam is directed **vertically downward; free air, especially small amounts, may not be visible.**

CALCIFICATIONS

⚠️ Abdominal calcifications are discussed in Chapter 16, *Recognizing Abnormal Calcifications.* There are two abdominal calcifications that should not be confused with pathologic calcifications.

- **Phleboliths** are small, rounded calcifications that represent calcified venous thrombi that occur with increasing age,

most often in the pelvic veins of women. They classically have a **lucent center**, which helps to differentiate them from ureteral calculi with which phleboliths can be confused (Fig. 13-18).
- **Calcification of the rib cartilages** occurs with advancing age and, while not a true abdominal calcification, can sometimes be confused for renal or biliary calculi when they overlie the kidney or region of the gallbladder. Calcified cartilage tends to have an **amorphous, speckled appearance** and the calcified cartilage will occur in an arc corresponding to that of the anterior rib cartilage as it sweeps back towards the sternum (Fig. 13-19).

ORGANOMEGALY

- **Conventional radiographic evaluation of soft tissue structures in the abdomen** (e.g., the liver, spleen, kidneys, gallbladder, urinary bladder, or soft tissue masses such as tumors or abscesses) **is limited** because these structures are **soft tissue densities** and they are **surrounded by other soft tissues or fluid** of similar density.
  - Only a **difference in density** between two adjacent structures **will render their outlines visible** on conventional radiographs.
- Still, conventional radiographs are easy to obtain and frequently the first study ordered in a patient with abdominal symptoms.

➡️ There **are two fundamental ways of recognizing the presence and estimating the size of soft tissue masses or organs** on conventional radiographs of the abdomen:

- The first is by **direct visualization of the edges of the structure,** which can only occur if it is surrounded by

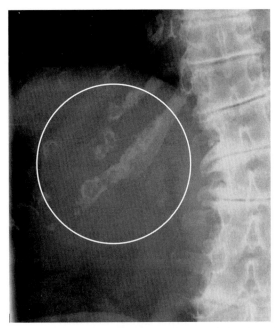

Figure 13-19 Calcified rib cartilages. Calcification of the rib cartilages (*white circle*) occurs with advancing age and, while not a true abdominal calcification, can sometimes be confused for calculi when it overlies the kidney or region of the gallbladder. Calcified cartilage tends to have an amorphous, mottled appearance. Calcified rib cartilages will occur along an arc corresponding to the sweep of the anterior ribs as they turn back toward the sternum.

something of a different density than soft tissue, like that of fat or free air.
- The second is to recognize **indirect evidence of the mass** or enlarged visceral organ by **recognizing pathologic displacement of air-filled loops of bowel**.

Liver

- **Normal**
  - The liver normally displaces all bowel gas from the right upper quadrant.
  - Occasionally, a **tonguelike projection of the right lobe** of the liver may extend to the iliac crest, **especially in females**. This is called a *Riedel lobe* and is normal (Fig. 13-20).
- **Enlarged liver**
  - An **enlarged liver might be suggested** from conventional radiographs if there is displacement of all bowel from the right upper quadrant **down to the iliac crest** and **across the midline** (Fig. 13-21).
  - **Conventional radiographs are notoriously poor for estimating the size of the liver**. Imaging evaluation of liver size is best made using CT, MRI, or ultrasound.

Spleen

- **Normal**
  - The adult **spleen is about 12 cm in length and usually does not project below the 12th posterior rib**. As a general rule, the **spleen is about as large as the left kidney**.
  - The **stomach bubble** (i.e., air in the gastric fundus) **usually nestles beneath the highest part of the left**

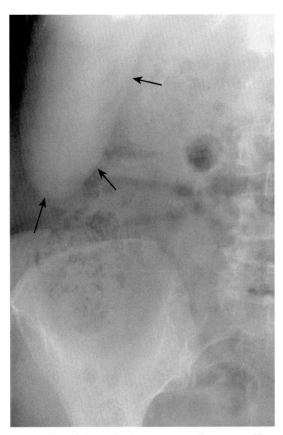

Figure 13-20 Riedel lobe of the liver. Occasionally, a tonguelike projection of the right lobe of the liver may extend to the iliac crest, especially in females. This is called a **Riedel lobe** and is normal (*solid black arrows*). Conventional radiographs are notoriously poor for estimating the size of the liver; CT, MRI, or US give a more accurate picture of liver size.

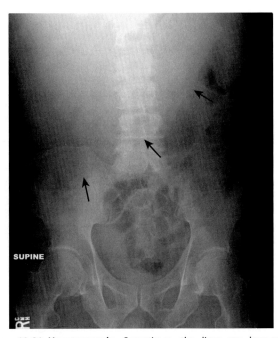

Figure 13-21 Hepatomegaly. Sometimes, the liver can become so enlarged it will be obvious even on conventional radiographs. An enlarged liver might be suggested from conventional radiographs if there is displacement of all bowel loops from the right upper quadrant down to the iliac crest and across the midline (*solid black arrows*), as in this patient with cirrhosis.

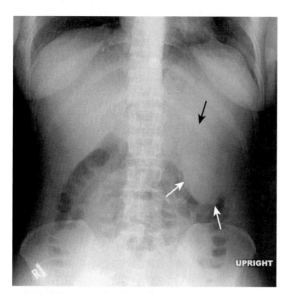

Figure 13-22 **Splenomegaly.** The spleen is about 12 cm in length and usually does not project below the 12th posterior rib. If the spleen (*solid white arrows*) projects well below the 12th posterior rib (*solid black arrow*) or displaces the stomach bubble toward or across the midline, the spleen is probably enlarged, as it is in this patient with leukemia.

hemidiaphragm about midway between the abdominal wall and the spine.

- **Enlarged spleen**
  - If the spleen projects well below the 12th posterior rib or displaces the stomach bubble toward or across the midline, the spleen is probably enlarged. (Fig. 13-22).

Kidneys

- **Normal**
  - Portions of the kidney outlines may be visible on conventional radiographs if there is an adequate amount of perirenal fat present.
  - The **kidney length is approximately the height of four lumbar vertebral bodies** or about **10 to 14 cm in size in an adult.**
  - The liver depresses the right kidney so that the **right kidney is usually lower in the abdomen than the left kidney** (Fig. 13-23).
  - The **left kidney is roughly the same length as the spleen.**
- **Enlarged kidney**
  - Usually only extremely enlarged kidneys or large renal masses will be recognizable on conventional radiographs by displacement of bowel gas (Fig. 13-24).

Urinary Bladder

- **Normal**
  - The bladder frequently is surrounded by **enough extravesical fat that at least the dome is visible** in most individuals as the top of an oval structure with its long axis parallel to the hips and the **base of the bladder just above the top of the symphysis pubis.**
  - The urinary bladder is about the size of a small cantaloupe when distended and about the size of a lemon when contracted (Fig. 13-25).

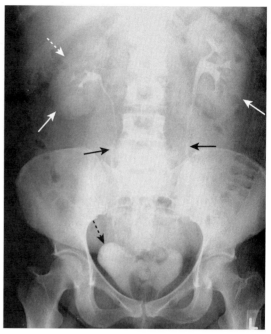

Figure 13-23 **Position of the kidneys.** This is one image from an intravenous urogram (intravenous pyelogram [IVP]) in which the patient receives an intravenous injection of iodinated contrast which is excreted by the kidneys. Both kidney outlines (*solid white arrows*), ureters (*solid black arrows*) and urinary bladder (*dotted black arrow*) can be seen. Other images of the kidneys, including oblique views, were often obtained to visualize the entire contour of the kidney. CT scans and CT urograms have largely replaced IVPs. The liver (*dotted white arrow*) normally depresses the right kidney more inferior than the left kidney.

- **Enlarged urinary bladder**
  - Bladder enlargement is usually recognized by displacement of bowel out of the pelvis by a soft tissue mass. Bladder outlet obstruction is much more common in men from enlargement of the prostate, so that a pelvic soft tissue mass is more likely to be a dilated bladder in a male than a female (Fig. 13-26).

Uterus

- **Normal**
  - The uterus usually sits atop the dome of the bladder. There is a lucency that is frequently produced by fat between the top of the bladder and the bottom of the uterus. The **normal uterus is about 8 cm by 4 cm by 6 cm.**
- **Enlarged uterus**
  - **Ultrasound** is the **best** tool for **evaluating the size of the uterus and ovaries.**
  - **Occasionally uterine enlargement,** when marked, **may be visible on conventional radiographs.**
  - The key to differentiating an enlarged uterus from a distended bladder is **identification of the lucency between the bladder and the uterus;** when the uterus is enlarged, the fat plane will be present; when the bladder is dilated, the fat plane will not be visible (see Fig. 13-26).

Psoas Muscles

- One or both of them may be visible if there is adequate extraperitoneal fat surrounding them. Inability to visualize

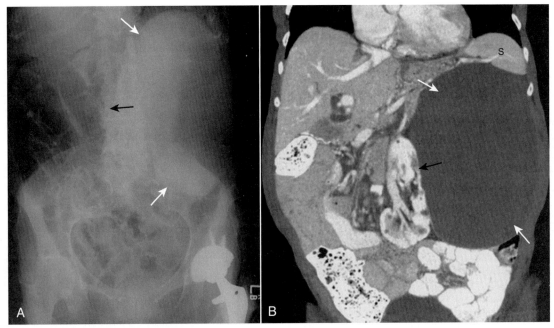

Figure 13-24 Enlarged kidney. Soft tissue masses or organomegaly can be diagnosed from a conventional radiograph either by visualizing the edge of the mass if there is fat or air surrounding it or by displacement of bowel. **A,** On the conventional radiograph, there is a soft tissue mass in the left upper quadrant (*solid white arrows*), which is displacing bowel to the right (*solid black arrow*). **B,** A coronal reformatted CT scan of the same patient demonstrates a large renal cyst (*solid white arrows*) arising from the left kidney (*solid black arrow*), displacing it and the surrounding bowel. The cyst is compressing the spleen (*S*).

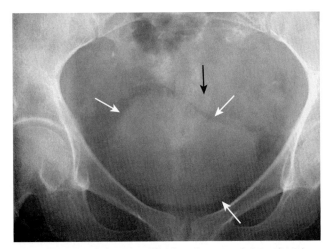

Figure 13-25 Normal urinary bladder. Close-up of the pelvis shows enough perivesical fat to make the outline of the urinary bladder visible (*solid white arrows*). In males, the sigmoid colon usually occupies the space just above the bladder (*solid black arrow*); in females, the soft tissue above the bladder may be either the uterus or sigmoid colon.

one or both psoas muscles is not a reliable indicator of retroperitoneal disease (see Fig. 13-1).

WEBLINK

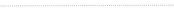

Registered users may obtain more information on Recognizing the Normal Abdomen: Conventional Radiographs on StudentConsult.com.

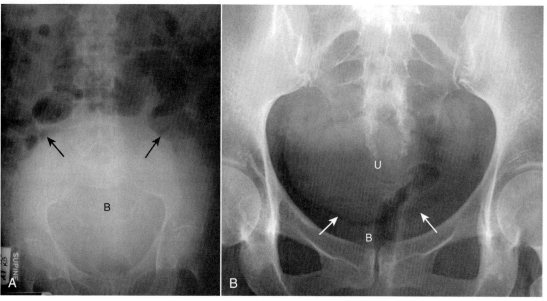

Figure 13-26 Distended urinary bladder and enlarged uterus. A, The distended bladder (*B*) is a soft tissue mass that ascends from the pelvis into the lower abdomen displacing the bowel into the midabdomen (*solid black arrows*). This was a 72-year-old man with bladder outlet obstruction from benign prostatic hypertrophy. **B,** The uterus (*U*) is slightly enlarged. It can be distinguished from the bladder because there is a fat plane (*solid white arrows*) seen between it and the urinary bladder (*B*) below it.

 TAKE-HOME POINTS

Recognizing the Normal Abdomen: Conventional Radiographs

Evaluation of the abdomen should focus on four main areas: the gas pattern, free air, soft tissue masses or organomegaly, and abnormal calcifications.

Air is normally present in the stomach and colon, especially the rectosigmoid, while a small amount of air (2-3 loops) may be seen in normal small bowel.

An air-fluid level is found normally in the stomach; two or three air fluid levels may be seen in nondilated small bowel, but usually no fluid is visible in the colon.

An acute abdominal series usually consists of: supine abdomen, prone abdomen (or its substitute, a lateral rectum view), upright abdomen (or its substitute, a left lateral decubitus view), and an upright chest (or its substitute, a supine chest).

The supine view of the abdomen is the general scout view for the bowel gas pattern and is useful for seeing calcifications and detecting organomegaly or soft tissue masses.

The prone view allows air, if present, to be seen in the rectosigmoid, which is important in the evaluation of mechanical obstruction of the bowel.

The upright abdomen may demonstrate air-fluid levels in the bowel or free intraperitoneal air.

The upright chest radiograph may demonstrate free air beneath the diaphragm, pleural effusion (which may provide a clue as to the presence and the nature of intraabdominal pathology), or pneumonia (which can mimic an acute abdomen).

CT, US, and MRI have essentially replaced conventional radiography in the assessment of organomegaly or soft tissue masses.

Chapter 14

Recognizing Bowel Obstruction and Ileus

- In Chapter 13, we discussed how to recognize the normal intestinal gas pattern.
- In this chapter, you'll learn how to recognize and categorize the four most common abnormal bowel gas patterns and their causes. These abnormal bowel gas patterns will appear the same whether imaged initially by conventional radiography or by CT scanning. CT is superior in revealing the location, degree, and cause of an obstruction and in demonstrating any signs of reduced bowel viability.
- Abnormalities of bowel function are suspected by the history and clinical findings.
- The key questions in assessing the bowel gas pattern on imaging studies are:
  - **Is air present in the rectum or sigmoid?**
  - **Are there dilated loops of small bowel?**
  - **Are there dilated loops of large bowel?**

ABNORMAL GAS PATTERNS

- Abnormal intestinal gas patterns can be divided into two main categories, each of which can be subdivided into two subcategories (Box 14-1).
- *Functional ileus* is one main category in which it is presumed that **one or more loops of bowel lose their ability to propagate the peristaltic waves of the bowel**, usually due to some **local irritation or inflammation**, and hence **cause a functional type of "obstruction"** proximal to the affected loop(s).
- There are **two kinds** of **functional ileus.**
  - *Localized ileus* (also called *sentinel loops*) affects only **one or two loops** of (usually **small**) bowel.
  - *Generalized adynamic ileus* affects **all loops of large and small bowel** and frequently the stomach.
- *Mechanical obstruction* is the other main category of abnormal bowel gas pattern. With mechanical obstruction, a **physical, organic, obstructing lesion prevents the passage of intestinal content** past the point of either the small or large bowel blockage.
- There are **two kinds** of **mechanical obstruction.**
  - *Small bowel obstruction* (frequently abbreviated SBO)
  - *Large bowel obstruction* (frequently abbreviated LBO)

LAWS OF THE GUT

- The bowel reacts to a mechanical obstruction in more or less predictable ways.
- Loops **proximal** to the **obstruction** soon become **dilated with air and/or fluid.**

- This can occur within a few hours of a complete small bowel obstruction.
- **Peristalsis will continue** (except in the loops of bowel involved in a functional ileus) in an attempt to propel intestinal contents through the bowel.
- Loops **distal** to an **obstruction** will eventually become **decompressed or airless,** as their contents are evacuated.
- In a mechanical obstruction, **the loop(s) that will become the most dilated** will either be the **loop of bowel with the largest resting diameter before the onset of the obstruction** (e.g., the **cecum** in the large bowel), or the **loop(s) of bowel just proximal to the obstruction.**
- Most patients with a mechanical obstruction will present with some form of **abdominal pain, abdominal distension,** and **constipation.**
  - Patients may present with **vomiting early** in the course of a **proximal small bowel obstruction** and **later** in the course of the illness with a **distal small bowel obstruction.**
- **Prolonged obstruction** with persistently elevated intraluminal pressures can lead to vascular compromise, **necrosis** and **perforation** in the affected loop of bowel.
- Let's look at each of the four abnormal bowel gas patterns in detail (Table 14-1). For each of the four abnormalities, we'll look at their **pathophysiology, causes,** key **imaging features,** and **diagnostic pitfalls.**

FUNCTIONAL ILEUS, LOCALIZED: SENTINEL LOOPS

- Pathophysiology
  - **Focal irritation** of a loop or loops of bowel **occurs most often from inflammation of an adjacent visceral organ,** e.g., pancreatitis may affect bowel loops in the left upper quadrant, diverticulitis in the left lower quadrant.
    - The **loop(s) affected** are almost always loops of **small bowel** and, because they **herald the presence of underlying pathology,** they are called *sentinel loops.*
  - The irritation causes these loops to lose their normal function and become aperistaltic, which in turn leads to **dilatation** of these loops.
  - Because **a functional ileus does not produce the degree of obstruction that a mechanical obstruction does,** some gas continues to pass through the defunctionalized bowel past the point of the localized ileus.
  - **Air** usually reaches and is **visible in the rectum or sigmoid.**

Box 14-1 Abnormal Bowel Gas Patterns

Functional Ileus
Localized ileus (sentinel loops)
Generalized adynamic ileus
Mechanical Obstruction
Small bowel obstruction (SBO)
Large bowel obstruction (LBO)

TABLE 14-1 ABNORMAL GAS PATTERNS—SUMMARY

	Air in Rectum or Sigmoid	Air in Small Bowel	Air in Large Bowel
Normal	Yes	Yes—1-2 loops	Rectum and/or sigmoid
Localized ileus	Yes	2-3 distended loops	Rectum and/or sigmoid
Generalized ileus	Yes	Multiple distended loops	Yes—distended
SBO	No	Multiple dilated loops	No
LBO	No	None—unless ileocecal valve incompetent	Yes—dilated

TABLE 14-2 CAUSES OF A LOCALIZED ILEUS

Site of Dilated Loops	Cause(s)
Right upper quadrant	Cholecystitis
Left upper quadrant	Pancreatitis
Right lower quadrant	Appendicitis
Left lower quadrant	Diverticulitis
Midabdomen	Ulcer or kidney/ureteral calculus

- **Causes of a localized ileus**
  - The **dilated loops of bowel tend to occur** in the **same anatomic area** as the **inflammatory or irritative process** of the adjacent abdominal organ, although this may not always be the case.
  - Table 14-2 summarizes **sites of a localized ileus and their most common cause.**
- **Key imaging features of a localized ileus**
  - On conventional radiographs, there are **one or two** *persistently dilated* loops of small bowel.
    - *Persistently* means that these **same loops remain dilated** on **multiple views** of the abdomen (supine, prone, upright abdomen) or on **serial studies** done over the course of time.
    - *Dilated* means the small bowel loops are **persistently larger than 2.5 cm.** Small bowel loops involved in a functional ileus **usually do not dilate as greatly as those which are mechanically obstructed.**
    - Infrequently, the sentinel loop may be **large bowel,** rather than small bowel. This can especially occur in the **cecum,** with diseases such as appendicitis.
  - There are **frequently air-fluid levels** seen in **sentinel loops.**
  - There is usually **gas in the rectum or sigmoid** in a localized ileus (Fig. 14-1).

 Pitfalls: Differentiating a localized ileus from an early SBO

- A localized ileus may resemble an *early* mechanical SBO, i.e., there may be a few dilated loops of small bowel with air in the colon seen in both. *Early* means the **patient has had symptoms for a day or two.** Patients who have had obstructive symptoms for a week or more usually no longer demonstrate imaging findings of an early obstruction.

 Solution. A combination of the clinical and laboratory findings and CT scanning of the abdomen that demonstrates the underlying pathology should differentiate localized ileus from small bowel obstruction.

FUNCTIONAL ILEUS, GENERALIZED: ADYNAMIC ILEUS

- **Pathophysiology**
  - In a generalized adynamic ileus, the **entire bowel is aperistaltic or hypoperistaltic.** Swallowed **air dilates and fluid fills all loops of both small and large bowel.**
  - A generalized adynamic ileus is almost always the **result of abdominal or pelvic surgery** in which the bowel is manipulated during the surgery.
- **Causes of a generalized adynamic ileus** are summarized in Table 14-3.
- **Key imaging features of a generalized adynamic ileus**
  - The **entire bowel is usually air-containing and dilated,** both large and small bowel. The stomach may be dilated as well.
  - The absence of peristalsis and the continued production of intestinal secretions usually produce **many long air-fluid levels in the bowel.**
  - Since this is not a mechanical obstruction, there **should be gas seen in the rectum or sigmoid.**
  - **Bowel sounds are frequently absent or hypoactive** (Fig. 14-2).

 Pitfalls: Recognizing a generalized adynamic ileus

- Patients do not present to the emergency department with a generalized adynamic ileus unless they are one or two days postoperative (abdominal or gynecologic surgery) or they have a severe electrolyte imbalance (e.g., hypokalemia).
- Many patients who have either **intestinal pseudo-obstruction** (see the end of this chapter) or **aerophagia** can be mistakenly identified as having a generalized ileus on abdominal radiographs.

MECHANICAL OBSTRUCTION: SMALL BOWEL OBSTRUCTION (SBO)

- **Pathophysiology**
  - A lesion, either inside or outside of the small bowel, obstructs the lumen.
  - Over time, **from the point of obstruction** *backward*, the **small bowel dilates** from continuously swallowed air

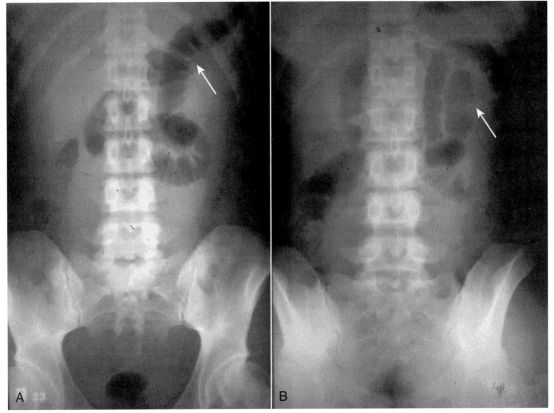

Figure 14-1 Sentinel loops from pancreatitis. A single, persistently dilated loop of small bowel is seen in the left upper quadrant (*solid white arrows*) on both the supine **(A)** and prone **(B)** radiographs of the abdomen. A sentinel loop or localized ileus often signals the presence of an adjacent irritative or inflammatory process. This patient had acute pancreatitis.

TABLE 14-3 CAUSES OF A GENERALIZED ADYNAMIC ILEUS

Cause	Remarks
Postoperative	Usually abdominal surgery
Electrolyte imbalance	Especially diabetics in ketoacidosis

and from intestinal fluid which continues to be produced by the stomach, pancreas, biliary system, and small bowel.

- **Peristalsis continues and may increase** in an effort to overcome the obstruction.
  - This can lead to high-pitched, hyperactive bowel sounds.
- As time passes, the **peristaltic waves empty the small bowel along with the colon of their contents from the point of obstruction** *forward.*
- If the obstruction is **complete** and if enough time has elapsed since the onset of symptoms, **there is usually no air found in the rectum or sigmoid.**
- Causes of a mechanical small bowel obstruction are summarized in Table 14-4 (Fig. 14-3).
- Key imaging features of mechanical small bowel obstruction
  - On conventional radiographs, **there are multiple dilated loops of small bowel** demonstrated proximal to the point of the obstruction (>2.5 cm).
    - As they begin to dilate, **small bowel loops** *stack up on* one another forming a *step-ladder* appearance, usually beginning in the left upper quadrant and

proceeding, depending on how distal the small bowel obstruction is, to the right lower quadrant (Fig. 14-4).
  - Generally speaking, **the more proximal the small bowel obstruction** (e.g., proximal jejunum), **the fewer the dilated loops** there will be; **the more distal the obstruction** (e.g., at the ileocecal valve), the **greater the number of dilated small bowel loops.**
- On upright or decubitus radiographs, there will usually be **numerous air-fluid levels present in the small bowel** proximal to the obstruction.
- If enough time has elapsed to decompress and empty the bowel distal to the point of obstruction, **there will be little or no gas found in the colon, especially the rectum.**

 In a mechanical small bowel obstruction, there should always be a **disproportionate dilatation of small bowel compared to the collapsed large bowel** (Fig. 14-5).

Pitfalls: Differentiating a partial SBO from a functional (localized) adynamic ileus

- An **intermittent,** (also known as a *partial* or *incomplete*) **mechanical small bowel obstruction** is one that **allows some gas to pass the point of obstruction,** at least at times. It can lead to a confusing picture because gas may pass into the colon long after the large bowel would be expected to be devoid of such gas. **Partial or incomplete small bowel obstruction** occurs **more often in patients** in whom **adhesions** are the etiology (Fig. 14-6).

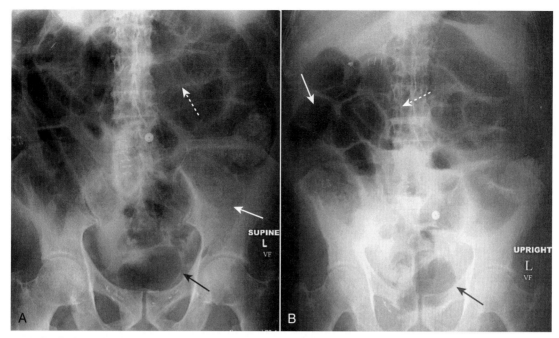

Figure 14-2 Generalized adynamic ileus, supine (A) and upright abdomen (B). There are dilated loops of large (*solid white arrows*) and small bowel (*dotted white arrows*) with gas seen down to and including the rectum (*solid black arrows*). The patient had undergone colon surgery the previous day.

TABLE 14-4 CAUSES OF A MECHANICAL SMALL BOWEL OBSTRUCTION

Cause	Remarks
Postsurgical adhesions	Most common cause of a small bowel obstruction; most frequently following appendectomy, colorectal surgery and pelvic surgery; transition point on small bowel CT without other identifying cause most likely represents adhesions
Malignancy	Primary malignancies of the small bowel are rare; secondary tumors such as gastric and colonic carcinomas and ovarian cancers may compromise the lumen of small bowel
Hernia	An inguinal hernia may be visible on conventional radiographs if air-containing loops of bowel are seen over the obturator foramen; easily seen on CT (see Fig. 14-3).
Gallstone ileus	May be visible on conventional radiographs or CT if air is seen in the biliary tree and (rarely) a gallstone is present in RLQ (see Chapter 15)
Intussusception	Ileocolic intussusception is the most common form and produces SBO
Inflammatory bowel disease	Thickening of the bowel wall may occur with compromise of the lumen in patients with Crohn disease; this is most likely to occur in the terminal ileum

- CT with or without oral contrast should be able to demonstrate a partial small bowel obstruction or identify the abnormality producing the sentinel loops (Fig. 14-7).
- **CT is the most sensitive study** for diagnosing the site and cause of a mechanical small bowel obstruction.
  - CT scans for bowel obstruction can be performed with or without oral contrast, utilizing the fluid already present in the bowel as contrast. Orally administered contrast (either barium or iodinated contrast) may help

in **identifying dilated loops** of bowel and in finding the *transition point* between the **proximal dilated** bowel and the **distal collapsed** bowel, but the oral contrast might also obscure important findings displayed by the use of intravenous contrast.
- **Intravenous contrast** is used for detecting **complications** of bowel obstruction such as **ischemia** and **strangulation**.

- The CT findings of a small bowel obstruction:
  - **Fluid-filled and dilated loops of small bowel** (>2.5 cm in diameter) proximal to the point of obstruction.
  - Identification of a *transition point*, which is where the **bowel changes caliber** from **dilated to normal** indicating the site of the obstruction. In the absence of identifying a mass or other obstructive cause at the transition point, the cause is almost certainly **adhesions** (Fig. 14-8).
  - **Collapsed small bowel or colon distal to the point of obstruction** (Fig. 14-9).
  - **Small-bowel feces sign.** Proximal to the transition point of a small bowel obstruction, intestinal debris and fluid may accumulate producing the appearance of fecal material in the small bowel. This is a sign of SBO (Fig. 14-10).
  - **Closed-loop obstruction** occurs when two points of the same loop of bowel are obstructed at a single location. The closed loop usually remains dilated and may form a U- or C-shaped structure. Most closed-loop obstructions are caused by adhesions. In the small bowel, a **closed-loop obstruction carries a higher risk of strangulation** of the bowel. In the large bowel, a closed-loop obstruction is called a *volvulus* (Fig. 14-11).
  - **Strangulation.** Vascular compromise can be identified by circumferential thickening of the wall of the bowel often with absence of normal wall enhancement following intravenous contrast administration. There may be associated edema of the mesentery and ascites (Fig. 14-12).

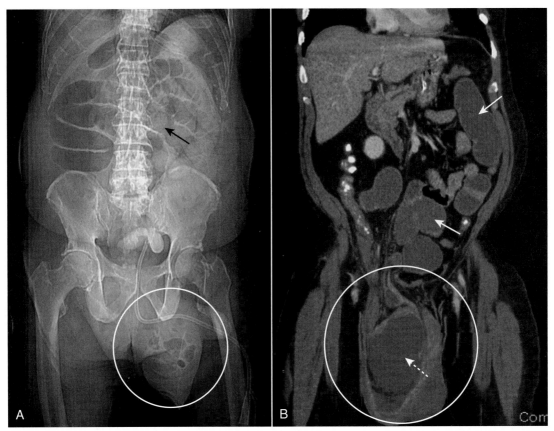

Figure 14-3 **Small bowel obstruction from inguinal hernia. A,** The scout image from a CT scan of the abdomen reveals dilated loops of small bowel (*solid black arrow*) caused by a left inguinal hernia (*white circle*). Loops of bowel should normally not be present in the scrotum. **B,** Coronal-reformatted CT scan on another patient shows multiple fluid-filled and dilated loops of small bowel (*solid white arrows*) from a right inguinal hernia (*white circle*) containing another dilated loop of small bowel (*dotted white arrow*).

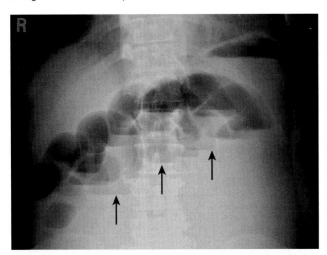

Figure 14-4 **Step-ladder appearance of obstructed small bowel.** As they begin to dilate, small bowel loops stack up, forming a step-ladder appearance usually beginning in the left upper quadrant and proceeding, depending on how distal the small bowel obstruction is, to the right lower quadrant (*solid black arrows*). The more proximal the small bowel obstruction (e.g., proximal jejunum), the fewer the dilated loops there will be; the more distal the obstruction (e.g., at the ileocecal valve), the greater the number of dilated small bowel loops. This was a distal small bowel obstruction caused by a carcinoma of the colon which obstructed the ileocecal valve.

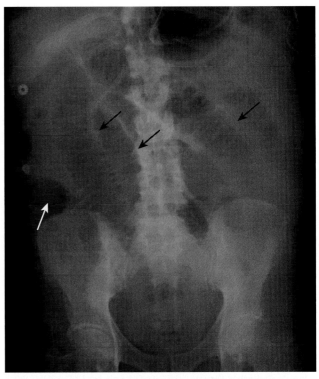

Figure 14-5 **Mechanical small bowel obstruction.** Even though there is still a small amount of air visible in the right colon (*solid white arrow*), the overall bowel gas pattern is one of disproportionate dilation of multiple loops of small bowel (*solid black arrows*) consistent with a mechanical small bowel obstruction. The obstruction was presumably secondary to adhesions.

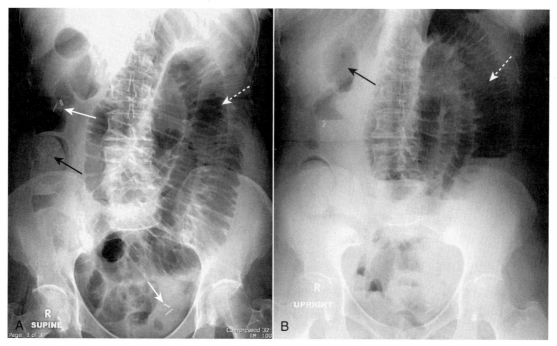

Figure 14-6 Partial small bowel obstruction, supine (A) and upright (B). A partial or incomplete mechanical small bowel obstruction allows some gas to pass the point of obstruction, possibly on an intermittent basis. This can lead to a confusing picture because gas may pass into the colon (*solid black arrows*) and be visible long after the large bowel would be expected to be devoid of gas. The important observation is that the small bowel is disproportionately dilated (*dotted white arrows*) compared to the large bowel, a finding suggestive of small bowel obstruction. Partial or incomplete small bowel obstructions occur more often in patients in whom adhesions are the etiology. Notice the clips (*solid white arrows*) attesting to prior surgery.

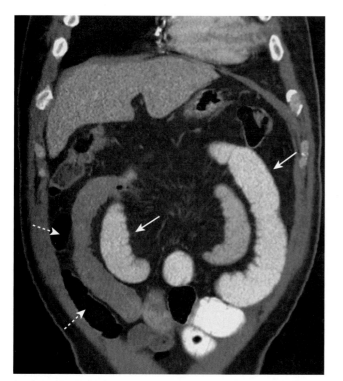

Figure 14-7 Partial small bowel obstruction. Coronal-reformatted CT scan with oral contrast shows dilated and contrast-containing loops of small bowel (*solid white arrows*). Although there is still air present in the collapsed colon (*dotted white arrows*), the disproportionate dilatation of small bowel identifies this as a small bowel obstruction.

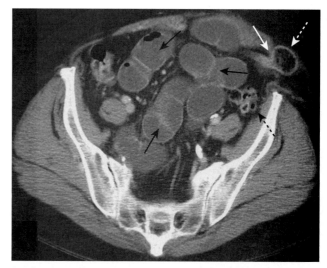

Figure 14-8 Small bowel obstruction due to Spigelian hernia. A Spigelian hernia occurs at the lateral edge of the rectus abdominis muscle at the semilunar line. This patient has a transition point (*solid white arrow*) as the small bowel enters the hernia (*dotted white arrow*). More proximally, there are multiple dilated loops of small bowel (*solid black arrows*) that indicate obstruction. The colon is beyond the point of obstruction and is collapsed (*dotted black arrow*).

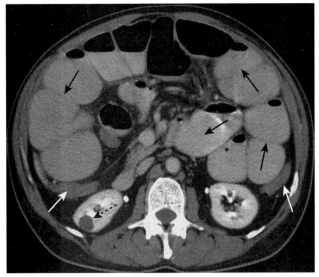

Figure 14-9 Small bowel obstruction, CT with oral and IV contrast. There are multiple fluid- and contrast-filled, dilated loops of small bowel demonstrated (*solid black arrows*), while the colon is collapsed (*solid white arrows*), indicating a small bowel obstruction. Bowel wall enhancement or lack thereof may be obscured by oral contrast, a drawback to the use of oral contrast. Incidentally noted is a right renal cyst (*dotted black arrow*).

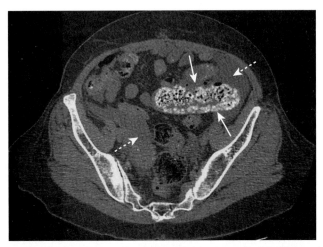

Figure 14-10 Small bowel feces sign. There is air mixed with debris and old oral contrast in a dilated loop of small bowel (*solid white arrows*). There are proximal fluid-containing, dilated loops of small bowel (*dotted white arrows*). The patient had a CT scan with oral contrast several days earlier for abdominal pain and returned for this noncontrast scan when symptoms persisted. Intestinal debris and fluid may accumulate in the loop usually just proximal to a small bowel obstruction and produce this finding which resembles fecal material in the colon.

MECHANICAL OBSTRUCTION: LARGE BOWEL OBSTRUCTION (LBO)

- Pathophysiology
  - A lesion, either inside or outside the colon, causes obstruction to the lumen.
  - Over time, from the point of obstruction *backward*, the **large bowel dilates** with the **cecum frequently attaining the greatest diameter** even if the obstruction is as far away as the sigmoid colon.
  - The large bowel normally functions to reabsorb water, so there are **usually few or no air-fluid levels seen in the obstructed colon.**

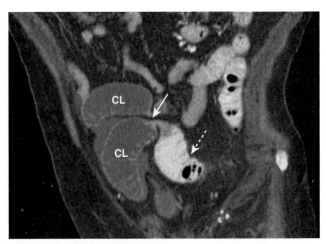

Figure 14-11 Closed-loop obstruction, CT. A loop of small bowel (*CL*) is obstructed twice at the same point of twist (*solid white arrow*) producing a closed loop. No oral contrast enters the closed loop but is present in a more proximal loop of small bowel (*dotted white arrow*). Closed-loop obstructions are important because of their higher incidence of necrosis from strangulation of the bowel.

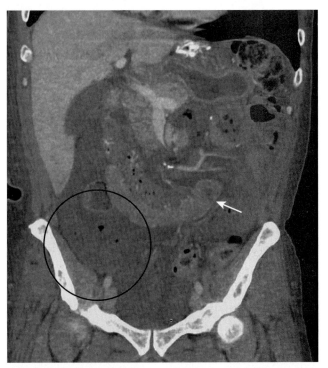

Figure 14-12 Bowel necrosis, contrast-enhanced CT. A dilated loop of small bowel demonstrates normal enhancement of the wall (*solid white arrow*) on this coronal reformat of a contrast-enhanced CT, while more distal, dilated loops of small bowel show no wall enhancement (*black circle*). This is an indication of vascular compromise of the distal loops with bowel necrosis.

- As time passes, continuing peristaltic waves from the point of obstruction *forward* empty the colon distal to the obstruction.
- There is usually little or no air found in the rectum in a mechanical large bowel obstruction.
- Causes of a mechanical large bowel obstruction are summarized in Table 14-5.

 Key imaging features of a mechanical large bowel obstruction

TABLE 14-5 CAUSES OF A MECHANICAL LARGE BOWEL OBSTRUCTION

Cause	Remarks
Tumor (carcinoma)	Most common cause of LBO; more frequently obstructs when it involves the left colon
Hernia	May be visible on conventional radiographs if air is seen over the obturator foramen
Volvulus	Either the sigmoid (more common) or cecum may twist on its axis and obstruct the colon and small bowel (Box 14-2)
Diverticulitis	Uncommon cause of colonic obstruction
Intussusception	Colocolic intussusception usually occurs because of a tumor acting as a lead point

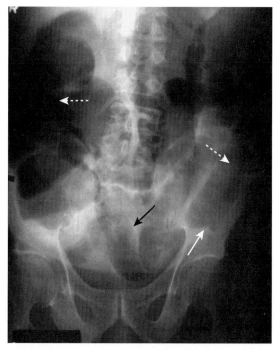

Figure 14-13 Mechanical large bowel obstruction. The entire colon is dilated (*dotted white arrows*) to a cut-off point in the distal descending colon (*solid white arrow*), the site of this patient's obstructing carcinoma of the colon. Some gas has passed backwards through an incompetent ileocecal valve and outlines a dilated ileum (*solid black arrow*). Notice that the large bowel is disproportionately dilated compared to the small bowel, a finding of large bowel obstruction.

- The **colon is dilated to the point of obstruction.**
  - Because there are a limited number of large bowel loops, they tend not to overlap each other (as do the loops of small bowel) **so it is sometimes possible to identify the site of obstruction** as the **last air-containing** segment of the colon (Fig. 14-13).
  - Regardless of the point of obstruction, **the cecum is often the most dilated segment of the colon. When the cecum reaches a diameter above 12-15 cm, there is danger of cecal rupture.**
- The **small bowel is not dilated** (unless the ileocecal valve becomes *incompetent*; see below).
- Because it is distal to the point of obstruction, **the rectum contains little or no air.**
- Since the large bowel functions to reabsorb water, **there are usually no or very few air-fluid levels present in the large bowel.**

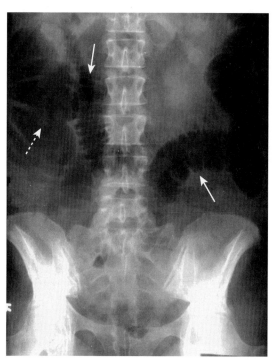

Figure 14-14 Large bowel obstruction masquerading as a small bowel obstruction. There are air-filled and dilated loops of small bowel (*solid white arrows*) seen in this patient who had a mechanical large bowel obstruction from a carcinoma of the middescending colon. The pressure in the colon was sufficient to open the ileocecal valve, which then allowed much of the gas in the colon to decompress backward into the small bowel. The cecum still contains air (*dotted white arrow*) and is dilated, a clue that this is really a large bowel obstruction. Abdominal CT can resolve the question of whether the large or small bowel is obstructed.

⚠ Pitfalls: How a LBO can mimic a SBO

- **So long as the ileocecal valve** prevents gas from reentering the small bowel in a retrograde direction (such an ileocecal valve is called **competent**), the colon will continue to dilate between the ileocecal valve and the point of colonic obstruction. **The small bowel is not dilated.**
  - But if the intracolonic pressure rises high enough and the **ileocecal valve opens** (such a valve is called **incompetent**), **then gas from the dilated large bowel decompresses backward into the small bowel,** much like the air escaping from a balloon.
  - This can produce a picture in which there is **disproportionate dilatation of the small bowel** compared to the **decompressed large bowel.** This **picture mimics that of a mechanical small bowel obstruction** (Fig. 14-14).
- **Solution**
  - Ask for a CT scan of the abdomen. It should show the site of obstruction in the colon rather than the small bowel.
- **Barium is not administered by mouth in a patient with a suspected large bowel obstruction** because water will be absorbed from the barium when it reaches the obstructed colon, increasing the viscosity of the barium and possibly leading to impaction.
- **Recognizing a large bowel obstruction on CT**
  - CT is obtained to identify the cause of the obstruction, assess for free intraperitoneal air and to identify

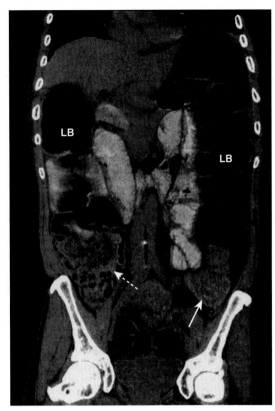

Figure 14-15 Large bowel obstruction from carcinoma of the colon. This coronal reformatted CT scan of the abdomen and pelvis shows dilated cecum (*dotted white arrow*) and large bowel (*LB*) to the level of the distal descending colon where a large soft tissue mass is identified (*solid white arrow*). This mass was surgically removed and was an adenocarcinoma of the colon.

associated lesions, such as metastases to the liver or lymph nodes.
- The large bowel is **dilated to the point of obstruction,** then normal in caliber distal to the obstructing lesion.
- The point of obstruction, frequently a carcinoma, can usually be located on CT as a **soft tissue mass.** Hernias containing large bowel are also easy to identify on CT. (Fig. 14-15).

VOLVULUS OF THE COLON

- Volvulus of the colon is a particular kind of large bowel obstruction that produces a striking and characteristic picture that is summarized in Box 14-2 (Fig. 14-16).

INTESTINAL PSEUDO-OBSTRUCTION (OGILVIE SYNDROME)

- **Ogilvie syndrome (acute intestinal pseudo-obstruction)** may occur in elderly individuals who are usually already hospitalized or at chronic bed rest.
  - Drugs with **anticholinergic effects, such as antidepressants, phenothiazines, antiparkinsonian agents, and narcotics,** may cause or exacerbate the condition.

Box 14-2 Volvulus: A Cause of Mechanical Large Bowel Obstruction

Either the cecum or the sigmoid colon can twist upon itself producing a mechanical obstruction known as a *volvulus*.

Sigmoid volvulus is more common and tends to occur in older men.

The volvulated sigmoid assumes a massive size rising up from the pelvis with the wall between the twisted loops of sigmoid forming a line that points from the left lower to the right upper quadrant.

The appearance of the dilated sigmoid has been likened to a **coffee bean** (see Fig. 14-16).

When the cecum volvulates, it usually moves across the midline into the left upper quadrant producing loops of bowel forming a line that characteristically points from the right lower to the left upper quadrant.

A contrast enema can be both diagnostic (the obstructed sigmoid produces a **beak sign**) and therapeutic as the hydrostatic pressure of the enema can sometimes decompress the volvulus.

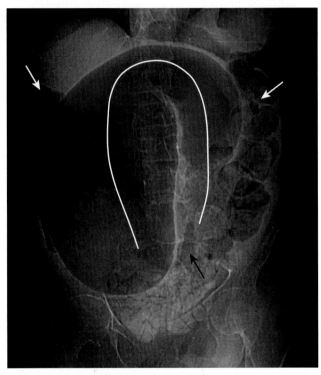

Figure 14-16 Sigmoid volvulus, supine abdomen. There is a massively dilated sigmoid colon (*solid white line*) twisted upon itself in the pelvis (*solid black arrow*). The dilated sigmoid has a coffee-bean shape. Since the point of obstruction is in the distal colon, there are air and stool present in the more proximal portion of the colon (*solid white arrows*). Volvulus can produce massively dilated loops of sigmoid colon.

- The syndrome is characterized by **a loss of peristalsis,** resulting in sometimes **massive dilatation of the entire colon resembling a large bowel obstruction** (Fig. 14-17).
  - Unlike a mechanical obstruction, **no obstructing lesion can be demonstrated** on CT or with barium enema. Unlike a generalized ileus, **patients have more marked abdominal distension,** and bowel sounds may be **normal or hyperactive** in almost half of patients with Ogilvie syndrome.
- The supine abdominal radiograph **shows marked bowel dilatation, almost always confined to the colon.**

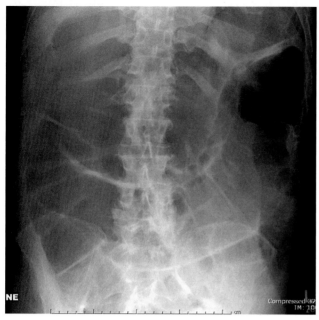

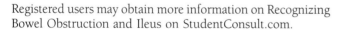

Figure 14-17 Ogilvie syndrome. Ogilvie syndrome (acute intestinal pseudo-obstruction) may occur in elderly individuals who are usually already hospitalized or at chronic bed rest. Drugs with anticholinergic effects may cause or exacerbate the condition. The syndrome is characterized by a loss of peristalsis, resulting in sometimes massive dilatation of the entire colon resembling a large bowel obstruction, as in this patient. Treatment is pharmacologic stimulation of the bowel.

- Management is **pharmacologic stimulation of colonic contractions,** usually with drugs such as neostigmine.

WEBLINK

Registered users may obtain more information on Recognizing Bowel Obstruction and Ileus on StudentConsult.com.

TAKE-HOME POINTS

Recognizing Bowel Obstruction and Ileus

Abnormal bowel gas patterns can be divided into two main groups: functional ileus and mechanical obstruction.

There are two varieties of functional ileus: localized ileus (sentinel loops) and generalized adynamic ileus. There are two varieties of mechanical obstruction: small bowel obstruction (SBO) and large bowel obstruction (LBO).

In mechanical obstruction, the gut reacts in predictable ways: loops proximal to the obstruction become dilated, peristalsis attempts to propel intestinal contents through the bowel and loops distal to the obstruction eventually are evacuated; the loop(s) that become the most dilated will either be the loop of bowel with the largest resting diameter or the loop(s) of bowel just proximal to the obstruction.

The key findings in a localized ileus (*sentinel loops*) are 2-3 dilated loops of small bowel with air in the rectosigmoid and an underlying irritative process that frequently is adjacent to the dilated loops.

Some causes of sentinel loops include pancreatitis (LUQ), cholecystitis (RUQ), diverticulitis (LLQ) and appendicitis (RLQ). All can be readily identified using ultrasound or CT.

The key findings in a **generalized adynamic ileus** are dilated loops of large and small bowel with gas in the rectosigmoid and long, air-fluid levels. Post-operative patients develop generalized adynamic ileus.

The key imaging findings in a **mechanical small bowel obstruction** are disproportionately dilated and fluid-filled loops of small bowel with little or no gas in the recto-sigmoid. CT is best at identifying the cause and site of obstruction or its complications.

The most common cause of a SBO is adhesions; other causes include hernias, intussusception, gallstone ileus, malignancy, and inflammatory bowel disease, such as Crohn disease.

A **closed-loop obstruction** is one in which two points of the bowel are obstructed in the same location producing the "closed-loop." In the small bowel, a closed-loop obstruction carries a higher risk of strangulation of the bowel. In the large bowel, a closed-loop obstruction is called a volvulus.

The key imaging findings in **mechanical LBO** include dilatation of the colon to the point of the obstruction and absence of gas in the rectum with no dilatation of the small bowel as long as the ileocecal valve remains competent. CT will often demonstrate the cause of the obstruction.

Causes of mechanical LBO include malignancy, hernia, diverticulitis, and intussusception.

Ogilvie syndrome is characterized by a loss of peristalsis, resulting in sometimes massive dilatation of the entire colon resembling a large bowel obstruction but without a demonstrable point of obstruction; it can sometimes be confused for a generalized adynamic ileus.

Chapter 15

Recognizing Extraluminal Air in the Abdomen

- Recognition of extraluminal air is an important finding that can have an immediate effect on the course of treatment.
- Air is normally not present in the peritoneal or extraperitoneal spaces, bowel wall, or biliary system.
  - **Air outside of the bowel** is called *extraluminal air.*
- **The four most common locations of extraluminal air:**
  - **Intraperitoneal (pneumoperitoneum)** (frequently called *free air*)
  - **Retroperitoneal air**
  - **Air in the bowel wall (pneumatosis intestinalis)**
  - **Air in the biliary system (pneumobilia)**

SIGNS OF FREE INTRAPERITONEAL AIR

 There are **three major signs of free intraperitoneal air** arranged below in the order in which they are most commonly seen:

- **Air beneath the diaphragm**
- **Visualization of both sides of the bowel wall**
- **Visualization of the falciform ligament**

Air Beneath the Diaphragm

- Air will rise to the highest part of the abdomen. Therefore, in the upright position, **free air will usually reveal itself under the diaphragm as a crescentic lucency that parallels the undersurface of the diaphragm** (Fig. 15-1).
  - The **size of the crescent** will be **roughly proportional to the amount of free air.**
    - The smaller the amount of free air, the thinner the crescent; the larger the amount of free air, the larger the crescent (Fig. 15-2).
- **While free air is best demonstrated on CT scans of the abdomen** because of its greater sensitivity in detecting very small amounts of free air (Fig. 15-3), most surveys of the abdomen begin with conventional radiographs. **Conventional radiographs serve as an important screening tool** on which many previously unsuspected cases of free air are discovered.

On conventional radiographs, **free air is best demonstrated with the x-ray beam directed parallel to the floor** (i.e., a horizontal beam) (see Figs. 13-14 and 13-15). **Small amounts of free air will not be visible on supine radiographs.**

- Free air is **easier to recognize under the right hemidiaphragm** because only the soft tissue density of the liver is usually located there. Free air is **more difficult to recognize under the left hemidiaphragm** because air-containing structures, such as the fundus of the stomach and the splenic flexure, already reside in that location and may mask the presence of free air (Fig. 15-4).
- If the patient is unable to stand or sit upright, then a view of the abdomen with the patient lying on his or her left side taken with a horizontal x-ray beam may show free air rising above the right edge of the liver. This is the **left lateral decubitus view** of the abdomen (Fig. 15-5).

⚠️ Pitfall: Chilaiditi syndrome

- Occasionally, colon may be interposed between the dome of the liver and the right hemidiaphragm and may be mistaken for free air, unless a **careful search** is made **for the presence of haustral folds** characteristic of the colon (Fig. 15-6).
- **Solution:** Obtain a left lateral decubitus view of the abdomen or, if necessary, a CT scan of the abdomen.

Visualization of Both Sides of the Bowel Wall

- In the **normal** abdomen, we visualize only the air **inside the lumen of the bowel, not the wall of the bowel itself.** This is because the wall is soft tissue density and surrounded by tissue of the same density.
- Introduction of **air into the peritoneal cavity enables us to visualize the wall of the bowel itself** since the wall is now surrounded on both inside and outside by air.
  - The **ability to see both sides of the bowel wall is a sign of free intraperitoneal air** called *Rigler sign.* Rigler sign usually requires large amounts of free air in order to be present (Fig. 15-7).
  - The sign can be seen on supine, upright, or prone films of the abdomen so long as an adequate amount of free air is present.

⚠️ Pitfall: When dilated loops of small bowel overlap each other, they may occasionally produce the mistaken impression that you are seeing both sides of the bowel wall (Fig. 15-8).

- **Solution:** Confirm the presence of free air with an upright view, left lateral decubitus view, or CT scan of the abdomen.

Visualization of the Falciform Ligament

- The **falciform ligament** courses over the **free edge of the liver anteriorly** just to the **right of the upper lumbar**

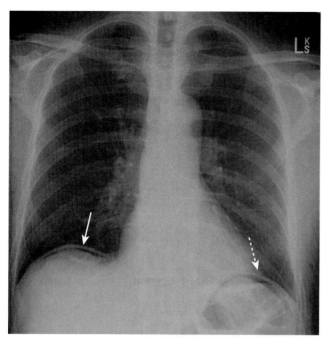

Figure 15-1 Free air beneath the diaphragm. There are thin crescents of air beneath both the right (*solid white arrow*) and left (*dotted white arrow*) hemidiaphragms representing free intraperitoneal air. The patient had undergone abdominal surgery 3 days earlier. Free air can remain for up to 7 days after surgery in an adult, but serial studies should demonstrate a progressively decreasing amount of air.

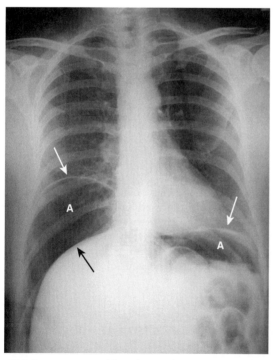

Figure 15-2 Large amount of free air. Upright view of the chest demonstrates a large amount of free air (*A*) beneath each hemidiaphragm (*solid white arrows*). The top of the liver (*solid black arrow*) is made visible by the air above it. The patient had a perforated gastric ulcer.

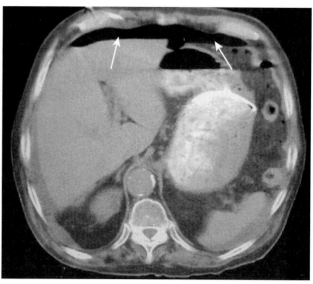

Figure 15-3 Free air seen on CT scan of the abdomen. Axial CT scan of the upper abdomen performed with the patient supine shows free air anteriorly (*solid white arrows*). The air is not contained within any bowel. Free intraperitoneal air will normally rise to the highest point of the abdomen which, in the supine position, is beneath the anterior abdominal wall.

spine. It contains a remnant of the obliterated umbilical artery.

- **It is normally invisible,** composed of soft tissue, and surrounded by tissue of similar density.
- When a relatively large amount of free air is present and the **patient is in the supine position, free air** may rise over the anterior surface of the liver, **surround the falciform ligament,** and **render it visible.**
- Visualization of the falciform ligament is aptly called the *falciform ligament sign* and is a sign of free air (Fig. 15-9).
- The curvilinear appearance of the falciform ligament, combined with the oval-shaped collection of air that collects beneath and distends the abdominal wall, has been likened to the appearance of a football with its laces and is called the *football sign.*
- Table 15-1 summarizes the **three major signs of free air.**

CAUSES OF FREE AIR

- **The most common cause of free intraperitoneal air is rupture of an air-containing loop of bowel,** either stomach, small, or large bowel.

➡ **Perforated peptic ulcer** is the most common cause of a perforated stomach or duodenum and is still the most common cause of free air.

- **Trauma,** whether iatrogenic or accidental, can also produce free air.
  - On rare occasions, endoscopy can lead to bowel perforation. Since insufflation of additional air into the bowel is a part of the procedure, there is frequently a large amount of free air present if such a perforation occurs.
  - **Free air following penetrating trauma** usually **implies a perforation of the bowel,** not free air generated simply by penetration of the abdominal wall itself.

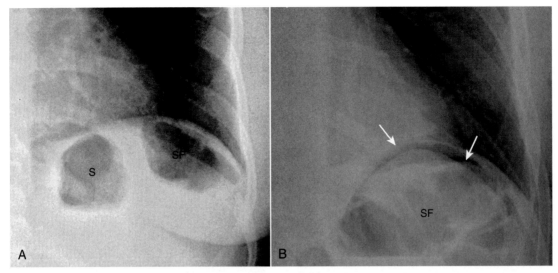

Figure 15-4 Normal left hemidiaphragm (A) and free air under hemidiaphragm (B). Close-up views of the left upper quadrant demonstrate the difficulty in recognizing free air beneath the left hemidiaphragm because of the normal location of gas-containing structures such as the stomach (*S*) and splenic flexure (*SF*). There is no free air seen in **(A)** but the other patient **(B)** does have a crescent of free air (*solid white arrows*). It is easier to recognize free air beneath the right hemidiaphragm because there is usually no air present above the liver on the right side.

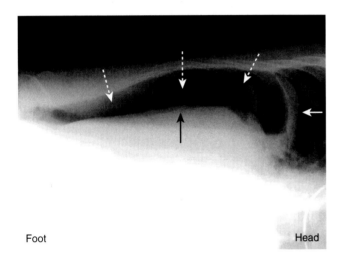

Figure 15-5 Left lateral decubitus view showing free air. Close-up of the right upper quadrant in a patient lying on his or her left side in the left lateral decubitus position shows a crescent of air (*dotted white arrows*) above the outer edge of the liver (*solid black arrow*), beneath the right hemidiaphragm (*solid white arrow*). The *head/foot* orientation of the patient is indicated. If the patient is unable to stand or sit up for an upright view of the abdomen, a left lateral decubitus view with a horizontal beam can substitute.

- **For several days following abdominal surgery (about 5-7 days)**, whether the surgery had been performed on the bowel or not, **it is normal to see free air** on post-operative studies. The **amount** of free air following surgery **should diminish with each successive study.**
- If free air persists for **longer than a week postoperatively** or if the **amount increases on successive studies**, then a complication either of the surgery or of the original disease itself should be considered.
- **Perforated diverticulitis and perforated appendicitis** usually produce walled-off abscess collections around the site of the perforation and rarely lead to significant amounts of free air.
- **Perforation of a carcinoma**, usually of the colon, is unusual but can also lead to free air.

SIGNS OF EXTRAPERITONEAL AIR (RETROPERITONEAL AIR)

- Unlike the collections of free intraperitoneal air that outline loops of bowel and usually move freely in the abdomen, **extraperitoneal air can be recognized** by certain other characteristics:
  - Streaky, linear appearance outlining extraperitoneal structures
  - A mottled, blotchy appearance (anterior pararenal space, especially)
  - Relatively fixed position, moving little if at all with changes in patient positioning
- Extraperitoneal air may outline extraperitoneal structures:
  - Psoas muscles
  - Kidneys, ureters, or urinary bladder
  - Aorta or inferior vena cava (Fig. 15-10)
  - Inferior border of the diaphragm by collecting in the subphrenic tissues
- **Extraperitoneal air may extend through a diaphragmatic hiatus into the mediastinum** (and produce *pneumomediastinum*) or **may extend to the peritoneal cavity** through openings in the peritoneum (and produce *pneumoperitoneum*).
- Box 15-1 summarizes the signs of extraperitoneal air.

CAUSES OF EXTRAPERITONEAL AIR

- **Extraperitoneal air is most frequently the result of bowel perforation** secondary to either:
  - **Inflammatory** disease (e.g., **ruptured appendix**), or
  - **Ulcerative** disease (e.g., **Crohn disease** of the ileum or colon)
- **Other causes of extraperitoneal air:**
  - **Blunt or penetrating trauma**
  - **Iatrogenic manipulation** (e.g., perforation of the bowel during **sigmoidoscopy**)

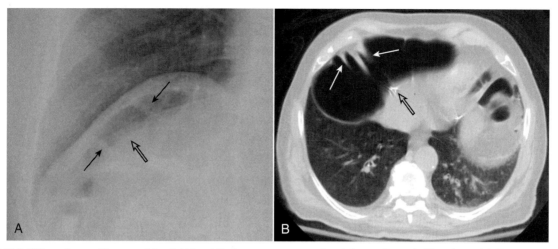

Figure 15-6 Chilaiditi syndrome. Close-up of the right hemidiaphragm on a conventional chest radiograph **(A)** and an axial CT scan at the level of the diaphragm **(B)** both demonstrate air beneath the diaphragm that could be confused for free air (*open black arrows* in both photos). Careful evaluation of this air demonstrates several haustral folds (*solid black arrows* in **[A]** and *solid white arrows* in **[B]**) which indicate this is a loop of colon interposed between the liver and the diaphragm (Chilaiditi syndrome) rather than free air.

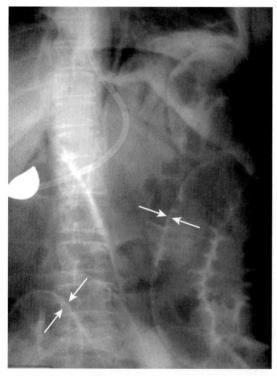

Figure 15-7 Rigler sign. When air fills the peritoneal cavity, both sides of the bowel wall will be outlined by air (*solid white arrows*) making the wall of the bowel visible as a discrete line. This is known as **Rigler sign** and indicates the presence of a pneumoperitoneum.

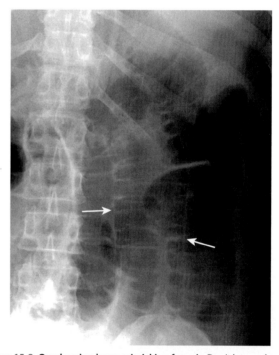

Figure 15-8 Overlapping loops mimicking free air. Don't let overlapping loops of dilated small bowel (*solid white arrows*) fool you into thinking you are seeing both sides of the bowel wall due to free air. If doubt exists about the presence of free air, confirmation may be obtained through an upright or left lateral decubitus view of the abdomen or a CT scan of the abdomen.

- **Foreign body** (e.g., perforation of extraperitoneal ascending colon by an ingested foreign body)
- **Gas-producing infection** originating in extraperitoneal organs (such as **perforated diverticulitis**)

SIGNS OF AIR IN THE BOWEL WALL

- Air in the bowel wall is called *pneumatosis intestinalis.*
- Air in the bowel wall is **most easily recognized when it is seen in profile** producing a **linear radiolucency** (black line) whose contour exactly parallels the bowel lumen (Fig. 15-11).
- **Air** in the bowel wall **seen** *en face* is **more difficult to recognize** but frequently has a **mottled appearance that resembles gas mixed with fecal material** (Fig. 15-12).
- Clues to help differentiate pneumatosis from fecal material:
  - **Presence of such mottled gas in an area of the abdomen unlikely to contain colon.**
  - **Lack of change** in the appearance of the mottled gas pattern over several images in **differing positions.**
- Table 15-2 summarizes the signs of air in the bowel wall.

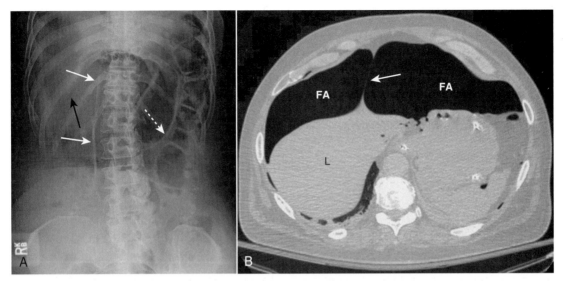

Figure 15-9 Falciform ligament sign. A, Free intraperitoneal air may surround the normally invisible falciform ligament on the anterior edge of the liver causing that thin, soft tissue structure to become visible (*solid white arrows*) just to the right of the upper lumbar spine. Notice also that both sides of the stomach wall are visible (Rigler sign) (*dotted white arrow*) and there is increased lucency in the right upper quadrant (*solid black arrow*) in this patient with a large pneumoperitoneum from a perforated gastric ulcer. **B,** The falciform ligament (*solid white arrow*) is outlined by free air (*FA*) on either side of it, anterior to the liver (*L*).

TABLE 15-1 THREE SIGNS OF FREE AIR

Sign	Remarks
Air beneath diaphragm	Requires patient to be in the upright or left lateral decubitus position and a horizontal x-ray beam unless massive in amount
Visualization of both sides of the bowel wall	Usually requires large amount of free air; will be visible in any position
Visualization of the falciform ligament	Usually requires large amounts of free air; patient is usually supine

Box 15-1 Signs of Extraperitoneal Air

Streaky, linear collections of air that outline extraperitoneal structures.

Mottled, blotchy collections of air that remain in a fixed position.

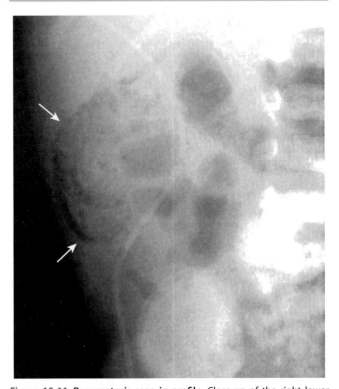

Figure 15-11 Pneumatosis seen in profile. Close-up of the right lower quadrant in an infant demonstrates a thin curvilinear lucency that parallels the lumen of the adjacent bowel (*solid white arrows*), an appearance characteristic of gas in the bowel wall seen in profile. In infants, the most common cause for this finding is necrotizing enterocolitis, a disease found mostly in premature infants in which the terminal ileum is most affected. Pneumatosis intestinalis is pathognomonic for necrotizing enterocolitis in infants.

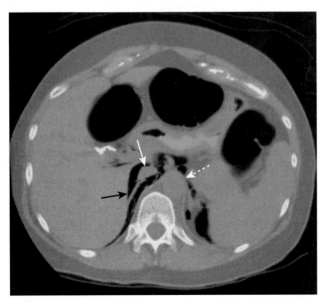

Figure 15-10 Extraperitoneal air seen on CT. Air is seen in the retroperitoneum (*solid black arrow*) on this axial CT scan of the upper abdomen. Air outlines the inferior vena cava (*solid white arrow*) and the aorta (*dotted white arrow*). Unlike free air, extraperitoneal air is streaky, relatively fixed in position, and outlines extraperitoneal structures such as the vena cava, aorta, psoas muscles, and kidneys.

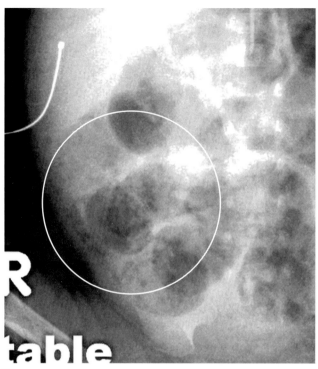

Figure 15-12 Pneumatosis seen *en face.* Close-up of the right lower quadrant in another infant shows multiple faint, mottled lucencies in the right lower quadrant (*white circle*), which is the appearance of pneumatosis intestinalis when seen *en face.* The density has the same appearance as air mixed with stool, but can be distinguished from stool because it occurs in areas stool might not be expected and it does not change over time. This infant also had necrotizing enterocolitis.

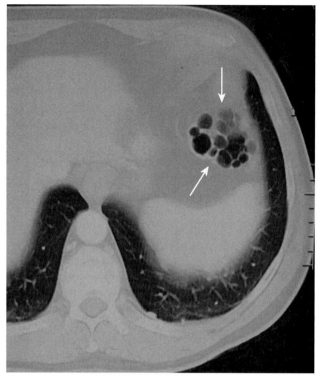

Figure 15-13 Pneumatosis cystoides intestinalis. Axial CT scan of the upper abdomen windowed for lung technique shows a cluster of air-containing cysts (*solid white arrows*) associated with the left colon, characteristic of pneumatosis cystoides intestinalis, a rare but benign condition in which air-containing cysts form in the submucosa or serosa of the bowel.

TABLE 15-2 SIGNS OF AIR IN THE BOWEL WALL

Sign	Remarks
Linear radiolucency paralleling the contour of air in the adjacent bowel lumen	Occurs when the air is seen in profile
Mottled appearance that resembles air mixed with fecal material	May occur in an area of the abdomen not expected to contain colon; won't change over time
Globular, cystlike collections of air that parallel the contour of the bowel	Unusual, benign condition usually affecting left side of colon

CAUSES AND SIGNIFICANCE OF AIR IN THE BOWEL WALL

- Pneumatosis intestinalis can be divided into two major categories.
  - A **rare, primary form** called *pneumatosis cystoides intestinalis,* which usually **affects the left colon,** producing **cystlike collections of air in the submucosa or serosa** (Fig. 15-13).
  - A **more common, secondary form,** which can occur in obstructive and necrotizing diseases:
    - **Chronic obstructive pulmonary disease—** presumably secondary to air from ruptured blebs dissecting through the mediastinum to the abdomen.
    - Diseases in which there is **necrosis of the bowel** wall such as:

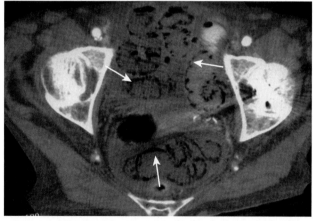

Figure 15-14 Necrosis of bowel from mesenteric ischemia. Axial CT image of the pelvis demonstrates multiple loops of bowel with punctate collections of air throughout their walls consistent with pneumatosis (*solid white arrows*). The patient had widespread ischemia of bowel from mesenteric vascular disease. Pneumatosis that results from bowel necrosis is an ominous sign.

- **Necrotizing enterocolitis** in infants
- **Ischemic bowel disease** in adults (Fig. 15-14).
  - **Obstructing lesions of the bowel** that raise intraluminal pressure:
    - **Hirschsprung disease** or **pyloric stenosis** in children
    - **Obstructing carcinomas** in adults

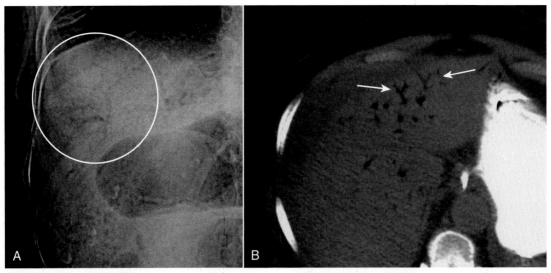

Figure 15-15 Portal venous gas. A, Numerous small black branching structures are visible over the periphery of the liver (*white circle*). This is air in the portal venous system, a finding most often associated with necrotizing enterocolitis in infants but which can also be seen in adults, usually with bowel necrosis. Unlike air in the biliary system, this air is peripheral rather than central and has numerous branching structures rather than the few tubular structures seen with pneumobilia. **B,** Close-up of axial CT scan through the liver shows air in the portal venous system (*solid white arrows*) in a patient with mesenteric vascular disease.

➡ Pneumatosis intestinalis **associated with diseases that produce necrosis of bowel** is usually a **more ominous prognostic sign** than pneumatosis associated with obstructing lesions of the bowel or chronic obstructive pulmonary disease.

- **Complications of pneumatosis intestinalis:**
  - **Rupture into the peritoneal cavity** leading to intraperitoneal free air (**pneumoperitoneum**).
  - Dissection of **air into the portal venous system** (Fig. 15-15).

SIGNS OF AIR IN THE BILIARY SYSTEM

- Air in the biliary system presents as **one or two tubelike, branching lucencies** in the **right upper quadrant overlying the central portion of the liver which conform to the location and appearance of the major bile ducts:** the common duct, cystic duct, and the hepatic ducts (Fig. 15-16).
- Sometimes, the gallbladder itself fills with air.
- Box 15-2 summarizes the signs of **air in the biliary system.**

CAUSES OF AIR IN THE BILIARY SYSTEM

- Gas in the biliary system **may be a "normal" finding** if the sphincter of Oddi, which guards the entrance of the common bile duct as it enters the duodenum, is open (said to be *incompetent*).
- Prior **sphincterotomy**, such as might be done to allow gallstones to exit from the ductal system into the bowel.
- **Prior surgery** that results in the **reimplantation of the common bile duct** into another part of the bowel (i.e., choledocho-enterostomy) is frequently accompanied by gas in the biliary ductal system.
- Pathologic conditions that can produce pneumobilia include **uncommon causes:**

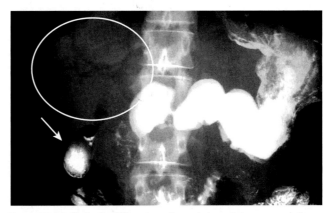

Figure 15-16 Air in the biliary tree. Frontal view of the upper abdomen from an upper gastrointestinal series demonstrates several air-containing tubular structures over the central portion of the liver consistent with air in the biliary system (*white circle*). There is also barium present in the gallbladder (*solid white arrow*). This patient had a history of a prior sphincterotomy for gallstones so that reflux of air and barium into the biliary system would be expected.

Box 15-2 **Signs of Air in the Biliary Tract**
Tubelike, branching lucencies in the right upper quadrant overlying the liver.
Tubular structures are central in location and few in number compared to portal venous air which is peripheral in location and fills innumerable vessels.
Gas in the lumen of the gallbladder.

➡ **Gallstone ileus**—in which a **gallstone erodes through the wall of the gallbladder** into the **duodenum,** usually producing a **fistula between the bowel and the biliary system.**

- The **gallstone impacts in the small bowel,** usually in the narrower terminal ileum, and produces a mechanical small bowel obstruction (unfortunately misnamed an "ileus") (Fig. 15-17).

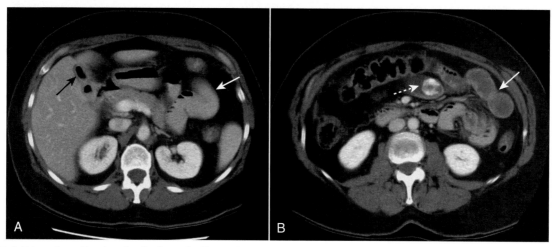

Figure 15-17 Gallstone ileus. The three key findings of gallstone ileus are present on this study. **A,** Axial CT scan of the upper abdomen shows air in the lumen of the gallbladder (*solid black arrow*) and dilated small bowel (*solid white arrow*) consistent with a mechanical small bowel obstruction. At a lower level, another axial CT scan of the abdomen (**B**) shows a large calcified gallstone inside the small bowel (*dotted white arrow*) and additional proximal, dilated loops of small bowel (*solid white arrow*). The gallstone had eroded through the wall of the gallbladder into the duodenum and then began a journey down the small bowel before becoming impacted and producing obstruction.

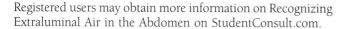

WEBLINK

Registered users may obtain more information on Recognizing Extraluminal Air in the Abdomen on StudentConsult.com.

 TAKE-HOME POINTS

Recognizing Extraluminal Air in the Abdomen

Gas in the abdomen outside of the normal confines of the bowel is called extraluminal air.

The four most common locations for extraluminal air are intraperitoneal (*pneumoperitoneum*—frequently called *free air*), retroperitoneal air, air in the bowel wall (*pneumatosis*), and air in the biliary system (*pneumobilia*).

The three key signs of pneumoperitoneum are air beneath the diaphragm, visualization of both sides of the bowel wall (*Rigler sign*), and visualization of the falciform ligament.

The most common causes of free air are perforated peptic ulcer, trauma whether accidental or iatrogenic, and perforated diverticulitis. Perforated appendicitis and perforation of a carcinoma, usually of the colon, are rare causes of free air.

The key signs of **extraperitoneal (retroperitoneal) air** are a streaky, linear appearance or a mottled, blotchy appearance outlining extraperitoneal structures and its relatively fixed position, moving little or not at all with changes in patient positioning.

Extraperitoneal air outlines extraperitoneal structures such as the psoas muscles, kidneys, aorta, and inferior vena cava.

Causes of extraperitoneal air include bowel perforation secondary to either inflammatory or ulcerative disease, blunt or penetrating trauma, iatrogenic manipulation, and foreign body ingestion.

The key signs of **air in the bowel wall** include linear radiolucencies paralleling the contour of air in the adjacent bowel lumen, a mottled appearance that resembles air mixed with fecal material, or uncommonly, globular, cystlike collections of air that parallel the contour of the bowel.

Causes of air in the bowel wall (*pneumatosis intestinalis*) include a rare primary form called *pneumatosis cystoides intestinalis* and a more common secondary form that includes diseases in which there is necrosis of the bowel wall such as necrotizing enterocolitis in infants and ischemic bowel disease in adults, as well as obstructing lesions of the bowel which raise intraluminal pressure such as Hirschsprung disease in children and obstructing carcinomas in adults.

Pneumatosis intestinalis associated with diseases that produce necrosis of bowel is usually a more ominous prognostic sign than pneumatosis associated with obstructing lesions of the bowel or chronic obstructive pulmonary disease.

Signs of **air in the biliary system** include tubelike, branching lucencies in the right upper quadrant overlying the liver, which are central in location and few in number, and gas in the lumen of the gallbladder.

Causes of pneumobilia include incompetence of the sphincter of Oddi, prior sphincterotomy, prior surgery that results in the reimplantation of the common bile duct into another part of the bowel, and gallstone ileus.

The three findings in **gallstone ileus** are air in the biliary system, small bowel obstruction, and visualization of the gallstone itself.

Chapter 16

Recognizing Abnormal Calcifications and Their Causes

- Soft tissue calcifications lend themselves to an intuitive approach that ties together a diverse group of diseases. While this chapter focuses primarily on abdominal calcifications, the same principles and approach apply to dystrophic calcifications found anywhere in the body.
- **Dystrophic calcification** is soft tissue calcification that occurs in tissue that is already **abnormal**. (**Metastatic calcification,** by contrast, is calcification in otherwise normal soft tissues due to disturbances in calcium/phosphorus metabolism.)
- On conventional radiographs, the **nature of most calcifications can be determined by examining** their **pattern of calcification** and their **anatomic location.**
- The same principles hold true for CT evaluation of calcifications except that the anatomic location is usually easier to determine on CT.

PATTERNS OF CALCIFICATION

- Calcifications **tend to occur in one of four distinct patterns,** depending on the type of structure that has calcified:
  - **Rimlike**
  - **Linear or tracklike**
  - **Lamellar (or laminar)**
  - **Cloudlike, amorphous, or popcorn**

RIMLIKE CALCIFICATION

- Rimlike calcification implies **calcification that has occurred in the wall of a hollow viscus.**
- Examples of structures that manifest rimlike calcifications:
  - Cysts—calcification in any one of these is relatively **uncommon.**
    - Renal cysts
    - Splenic cysts
    - Extraabdominal sites
      - **Mediastinal cysts,** such as pericardial and bronchial cysts (Fig. 16-1).
      - **Popliteal cysts** (Baker cysts)
  - Aneurysms
    - **Aortic aneurysm.** CT and US are used to identify and characterize abdominal aortic aneurysms. On conventional radiographs, such aneurysms are most easily recognized on a lateral radiograph of the lumbar spine. The abdominal aorta should normally measure <3 cm in diameter (Fig. 16-2).

- **Splenic artery** or **renal artery** aneurysms—usually secondary to atherosclerosis.
- **Extraabdominal sites**
  - Femoral artery aneurysms
  - Cerebral aneurysms
- **Saccular organs, such as the gallbladder or urinary bladder**
  - **Porcelain gallbladder**—an uncommon entity (named after the gross appearance of the gallbladder, which resembles porcelain) that occurs with chronic inflammation of and stasis in the gallbladder and is associated with gallstones and an increased incidence of carcinoma of the gallbladder (Fig. 16-3).
  - **Urinary bladder**—calcification of the wall is an uncommon occurrence in diseases such as schistosomiasis, bladder cancer, and tuberculosis.
- Table 16-1 highlights key facts about rimlike calcifications.

LINEAR OR TRACKLIKE CALCIFICATION

- Linear or tracklike calcifications imply **calcification that has occurred in the walls of tubular structures** (Fig. 16-4).
- Examples include calcifications in the walls of:
  - Arteries
    - **Common in atherosclerosis** and seen anywhere in the body.
    - **Walls of veins do not calcify.** In veins, **long, linear thrombi** or **small, focal thrombi** (the latter called *phleboliths*) may calcify (see Fig. 13-18).
  - Tubular structures
    - **Fallopian tubes and vas deferens**—seen more often in diabetics (Fig. 16-5).
    - **Ureter**—uncommon finding seen in schistosomiasis and even more rarely in tuberculosis.
- Table 16-2 highlights key facts about linear or tracklike calcifications

LAMELLAR OR LAMINAR CALCIFICATION

- **Lamellar** (or laminar) **calcifications imply calcification that forms around a nidus inside a hollow lumen** (Fig. 16-6).
  - A "hollow lumen" refers to a structure such as the gallbladder or urinary bladder.
  - **Calcification in concentric layers** begins with a central nidus around which alternating layers of calcified and

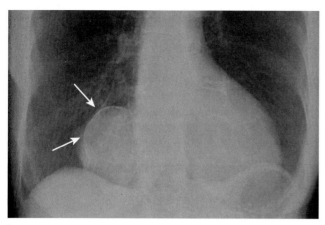

Figure 16-1 Calcified pericardial cyst. There is a rimlike calcification (*solid white arrows*) that identifies the structure containing the calcification as cystic or saccular. The calcification is in the right cardiophrenic angle, an ideal location for pericardial cysts. Pericardial cysts are usually asymptomatic and discovered when a chest radiograph is obtained for another reason.

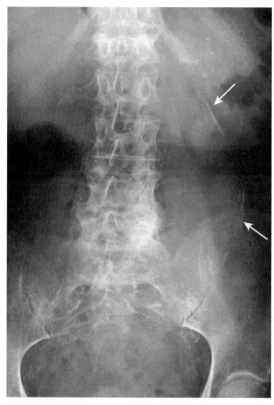

Figure 16-2 Calcified aortic aneurysm. Calcification in the wall of the abdominal aorta is a common finding in atherosclerosis, especially in those with diabetes mellitus. In this patient, the aorta is enlarged and demonstrates a rimlike calcification (*solid white arrows*). The opposing wall is also calcified, but overlaps the spine. An aneurysm is present when the diameter of the abdominal aorta exceeds its normal diameter by more than 50%.

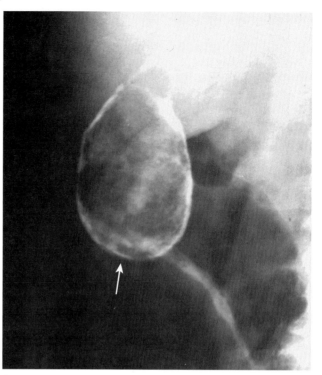

Figure 16-3 Calcified gallbladder wall. The rimlike calcification (*solid white arrow*) identifies this as occurring in the wall of a cyst or saccular organ. The calcification is in the right upper quadrant, the location of the gallbladder. This is a **_porcelain gallbladder_**, an uncommon entity (named after the gross appearance of the gallbladder which resembles porcelain) that occurs with chronic inflammation and stasis and is associated with gallstones and an increased incidence of carcinoma of the gallbladder.

TABLE 16-1 RIMLIKE CALCIFICATIONS

Organ of Origin	Remarks
Renal cyst	Thick and irregular calcifications, though uncommon, may indicate the presence of renal cell carcinoma.
Splenic cysts	May be a manifestation of hydatid cyst, old trauma, or prior infection.
Aortic aneurysms	Occurs more often in diabetics with advanced atherosclerosis.
Gallbladder	Associated with chronic stasis; called *porcelain gallbladder* for its gross appearance; higher incidence of carcinoma of the gallbladder.

noncalcified material form due to the prolonged movement of the stone within the hollow viscus.

- Lamellar or laminated calcifications are usually called *stones* or *calculi* (singular: calculus) and include **renal and ureteral calculi.**
  - Conventional radiographs are only about 50% to 60% sensitive for displaying renal calculi despite the fact that about 90% of renal calculi contain calcium (Fig. 16-7).
  - Unenhanced, multislice spiral CT scans (*stone searches*) have replaced conventional radiography in the search for renal and ureteral calculi and their complications.
  - A **negative CT stone search study has a negative predictive value of 98%.**
  - Besides urinary tract calculi, CT scans detect **symptomatic lesions in other organ systems** in almost one third of patients in whom a stone search study is conducted.
- **Recognizing a calculus on a stone search study** (all signs discussed are on the symptomatic side):
  - The **direct finding** is a calcific density in the ureter, at the ureterovesical junction or in the bladder.
  - **Indirect findings include** signs of **obstruction** such as **dilatation of the ureter** or **intrarenal collecting**

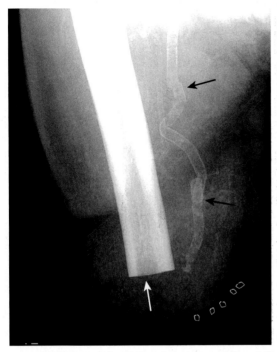

Figure 16-4 Calcified arterial wall. There is linear or tracklike calcification present (*solid black arrows*), which implies calcification that has occurred in the walls of tubular structures. In the leg, this is calcification in the femoral artery. Such wall calcification occurs in arteries, not veins, and is usually secondary to atherosclerosis, frequently associated with diabetes, or in patients with chronic renal disease. This patient obviously suffered one of the complications of diabetes and has had an above-the-knee amputation (*solid white arrow*) of a formerly gangrenous leg.

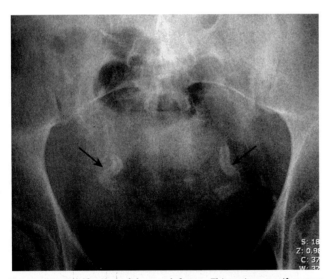

Figure 16-5 Calcification of the vas deferens. This patient manifests two tracklike calcifications (*solid black arrows*) symmetrically on each side of the urinary bladder that end in the urethra in this man who also has an enlarged prostate which is elevating the base of the bladder. This type of calcification identifies it as occurring in the wall of a tubular structure. The location identifies it as calcification in the walls of the vas deferens, which occurs more commonly and earlier in diabetics than as a natural degenerative process.

 system or overall **enlargement of the kidney** and signs of **inflammation** such as **perinephric stranding** (Fig. 16-8).
- **Gallstones.** Ultrasound is the study of choice (see Chapter 19). Only about 10% to 15% of gallstones contain

TABLE 16-2 LINEAR OR TRACKLIKE CALCIFICATIONS

Organ of Origin	Remarks
Walls of smaller arteries	Mostly seen in atherosclerosis accelerated by diabetes and renal disease
Fallopian tubes or vas deferens	Usually accelerated by diabetes
Ureters	Uncommon occurrence described with schistosomiasis and rarely TB

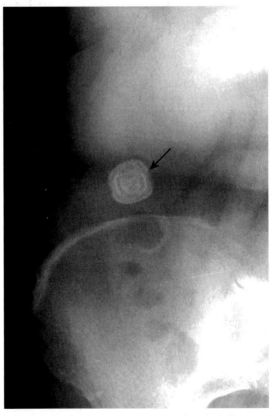

Figure 16-6 Calcified gallstone. There is a lamellated calcification present in the right upper quadrant (*solid black arrow*). The lamination identifies it as a calculus that has formed in a hollow viscus. The anatomic location places it in the gallbladder. Notice the alternating rings of calcified and noncalcified material that form as the stone moves about in the gallbladder lumen.

enough calcification to be visible on conventional radiographs (Fig. 16-9).
- **Bladder stones** usually develop secondary to chronic bladder outlet obstruction. They are very prone to develop lamination (Fig. 16-10).
- Table 16-3 highlights key facts about laminated or lamellar calcifications

CLOUDLIKE, AMORPHOUS, OR POPCORN CALCIFICATION

- Cloudlike, amorphous, or popcorn calcification is calcification that has formed inside of a solid organ or tumor. Examples include:
  - **Body of the pancreas**—pathognomonic for chronic pancreatitis (Fig. 16-11).

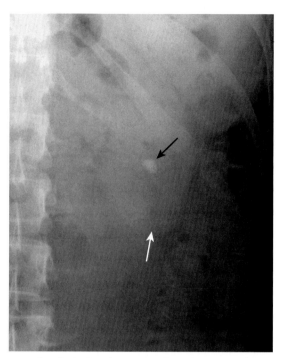

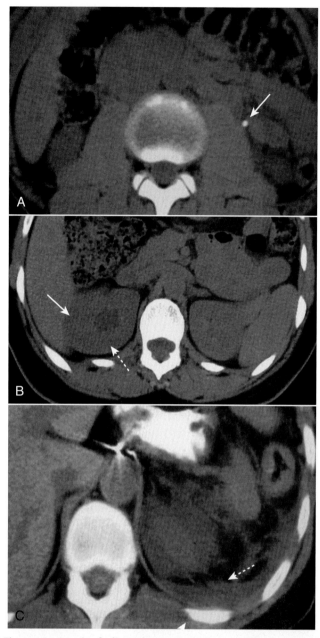

Figure 16-7 Renal calculus. There is a small calcification (*solid black arrow*) that overlies the shadow of the left kidney (*solid white arrow*) on this close-up of a conventional abdominal radiograph. Although the stone is too small to recognize lamination, its location suggests a renal calculus. Because of its greater sensitivity, a CT stone search has essentially replaced conventional radiography for the identification of renal and ureteral calculi.

- **Leiomyomas of uterus.** Uterine fibroids or leiomyomas very commonly degenerate and calcify over time (Fig. 16-12).

 Pitfall: Solid masses that have rimlike calcification

- Sometimes a **solid tumor will outgrow its blood supply, and the center of the tumor will undergo necrosis** leaving only a viable "outer shell."
- The subsequent calcification will be **more rimlike than amorphous.**
  - Uterine fibroids are especially prone to this appearance (Fig. 16-13).
- **Lymph nodes**—can calcify anywhere in the body, mostly due to prior granulomatous infection such as old tuberculosis.
- **Mucin-producing adenocarcinomas** of the stomach, ovary, and colon. Their metastases may also calcify (Fig. 16-14).
- **Soft tissue calcification**—can occur as a result of prior trauma or from deposition of crystal salts in the soft tissues (Fig. 16-15).
- Table 16-4 highlights key facts about amorphous, cloud-like, or popcorn calcifications.
- Table 16-5 summarizes the key findings of the four patterns of abnormal calcification.

No matter what its cause, the presence of calcification implies a process that is subacute or chronic.

Figure 16-8 Imaging findings of ureteral calculi, three different patients. A, A calcified stone is seen in the left ureter (*solid white arrow*). **B,** Hydronephrosis is present on the right (*dotted white arrow*) with overall enlargement of the right kidney (*solid white arrow*). **C,** There is considerable perinephric stranding (*dotted white arrows*) and fluid that has leaked from the kidney (*solid white arrow*), most likely from a rupture of one of the renal fornices.

LOCATION OF CALCIFICATION

- Identifying the **pattern** of calcification helps in identifying the **type of structure in which it has formed.**
- Identifying the anatomic **location** of the calcification helps to identify its **organ or tissue of origin.** Combining the **type** of calcification with its **anatomic location** should provide the keys to the **cause** of most pathologic calcifications.
- Table 16-6 summarizes some of the possibilities in the abdomen.

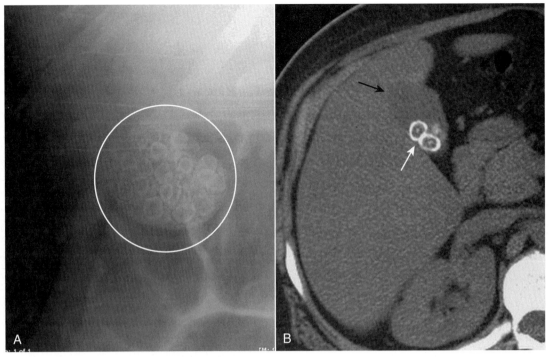

Figure 16-9 Gallstones, conventional radiograph (A) and axial CT scan (B). A, There are multiple laminated calcifications (*white circle*) that have interlocking edges, suggesting that they all formed in a hollow viscus in proximity to each other. These are called **faceted stones** for their characteristic shapes. **B,** A close-up view of an unenhanced axial CT scan of the right upper quadrant shows several gallstones (*solid white arrow*), two of which clearly have a central nidus surrounded by laminated, concentric rings of noncalcified and calcified material. The gallbladder (*solid black arrow*) contains bile fats and is less dense than the liver.

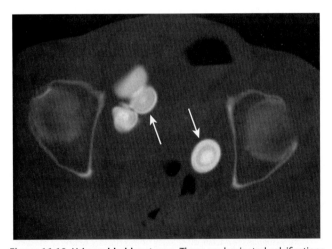

Figure 16-10 Urinary bladder stones. There are laminated calcifications (*solid white arrows*) seen on this axial CT scan through the level of the pelvis and windowed to show the laminations better. The laminations imply that these calcifications have formed inside of a hollow viscus. The anatomic location of these calculi places them in the urinary bladder.

TABLE 16-3 LAMINAR OR LAMELLATED CALCIFICATIONS

Organ of Origin	Remarks
Kidney	Most calcified renal stones are composed of calcium oxalate crystals; mostly form due to stasis or infection.
Gallbladder	Most calcified gallstones are calcium bilirubinate; they form due to chronic infection and stasis.
Urinary bladder	Most bladder calculi contain urate crystals; they form most often from outlet obstruction.

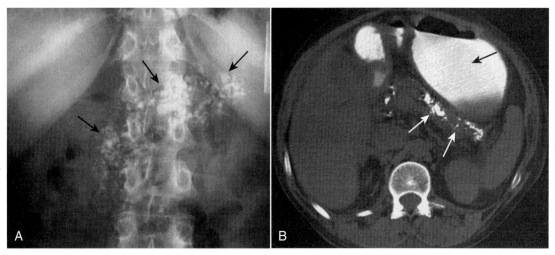

Figure 16-11 **Chronic calcific pancreatitis, conventional radiograph (A) and axial CT scan (B). A,** A close-up view of the left upper quadrant of a conventional radiograph of the abdomen shows amorphous calcifications (*solid black arrows*) implying calcification in a solid organ or tumor. The anatomic distribution of the calcification corresponds to the pancreas. **B,** In another patient, a nonenhanced image of the upper abdomen shows calcifications distributed along the course of the body and tail of the pancreas (*solid white arrows*). There is oral contrast seen in the stomach (*solid black arrow*). These calcifications are pathognomonic of chronic pancreatitis, a chronic and irreversible disease that leads to atrophy of the gland and diabetes, occurring mostly secondary to alcoholism.

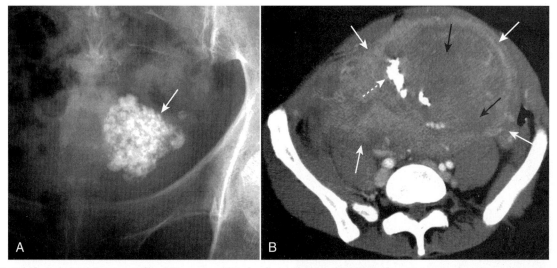

Figure 16-12 **Calcified uterine leiomyoma (fibroid) on conventional radiograph (A) and CT (B). A,** There is an amorphous (or popcorn, if you're hungry) calcification (*solid white arrow*) visible in the pelvis of this 48-year-old female. The type of calcification suggests formation in a solid organ or tumor. This is the anatomic location and the classical appearance of calcified uterine leiomyomas (fibroids). **B,** Another patient has large uterine fibroids (*solid white arrows*), portions of which have necrosed (*solid black arrows*) and calcified (*dotted white arrow*). Ultrasound is the study of choice in diagnosing uterine fibroids.

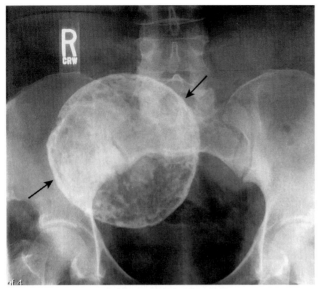

Figure 16-13 Calcified rim in uterine leiomyoma. This is a rimlike calcification in the pelvis of a female patient (*solid black arrows*), so that it would be appropriate to consider that this calcification formed in the wall of a hollow viscus or saccular structure. In fact, this is a characteristic pattern of calcification in the outer wall of a degenerated uterine leiomyoma (fibroid). Cystic lesions of the ovary might produce this appearance, and ultrasound of the pelvis would be the study of choice to identify the organ of origin.

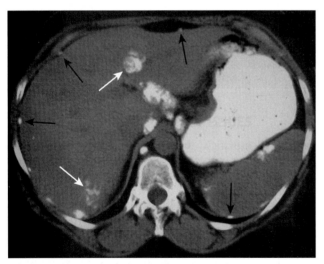

Figure 16-14 Calcified ovarian metastases. An unenhanced axial CT scan of the upper abdomen shows multiple amorphous calcifications, some within the liver (*solid white arrows*) and others that stud the peritoneal surface of the abdomen (*solid black arrows*). This patient had a mucin-producing adenocarcinoma of the ovary that metastasized to the peritoneum and liver. Mucin-producing tumors of the stomach and colon can also produce calcified metastases, but ovarian malignancy would be the most common to metastasize to the peritoneum.

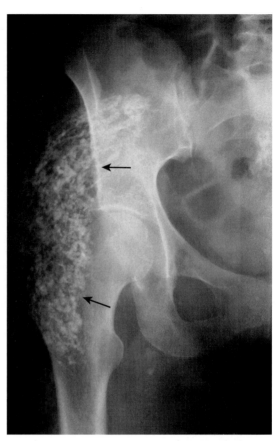

Figure 16-15 Dystrophic calcification in a calcified hematoma. There are amorphous calcifications demonstrated in the soft tissues overlying the right hip (*solid black arrows*) suggesting these calcifications have formed within a solid structure. The patient had a history of prior trauma to this region. Heterotopic ossification, which would have a similar appearance, also can form in soft tissues following trauma but it usually is more organized with distinct cortices and trabeculae.

TABLE 16-4 AMORPHOUS, CLOUDLIKE, OR POPCORN CALCIFICATIONS

Organ of Origin	Remarks
Pancreas	Chronic pancreatitis, frequently secondary to alcoholism
Uterine fibroids (leiomyomas)	Degenerating fibroids calcify
Mucin-producing tumors	Mucin-producing tumors of the ovary, stomach, or colon may calcify as can their metastases
Meningioma	Benign, extraaxial brain tumor of older individuals that calcifies about 20% of the time

TABLE 16-5 IDENTIFYING THE FOUR TYPES OF ABNORMAL CALCIFICATIONS

Type of Calcification	Implies	Examples
Rimlike	Formed in wall of hollow viscus	Cysts, aneurysms, gallbladder
Linear or tracklike	Formed in walls of tubular structures	Ureters, arteries
Lamellar or laminar	Formed in stones	Renal, gallbladder, and bladder calculi
Amorphous, cloudlike, popcorn	Forms in a solid organ or tumor	Uterine fibroids, some mucin-producing tumors

TABLE 16-6 LOCATION, LOCATION, LOCATION

Anatomic Quadrant in the Abdomen	Pattern of Calcification	Possible Organ of Origin	Cause
RUQ	Rimlike	Gallbladder wall	Chronic infection
	Tracklike	Hepatic artery	Atherosclerosis
	Laminated	Gallbladder	Gallstones
	Amorphous	Head of pancreas	Chronic pancreatitis
LUQ	Rimlike	Splenic cyst	Amebic infection
	Tracklike	Splenic artery	Atherosclerosis
	Laminated	Kidney	Renal stone
	Amorphous	Tail of pancreas	Chronic pancreatitis
RLQ	Rimlike	Iliac artery	Iliac artery aneurysm
	Tracklike	Iliac artery	Atherosclerosis
	Laminated	Appendix	Appendicolith
	Amorphous	Uterus	Fibroids
LLQ	Rimlike	Iliac artery	Iliac artery aneurysm
	Tracklike	Iliac artery	Atherosclerosis
	Laminated		
	Amorphous	Uterus or ovaries	Ovarian tumor

WEBLINK

Registered users may obtain more information on Recognizing Abnormal Calcifications and Their Causes on StudentConsult.com.

TAKE-HOME POINTS

Recognizing Abnormal Calcifications and Their Causes

Calcifications can be characterized by the pattern of their calcification and their anatomic location.

Four distinct patterns of calcifications are rimlike, linear or tracklike, lamellar (or laminar), and cloudlike (amorphous or popcorn).

Rimlike calcifications imply calcification that has occurred in the wall of a hollow viscus.

Examples of rimlike calcifications include cysts, aneurysms, or saccular organs such as the gallbladder.

Linear or tracklike calcifications imply calcification that has occurred in the walls of tubular structures.

Examples of tracklike calcifications include the walls of arteries and tubular structures such as the ureters, Fallopian tubes, and vas deferens.

Lamellar (or laminar) calcifications imply calcification that forms around a nidus inside a hollow lumen.

Examples of lamellar calcifications include renal calculi, gallstones, and bladder stones.

Cloudlike, amorphous, or popcorn calcification is calcification that has formed inside of a solid organ or tumor.

Examples of amorphous or popcorn calcifications include calcifications in the pancreas, leiomyomas of the uterus, lymph nodes, mucin-producing adenocarcinomas, and dystrophic, soft-tissue calcifications.

Combining the type of calcification with its anatomic location should provide the key to the etiology of most pathologic calcifications. CT scans are especially useful in identifying the type and location of abnormal calcifications.

Chapter 17

Recognizing the Imaging Findings of Trauma

- Trauma is the leading cause of death, hospitalization, and disability in Americans from the age of 1 year through age 45. The major imaging findings of most organ system's trauma will be discussed as a group in this chapter. Table 17-1 summarizes some of the traumatic injuries that are discussed in other chapters.
- Trauma-related injuries are divided into the two major mechanisms which produce them.
  - **Blunt trauma** is usually the result of motor vehicle accidents and is the more common of the two.
  - **Penetrating trauma** is usually the result of accidental or criminal stabbings and gunshot wounds.

CHEST TRAUMA

- Chest injuries in trauma patients are **very common** and are responsible for one out of four trauma-related deaths. The overwhelming majority of chest trauma is the result of motor vehicle accidents.

Rib Fractures

- The severity of underlying visceral injury is usually more important than the rib fractures themselves, but their presence might provide clues to unsuspected pathology.
- Fractures of the **first three ribs** are relatively **uncommon** and, if they occur following blunt trauma, **indicate a sufficient amount of force** to produce other internal injuries (Fig. 17-1).
- Fractures of **ribs 4-9 are common** and important if they are displaced (pneumothorax) or if there are two fractures in each of three or more contiguous ribs (*flail chest*).
  - **Flail chest** is almost always accompanied by a pulmonary contusion (see below). Because of the severity of the injuries with which it is usually associated, a flail chest has a significant mortality (Fig. 17-2).
- Fractures of **ribs 10-12** may indicate the presence of **underlying trauma** to the **liver** (right side) or the **spleen** (left side), especially if they are displaced.
- In cases of minor trauma, it is **not unusual for rib fractures to be undetectable on the initial examination** but to become visible in several weeks after callus begins to form.

Pulmonary Contusions

- Pulmonary contusions are the most frequent complications of blunt chest trauma. They **represent hemorrhage into the lung,** usually at the point of impact.

- **Recognizing a pulmonary contusion**
  - The history of trauma is of paramount importance as contusions present as airspace disease that is indistinguishable from other airspace diseases like pneumonia or aspiration.
  - Contusions tend to be peripherally placed and frequently occur at the point of maximum impact. Air bronchograms are usually not present because blood fills the bronchi as well as the airspaces (Fig. 17-3).
- Classically, they **appear within 6 hours after the trauma** and, because blood in the airspaces tends to be reabsorbed quickly, **disappear within 72 hours,** frequently sooner.
- Airspace disease that **lingers more than 72 hours** should **raise suspicions** of another process such as **aspiration pneumonia** or a **pulmonary laceration.**

Pulmonary Lacerations (Hematoma or Traumatic Pneumatocele)

- Pulmonary hematomas **result from a laceration of the lung parenchyma** and, as such, may accompany more severe **blunt trauma** or **penetrating chest trauma.**
- A pulmonary laceration is also called a *traumatic pneumatocele* or *hematoma.*
- They are sometimes masked by the airspace disease from a surrounding pulmonary contusion, at least for the first few days until the contusion resolves.
- **Recognizing a pulmonary laceration**
  - Their **appearance will depend on whether they contain blood and, if so, how much** blood fills the laceration.
  - If they are **completely filled with blood,** they will appear as a solid, **ovoid mass.**
  - If they are **partially filled with blood** and **partially filled with air,** they may contain a visible **air-fluid level** or demonstrate a *crescent sign* as the blood begins to form a clot and pull away from the wall of the laceration.
  - If they are **completely filled with air,** they will appear as an **air-containing, cystlike structure** in the lung (Fig. 17-4).
- Unlike pulmonary contusions that clear rapidly, **pulmonary lacerations,** especially if they are blood filled, **may take weeks or months to completely clear.**

AORTIC TRAUMA

- Trauma to the aorta is most frequently the result of **deceleration injuries in motor vehicle accidents.** Although the survival rates are improving, **most patients** with rupture

TABLE 17-1 OTHER MANIFESTATIONS OF TRAUMA

Injury	Discussed in
Pleural effusion/hemothorax	Chapter 6
Aspiration	Chapter 7
Pneumothorax, pneumomediastinum and pneumopericardium	Chapter 8
Fractures and dislocations	Chapter 22
Head trauma	Chapter 25

of the thoracic aorta **die before reaching the hospital** and, of those who survive an aortic injury, the likelihood of death increases the longer the abnormality remains untreated. Only those with **incomplete** tears in which the **adventitial lining prevents exsanguination (producing a *pseudoaneurysm*)** survive to be imaged.

■ The most common site of injury is the **aortic isthmus**, which is the portion of the **aorta just distal to the origin of the left subclavian artery.** Seat-belt injuries may involve

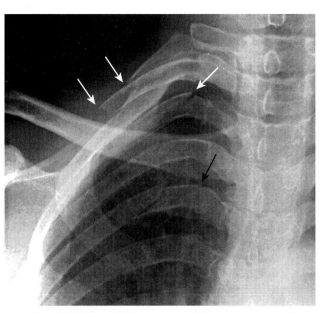

Figure 17-1 Rib fractures. Rib fractures are important primarily for the complications they might produce or the unsuspected pathology they might herald. Fractures of the first three ribs (*solid white arrows*) are relatively uncommon; following blunt trauma, their presence is a clue that the force to the chest may have been sufficient to produce other internal injuries. Don't mistake the normal costovertebral junction (*solid black arrow*) for a fracture.

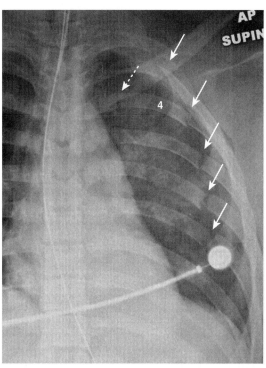

Figure 17-2 Flail chest. There are two or more fractures (*dotted white arrow* demonstrates second fracture in *rib 4*) present in more than three contiguous ribs (*solid white arrows*). The airspace disease in the left lung is an underlying pulmonary contusion, which almost always accompanies a flail chest.

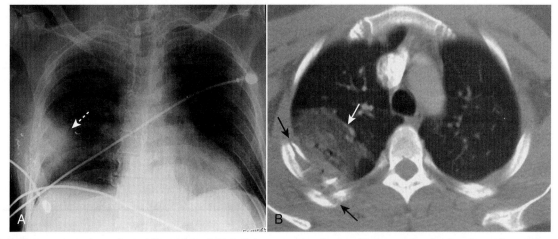

Figure 17-3 Pulmonary contusions, chest radiograph and CT. A, Pulmonary contusions tend to be peripherally placed most frequently at the point of maximum impact (*dotted white arrow*). Air bronchograms are usually not present because blood fills the bronchi as well as the airspaces. **B,** A second patient, who was in an unrestrained passenger in an automobile accident, also has a large contusion (*solid white arrow*) associated with multiple rib fractures (*solid black arrows*).

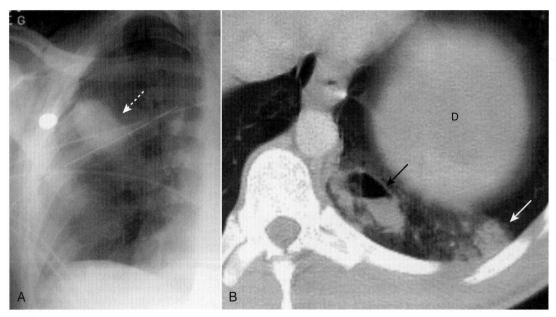

Figure 17-4 Pulmonary lacerations, conventional radiograph, and CT. Lacerations are sometimes masked, at least for the first few days, by the airspace disease in a surrounding pulmonary contusion. **A,** If they are completely filled with blood, they will appear as an ovoid mass (*dotted white arrow*). **B,** If they are partially filled with blood and partially filled with air, they may contain a visible air-fluid level (*solid black arrow*). Unlike the neighboring pulmonary contusion (*solid white arrow*), pulmonary lacerations, especially if they are blood filled, may take weeks or months to completely clear. The top of the left hemidiaphragm (*D*) is seen in this image.

the abdominal aorta, but such injuries are far less common than the deceleration injuries to the thoracic aorta.

- Only emergency surgery will prevent approximately 50% of patients with blunt aortic injuries from dying within the first 24 hours if left untreated.
- **Recognizing aortic trauma**
  - **Findings seen on conventional radiographs of the chest** are the same as those discussed under **Aortic Dissection** in Chapter 9. A completely **normal chest radiograph** has a relatively **high negative predictive value** for aortic injury, but an **abnormal chest x-ray** has a relatively **low positive predictive value (78%).**
    - "Widening of the mediastinum" is usually a **poor means of establishing the diagnosis** because it is difficult to assess on a supine, portable chest radiograph and it is commonly overinterpreted. There may also be **loss of the normal shadow of the aortic knob, a left apical pleural cap** of fluid or blood, a **left pleural effusion or deviation of the trachea or esophagus to the right** (Fig. 17-5).
  - **Findings on contrast-enhanced CT scans of the chest** (Fig. 17-6):
    - Under most circumstances, suspected aortic injuries are now studied using **multidetector CT** that allows for rapid image acquisition in one breath-hold and appropriately timed contrast delivery to the aorta **(CT angiography).** Most experts agree that a negative CT angiogram obviates the need for angiography. The findings are **frequently subtle** and require experience to recognize, as those patients with the more obvious findings may not have survived to be imaged.
      - **Aortic intimal flap.** A lucent defect in the contrast column of the aorta arising from a **tear** in the intima and media.

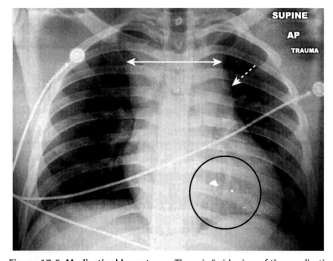

Figure 17-5 Mediastinal hematoma. There is "widening of the mediastinum" (*double white arrow*), an inexact finding on an AP supine, portable chest radiograph. More importantly, the shadow of the aortic knob is obscured by something of soft tissue density (*dotted white arrow*). Because the patient had been shot (bullet fragments in the *black circle*), these findings led to a request for a CT scan of the chest which demonstrated a large mediastinal hematoma.

- **Contour or caliber abnormalities.** Abrupt change in the smooth contour or size of the aorta at the point of injury.
- **Periaortic hematoma.** Delineation of a **contrast-filled collection outside of the normal confines of the aorta** representing *pseudoaneurysm* or extravasation.
- **Mediastinal hematoma.** Increased attenuation in the mediastinum from an admixture of blood and normal fat. May be present in the absence of an aortic injury, presumably due to small vessel trauma.

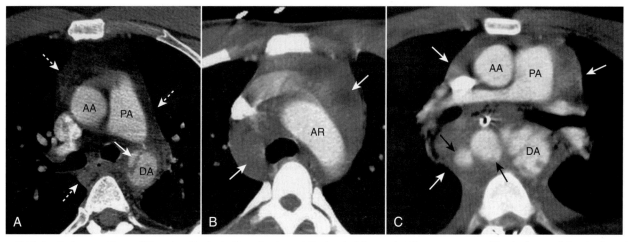

Figure 17-6 Aortic trauma, three different patients. A, There is a tear at the level of the aortic isthmus represented by the lucent defect in the wall of the descending aorta (*solid white arrow*). A mediastinal hematoma is also present (*dotted white arrows*). **B,** There is a large mediastinal hematoma (*solid white arrows*). **C,** There are periaortic hematomas containing extravasated blood (*solid black arrows*) and a large mediastinal hematoma (*solid white arrows*). (*AA* = ascending aorta; *AR* = aortic arch; *DA* = descending aorta; *PA* = pulmonary artery.)

- **Hemopericardium**. Fluid of high-attenuation (i.e., blood) in the pericardial sac indicates a significant injury to the aorta or heart itself.
- Patients with **equivocal** CT findings may go on to a catheter study of the aorta (**aortography**).

ABDOMINAL TRAUMA

- The role of advanced imaging techniques deserves special mention in abdominal trauma. Radiology has made a significant impact on the lives of traumatized patients by distinguishing those patients who can be managed conservatively from those who need surgical or other interventions and by helping to direct the most appropriate intervention for those who need it.
- **CT is the study of choice in abdominal trauma.**
  - **Intravenous contrast is always used** (unless contraindicated) to identify devascularized areas, hematomas, active extravasation of blood, or extraluminal urine (after contrast has passed through the kidneys).
    - If a **head CT is to be done** as well, it should be **done first** before contrast is injected for the abdomen.
  - **Oral contrast** is usually not administered. **Rectal contrast** is occasionally administered in penetrating trauma to search for a bowel laceration.
  - It is always best to consult with the radiologist so as to tailor the best study to fit the patient's needs.
  - In some emergency settings, a quick abdominal ultrasound is used in unstable trauma patients to evaluate for hemoperitoneum (Box 17-1).
- The most commonly affected solid organs in **blunt** abdominal trauma (in order of decreasing frequency) are the **spleen, liver, kidney, and urinary bladder.**
- Traumatic injuries to each of them will be discussed under each organ.

Liver

- The liver is discussed first because it is actually the **most frequently injured organ** if both penetrating and blunt

traumas are included together. The liver is the largest intraabdominal organ and is fixed in position, making it especially susceptible to injury. Injuries to the liver account for the **majority of deaths from abdominal trauma.**
- The posterior aspect of the **right lobe** is **injured most frequently**. Most hepatic injuries are associated with blood in the peritoneal cavity (*hemoperitoneum*).
- **Contrast-enhanced CT is the study of choice** and, because of its ability to demonstrate both the nature and extent of the trauma, the overwhelming majority of patients with liver trauma are now managed conservatively and do not require surgery.
- CT findings in hepatic trauma (Fig. 17-7):
  - **Subcapsular hematoma.** Lenticular fluid collections that conform to the shape of the outer contour of the liver but which frequently flatten the adjacent liver parenchyma. Most occur anterolaterally over the right hepatic lobe.
  - **Lacerations.** Most common finding. Irregularly marginated, low attenuation, linear or branching defects, usually at the periphery. "Fracture" is a term that has been used to describe a laceration that avulses a section of the liver.
  - **Intrahepatic hematomas.** Focal, high attenuation lesions first caused by blood; hematomas may progress to low attenuation, masslike lesions filled with serous fluid.
  - **Wedge-shaped defects.** Devascularized sections of liver parenchyma that do not contrast-enhance.
  - **Contusions.** A term used to describe an area of minimal parenchymal hemorrhage; they are lower in attenuation than the surrounding liver and have indistinct margins.

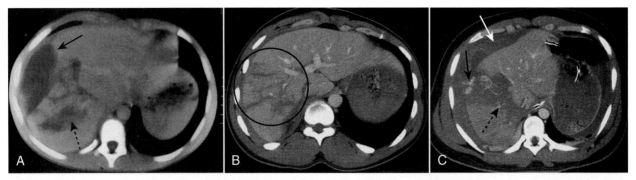

Figure 17-7 Hepatic trauma, three different patients. A, There is a lenticular fluid collection involving the lateral portion of the right lobe of the liver that represents a subcapsular hematoma (*solid black arrow*). A laceration of the right lobe is also present (*dotted black arrow*). **B,** There are multiple lacerations of the right lobe of the liver (*black circle*). **C,** Active extravasation of contrast-enhanced blood (*solid black arrow*) is seen from a large intrahepatic laceration with hematoma (*dotted black arrow*) and there is both subcapsular blood and hemoperitoneum (*solid white arrow*).

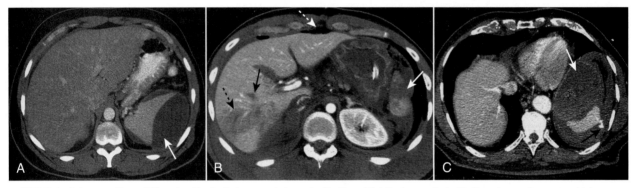

Figure 17-8 Splenic trauma, three different patients. A, A crescent-shaped collection of fluid is demonstrated in the subcapsular space which compresses the normal splenic parenchyma representing subcapsular hematoma (*solid white arrow*). **B,** This patient has a splenic (*solid white arrow*) and hepatic (*solid black arrow*) laceration and a large hepatic contusion (*dotted black arrow*). There is also pneumoperitoneum (*dotted white arrow*). **C,** Active extravasation of contrast-enhanced blood (*solid black arrow*) is shown along with a large intrasplenic hematoma (*solid white arrow*).

- **Pseudoaneurysms and acute hemorrhages.** Irregular collections of high attenuation, extravasated contrast that often require angiography with embolization or surgery.

Spleen

- Splenic trauma is usually caused by **deceleration injuries** in unrestrained occupants of motor vehicle collisions, by a fall from a height, or a pedestrian being struck by a motor vehicle.
- Because the **spleen is the most highly vascular organ**, hemorrhage represents the most serious complication of trauma. Despite its vascular nature and the delayed presentation of many splenic injuries, **most splenic trauma is treated conservatively** (nonsurgically).
- **CT is the study of choice for evaluating splenic trauma**. Findings include (Fig. 17-8):
  - **Contusion.** Alterations in the normal homogeneous appearance of the spleen, including mottled areas of low attenuation.
  - **Subcapsular hematoma.** Low-attenuation, crescent-shaped collection of fluid in the subcapsular space which frequently compresses the normal splenic parenchyma.
  - **Laceration.** Irregular, low-attenuation defect that typically transects the spleen.
  - **Intraparenchymal hematoma.** Lacerations filled with blood; they are intrasplenic, rounded areas of low attenuation which may have a mass effect and enlarge the spleen.

- **Intraperitoneal fluid or blood.** Hemoperitoneum occurs with almost all splenic injuries, including small amounts of blood in the pelvis. Its presence does not necessarily indicate active hemorrhage.

Kidneys

- Motor vehicle accidents are the most common cause of blunt abdominal trauma to the kidneys in the United States. Almost all patients with renal trauma will have **hematuria.**
- **Contrast-enhanced CT is the study of first choice** and has almost completely replaced the intravenous urogram and standard cystogram.
- CT findings in renal trauma (Fig. 17-9):
  - **Contusion.** Ill-defined, patchy, low-attenuation areas in the contrast-enhanced kidney.
  - **Subcapsular hematoma.** Crescentic or elliptical densities that compress the denser underlying renal parenchyma.
  - **Perinephric hematoma.** Ill-defined fluid collection surrounding the kidney confined by Gerota's fascia.
  - **Laceration.** Low-attenuation linear or branching defects in the renal parenchyma. More severe lacerations may extend through the renal hilum into the collecting system, renal artery, or vein. "Fracture" is a term that may be used when the laceration connects the hilum with the cortex.
  - **Vascular injuries.** If the injury is arterial, there may be no flow to the kidney and hence, no contrast-

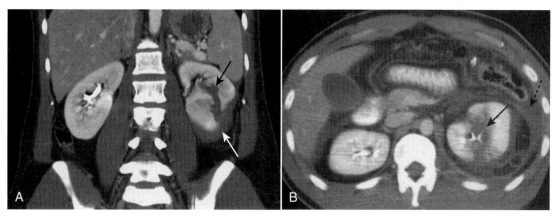

Figure 17-9 Renal trauma, two different patients. A, Coronal-reformatted, contrast-enhanced CT scan shows a low-attenuation linear defect representing a renal laceration (*solid black arrow*) and a subcapsular hematoma (*solid white arrow*). **B,** Axial CT scan on another patient also shows a renal laceration (*solid black arrow*) and a perinephric hematoma (*dotted black arrow*).

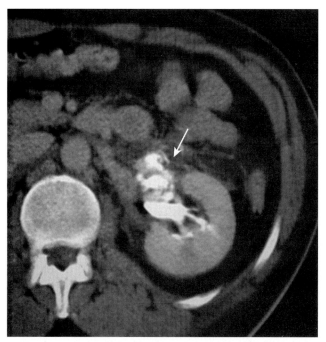

Figure 17-10 Tear of proximal ureter. There is a tear of the ureter at the level of the left ureteropelvic junction demonstrated by extraluminal contrast (*solid white arrow*) representing contrast-containing urine that is leaking from the collecting system.

enhancement. Vascular injuries may also produce wedge-shaped defects in the kidney.
- **Injuries to the collecting system.** Extraluminal contrast arising from the renal pelvis or ureter (Fig. 17-10).

Shock Bowel

- Shock bowel usually occurs with **blunt abdominal trauma** in which there is **severe hypovolemia and profound hypotension,** with complete reversibility of these findings following resuscitation.
- **Recognizing shock bowel on CT**
  - Diffuse thickening of the small bowel wall with increased enhancement.
  - Fluid-filled and dilated loops of bowel.
  - Other findings include a small inferior vena cava (<1 cm) and aorta (<6 mm) and decreased perfusion of the spleen (Fig. 17-11).

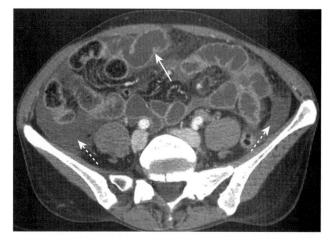

Figure 17-11 Shock bowel. Marked enhancement of the bowel wall is seen with multiple dilated and fluid-filled loops (*solid white arrow*). There is also retroperitoneal fluid present (*dotted white arrows*). Shock bowel usually occurs with severe hypovolemia and profound hypotension.

PELVIC TRAUMA

Rupture of the Urinary Bladder

- About **70% of bladder ruptures occur with pelvic fractures,** and about **10% of patients with pelvic fractures have an associated rupture of the bladder.**
- Bladder ruptures are best demonstrated by a **CT cystogram** in which contrast is infused under gravity through a Foley catheter into the bladder, but they can also be well-demonstrated by **antegrade filling of the bladder** from renal excretion of intravenously injected contrast.
- There are **two major types of bladder rupture** (Fig. 17-12):
  - **Extraperitoneal**—more common (80%)
    - Usually the **result of a pelvic fracture** with **direct puncture** of the bladder.
    - Extraluminal contrast **remains around the bladder,** especially the retropubic space.
  - **Intraperitoneal rupture**—less common
    - Usually the **result of a forceful blow to the pelvis with a distended bladder,** especially in children.
    - Rupture usually occurs at the **dome** of the bladder adjacent to the peritoneal cavity.

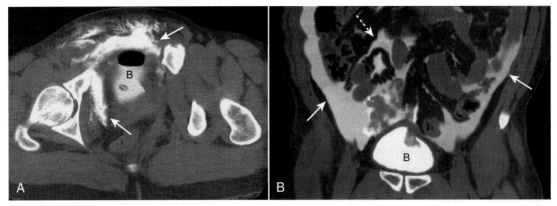

Figure 17-12 Bladder ruptures, extraperitoneal and intraperitoneal. A, Contrast-containing urine (*solid white arrows*) has leaked into the extraperitoneal spaces after being instilled into a perforated bladder following pelvic fractures. Contrast, the tip of a Foley catheter, and air are seen inside of the partially filled urinary bladder (*B*). **B,** Intraperitoneal bladder ruptures are less common and may occur with blunt trauma. The contrast flows freely away from the bladder (*B*) up the paracolic gutters (*solid white arrows*) and outlines loops of bowel (*dotted white arrow*).

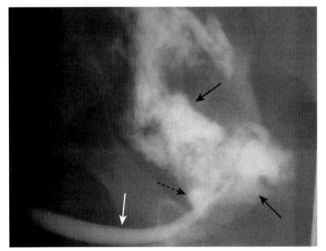

Figure 17-13 Urethral trauma. Contrast instilled retrograde through the penile urethra (*solid white arrow*) is seen to leak from the posterior urethra secondary to a perforation (*dotted black arrow*) and collects outside of the urinary system in the perineum and extraperitoneal bladder spaces (*solid black arrows*).

- Contrast runs freely through **the peritoneal cavity, surrounds bowel, and extends into the paracolic gutters.**

Urethral Injuries

- Urethral injuries are associated with significant pelvic trauma in **males,** most often **blunt trauma.**
- Urethral injuries should be investigated when there are **straddle fractures** of the pelvis or **penetrating injuries** in the region of the urethra. **Hematuria, blood at the urethral meatus,** and **inability to void** are suggestive clinical findings.
- Imaging is done most often using **retrograde urethrography (RUG),** in which contrast is instilled retrograde at the urethral meatus with retrograde filling of the urethra. This is done before insertion of a Foley catheter into the bladder.
- The **most common injury** is a rupture of the **posterior urethra** through the urogenital diaphragm into the proximal bulbous urethra.

- Extraluminal contrast can be seen outside of the urethra in the pelvis and perineum (Fig. 17-13).

WEBLINK

Registered users may obtain more information on Recognizing the Imaging Findings of Trauma on StudentConsult.com.

TAKE-HOME POINTS

Recognizing the Imaging Findings of Trauma

Trauma is generally divided into **blunt** and **penetrating** trauma. Most trauma-related injuries are due to blunt trauma, motor vehicle accidents contributing the majority.

CT has had a profound impact in traumatized patients by distinguishing those patients who can be managed conservatively from those who need surgical or other interventions.

Rib fractures may herald more serious internal injuries such as lacerations of the liver or spleen or pneumothoraces. Most occur in ribs 4-9.

Pulmonary contusions are the most common manifestation of blunt chest trauma and represent hemorrhage into the lung, usually at the point of impact. They classically clear in a few days.

Pulmonary lacerations are tears in the lung parenchyma that may contain fluid or air. Their presence may be hidden by a surrounding contusion, and they typically take longer than a contusion to clear.

Aortic injuries usually occur at the isthmus, require rapid recognition for optimum survival, and on contrast-enhanced CT may take the form of intimal flaps, contour abnormalities, or hematomas.

The most commonly affected solid organs in blunt abdominal trauma (in order of decreasing frequency) are the spleen, liver, kidney, and urinary bladder.

The **liver** is commonly injured in both blunt and penetrating trauma, and its injuries account for the majority of the deaths from abdominal trauma. It may demonstrate lacerations, hematomas, wedge-shaped defects, pseudoaneurysms, and acute hemorrhage.

Because the **spleen** is highly vascular, hemorrhage is the most serious sequela of splenic trauma, whose findings include hematomas, lacerations, and contusions.

Patients who have had **renal trauma** almost all have hematuria and may show contusions, lacerations, hematomas, or vascular pedicle injuries on CT. They may also demonstrate extraluminal contrast from an injury to the renal pelvis or ureter.

Shock bowel is a consequence of profound hypotension and shows diffuse small bowel wall thickening with enhancement of dilated and fluid-filled loops on CT.

Bladder ruptures may be either extraperitoneal (more common) or intraperitoneal, the former demonstrating extraluminal contrast surrounding the bladder, and the latter showing contrast flowing freely in the peritoneal cavity.

Urethral injuries occur almost exclusively in males, are frequently associated with pelvic fractures, and usually involve the posterior urethra where extraluminal contrast may be seen in the perineum or extraperitoneally in the pelvis.

Chapter 18

Recognizing Gastrointestinal, Hepatic, and Urinary Tract Abnormalities

- In this chapter, you'll learn how to recognize some of the most common abnormalities of the gastrointestinal (GI) tract from the esophagus to the rectum. We'll also discuss selected hepatic abnormalities. Chapter 19 on ultrasound will describe some of the more common biliary and pelvic abnormalities.
- CT, ultrasound, and MRI have essentially replaced conventional radiography and, in some instances, barium studies for the evaluation of the GI tract and the visceral abdominal organs.

BARIUM STUDIES OF THE GASTROINTESTINAL TRACT

- During the performance of barium studies, fluoroscopic spot films and overhead films are usually obtained by the radiologist and radiologic technologist in several projections for whatever part of the GI tract is being studied, depending on the **nature of the abnormality** and the **mobility of the patient.**
- As you go through this chapter, you will probably want to refer to the two tables in this chapter, one on **terminology** used in describing studies of the GI tract (Table 18-1) and the other on **basic principles in GI radiology** (Table 18-2), both of which will prove helpful in understanding the terms and concepts used here.

ESOPHAGUS

- Single- and double-contrast examinations of the esophagus are performed with the patient drinking liquid barium either by itself (*single contrast*) or accompanied by a gas-producing agent that provides the "air" in a *double-contrast examination.* Since both the single- and double-contrast techniques have their own strengths, many esophagrams are routinely performed using both techniques, called a *biphasic examination.*
- *Video esophagography* (video swallowing function) is a study of the **swallowing mechanism,** usually performed with fluoroscopy and frequently captured dynamically—digitally, on videotape, or on film. This is the study of choice for diagnosing and documenting *aspiration,* in which ingested substances pass into the trachea below the level of the vocal cords (Fig. 18-1).
- **Fluoroscopic observation** of the esophagus can also **reveal abnormalities in esophageal motility.** For example, *tertiary waves* are a common but nonspecific abnormality of esophageal motility, representing disordered and non-propulsive contractions of the esophagus. They can be observed fluoroscopically and captured on spot images (Fig. 18-2).

Esophageal Diverticula

- Diverticula of the GI tract are **usually produced when the mucosal and submucosal layers herniate through a defect in the muscular layer** of the bowel wall. Wherever they occur in the GI tract, diverticula produce an **outpouching** that projects beyond the borders of the lumen.

> Esophageal **diverticula occur in three locations:** the **neck, around the carina,** and **just above the diaphragm.** In the neck, the diverticulum is posteriorly located and is called a *Zenker diverticulum.* Diverticula at the level of the carina may be due to extrinsic inflammatory disease like tuberculosis (*traction diverticula*); diverticula just above the esophagogastric junction are called *epiphrenic diverticula* (Fig. 18-3).

Esophageal Carcinoma

- Esophageal carcinoma continues to have a very **poor prognosis** as more than **50% of patients will have metastases upon initial presentation.** The **lack of an esophageal serosa** and a **rich supply of lymphatics** aid in the extension and dissemination of esophageal carcinoma. A combination of long-term alcohol and tobacco use are associated with a higher risk of esophageal carcinoma.
- Esophageal malignancies are either **squamous cell carcinomas** or **adenocarcinomas,** the latter of which are **increasing in prevalence.** Adenocarcinomas arise in esophageal epithelium that has undergone **metaplasia** from **squamous to columnar epithelium** (*Barrett esophagus*), a process in which **gastroesophageal reflux (GERD) plays a major role.**
- Barium esophagrams are **frequently the initial study** in patients with symptoms, like dysphagia, that suggest this diagnosis.
- Esophageal carcinomas may **appear in one or more of several forms,** including an **annular-constricting lesion, polypoid mass, a superficial, infiltrating lesion or ulceration,** and **irregularity of the wall.** Most often, they present as a mixture of several of these patterns (Fig. 18-4).

Hiatal Hernia and Gastroesophageal Reflux (GERD)

- Hiatal hernias are divided into the **sliding type** (almost all) in which the **esophagogastric (EG) junction lies above the diaphragm** or the **paraesophageal type (1%)** in which a **portion of the stomach herniates through the**

TABLE 18-1 TERMINOLOGY

Term	Definition
Fluoroscopy	Utilization by the radiologist of special x-ray-producing equipment to observe in real time the dynamic movement of the bowel and to optimally position the patient so as to obtain diagnostic images frequently referred to as "spot films"; in this chapter, the term is used in reference to utilizing x-rays to image the GI tract.
Barium	Barium sulphate in suspension is an inert, radiopaque material prepared in liquid form to study the intraluminal anatomy of the GI tract.
Single contrast/double contrast/biphasic examination	A single-contrast (also called **full-column**) study usually refers to a GI imaging procedure in which only barium is used as the contrast agent; double contrast (sometimes called **air contrast**) usually refers to a study of the GI tract using both thicker barium and air; a **biphasic examination** is used to study the upper gastrointestinal tract and utilizes an initial double contrast study followed by a single contrast agent to optimize the study.
Filling defect	A lesion, usually of soft tissue density, that protrudes into the lumen and displaces the intraluminal contrast (e.g., a polyp is a filling defect).
Ulcer	Refers to a persistent collection of contrast that projects outward from the contrast-filled lumen and originates either through a break in the mucosal lining (as in gastric ulcer) or in a GI mass (as in an ulcerating malignancy).
Diverticulum	Refers to a persistent collection of contrast that projects outward from the contrast-filled lumen of the GI tract like an ulcer; unlike an ulcer, the mucosa of a diverticulum is intact; false diverticula represent outpouchings of mucosa and submucosa through the muscularis.
Spot films and overhead films	Spot films usually refer to static images obtained by the radiologist who utilizes fluoroscopy to position the patient for the optimum image; *overhead films* is a term which refers to additional images obtained by the radiologic technologist to complement fluoroscopic spot films using an x-ray tube mounted on the ceiling of the radiographic room (thus, the term *overhead*).
Intraluminal, intramural, extrinsic	Intraluminal (sometimes shortened to luminal) lesions are generally those that arise from the mucosa, like polyps and carcinomas; intramural (sometimes shortened to mural) lesions are those that arise from the wall, in this chapter from the GI tract, such as leiomyomas and lipomas; extrinsic lesions arise outside of the GI tract, e.g., serosal metastases or endometriosis implants.
En face and in profile	When you look at a lesion directly "head-on," you are seeing it *en face*; a lesion seen tangentially (from the side) is seen in profile; except for those that are perfect spheres, lesions will have a different shape when viewed *en face* and in profile.

TABLE 18-2 COMMON PRINCIPLES FOR ALL BARIUM STUDIES

Term	Definition
Fully distended vs. collapsed	Only loops that are fully distended by contrast can be accurately evaluated no matter what part of the GI tract is being studied; evaluating certain criteria (such as wall thickness) using collapsed loops may introduce errors of diagnosis.
Change and distensibility	Over time (usually measured in seconds), the walls of all of the GI luminal structures, from esophagus to rectum, change in contour, distending and ballooning outward with increasing volumes of barium and air. Change and distensibility are normal.
Rigid, stiff, fixed, nondistensible	If the bowel wall is infiltrated by tumor, blood, edema, or fibrous tissue, for example, the bowel may lose its ability to change and distend; this lack of distensibility is variously called **rigidity, stiffening, fixed, nondistensible**. This is abnormal.
Irregularity	Except for the normal marginal indentations caused by the folds in the stomach, small bowel, and colon, the walls of the entire GI tract appear relatively smooth and regular; diseases can produce ulceration, infiltration, and nodularity with resultant irregularity of the wall.
Persistence	Almost without exception, an apparent abnormality must be seen on more than one image to be considered a pathologic finding; transient changes in the GI tract caused by peristalsis, ingested food, the presence of stool, or incompletely distended loops of bowel will disappear over time, but true abnormalities will remain constant and persistent.

esophageal hiatus but the EG junction remains below the diaphragm. In general, hiatal hernias increase in incidence with age.

- Most hiatal hernias are asymptomatic, but there is an association between the presence of some hiatal hernias and clinically significant *gastroesophageal reflux.*
  - Gastroesophageal reflux **also occurs in patients without** any visible **hiatal hernia**, usually due to some dysfunction of the lower esophageal sphincter, which normally acts to prevent gastric acid from repeatedly refluxing into the esophagus.

 The radiologic findings of hiatal hernia include a bulbous area of the distal esophagus containing oral

contrast at the level of the diaphragm with **failure of the esophagus to narrow** on multiple images **as it passes through the esophageal hiatus, extension of multiple gastric folds above the diaphragm**, and sometimes visualization of a thin, circumferential filling defect in the distal esophagus called a *Schatzki ring.*

- A Schatzki ring **marks the position of the esophagogastric junction** so that its appearance above the diaphragm indicates the presence of a sliding hiatal hernia (Fig. 18-5).

- **Gastroesophageal reflux may be evident during fluoroscopy** when barium is seen to move from the stomach retrograde into the esophagus, but reflux is intermittent so

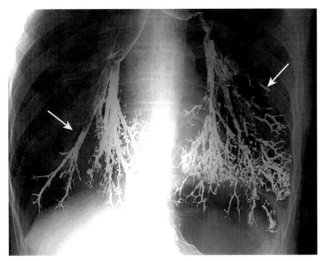

Figure 18-1 Aspiration, barium gone wild. Frontal radiograph of the lung bases demonstrates high density material outlining the tracheobronchial tree (*solid white arrows*). The material is barium that was aspirated into the lung during an upper gastrointestinal series. Barium is inert and did not cause any additional symptoms that the patient wasn't already experiencing from aspirating his own secretions. It will take some time, but most of this barium will be reabsorbed, most likely leaving only a small amount remaining.

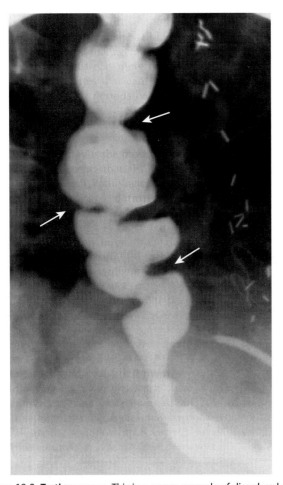

Figure 18-2 Tertiary waves. This is a severe example of disordered and nonpropulsive waves of contraction in the esophagus called tertiary waves (*solid white arrows*). The term **corkscrew-esophagus** is sometimes applied to this appearance. Tertiary waves are a nonspecific and very common abnormality that increases in frequency with advancing age.

that it may not occur during the course of the examination. The absence of reflux during the study **does not exclude reflux**, and demonstration of reflux **does not necessarily indicate the patient has the complications of GERD, i.e., esophagitis, stricture, and Barrett esophagus**.

STOMACH AND DUODENUM

- Today, the lumen of the stomach is most often studied by upper endoscopy; the wall thickness and structures outside of the stomach are studied by CT examination of the abdomen with oral contrast. Nevertheless, biphasic upper gastrointestinal (UGI) examinations, which include a study of the esophagus, stomach, and duodenum, remain a sensitive, cost-effective, readily available, and noninvasive examination.

Gastric Ulcers

- In the United States, the **incidence of gastric ulcer disease has been declining**. In adults, infection with *Helicobacter pylori* accounts for almost three out of four cases of gastric ulcer disease. Nonsteroidal anti-inflammatory agents account for most of the rest.

▶ Most ulcers occur on the **lesser curvature** or **posterior wall** in the region of the body or antrum. About **95% of all gastric ulcers are benign**. The other **5% will represent ulcerations in gastric malignancies** (Fig. 18-6).

Gastric Carcinoma

- There has been a dramatic **decline in the incidence of gastric carcinomas in the United States**. The **mortality, however, remains quite high** as they are frequently not diagnosed until after they have spread. Most gastric carcinomas (actually, they are adenocarcinomas) **occur in the distal third of the stomach** along the **lesser curvature**.
- Double-contrast UGI images and CT scans of the abdomen can demonstrate gastric carcinomas. CT is utilized for staging the extent of the tumor and degree of spread.
- Gastric carcinomas may be **polypoid, infiltrating** (i.e., *linitis plastica*), **or ulcerative** in form (Fig. 18-7).
- There are other mass lesions that may resemble gastric carcinoma, including *leiomyomas*, a benign, wall lesion that characteristically ulcerates, and *lymphoma*, which may produce diffusely thickened folds or multiple masses in the stomach.

Duodenal Ulcer

▶ **Duodenal ulcers are two to three times more common than gastric ulcers**. Almost all duodenal ulcers occur in the **duodenal bulb**, the majority on the **anterior wall** of the bulb. They are **overwhelmingly caused by** *H. pylori* infection (85%-95%).

- Double-contrast UGI series have a sensitivity that exceeds 90% in detecting duodenal ulcers (Fig. 18-8).

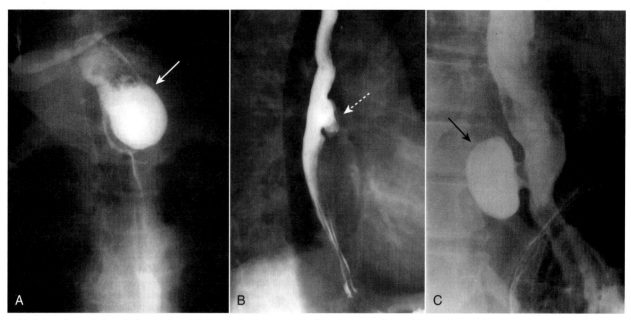

Figure 18-3 **Esophageal diverticula.** Esophageal diverticula characteristically occur **(A)** in the neck from a localized weakness in the posterior wall of the hypopharynx **(*Zenker diverticulum*)** (*solid white arrow*); in the mid-esophagus **(B)** from extrinsic disease like TB that causes fibrosis, which pulls on the esophagus forming a ***traction diverticulum*** (*dotted white arrow*); or **(C)** just above the diaphragm in the distal esophagus (***epiphrenic diverticulum***) (*solid black arrow*). Only the traction diverticulum is a ***true*** diverticulum in that it contains all layers of the esophagus; the Zenker and epiphrenic are ***false*** or ***pseudodiverticula*** because the mucosa and submucosa herniate through a defect in the muscular layer.

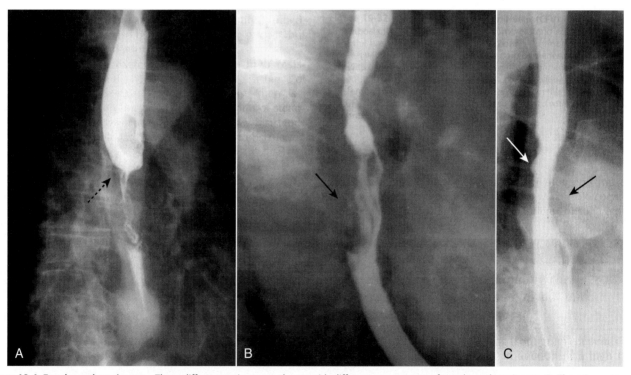

Figure 18-4 **Esophageal carcinomas.** Three different patients are shown with different appearances of esophageal carcinoma. **A,** There is an ***annular constricting*** lesion of the mid-esophagus (*dotted black arrow*)—the tumor encircles the normal lumen and obstructs it, in this case. **B,** A ***polypoid mass*** that arises from the right lateral wall of the esophagus displaces the barium around it (*solid black arrow*). **C,** The wall is irregular and rigid and contains a small ***ulceration*** (*solid white arrow*); the aortic knob is producing a normal indentation on the opposite wall of the esophagus (*solid black arrow*).

■ Complications of duodenal ulcers, best demonstrated by CT, include **obstruction, perforation** (into the peritoneal cavity), **penetration** (such as into the pancreas), or **hemorrhage** (Fig. 18-9).

SMALL AND LARGE BOWEL

General Considerations

■ Opacification and distension of the bowel lumen is necessary for proper evaluation of the bowel no matter what imaging modality is used.

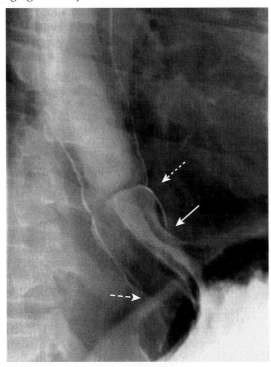

Figure 18-5 Sliding hiatal hernia. There is a bulbous collection of contrast representing the stomach herniated above the diaphragm. There are gastric folds present in the hernia, identifying it as part of the stomach (*solid white arrow*). Notice the esophagus does not narrow as it normally does when passing through the esophageal hiatus (*dashed white arrow*). Just above the hernia is a thin, weblike filling defect characteristic of a **Schatzki ring** (*dotted white arrow*). The Schatzki ring marks the level of the esophagogastric junction.

⚠ **Collapsed or unopacified loops of bowel can introduce errors of diagnosis** related to our inability to first visualize and then to differentiate real from artifactual findings or to accurately characterize the abnormality even if recognized. On CT scans of the abdomen and pelvis, unopacified loops of bowel may mimic masses or adenopathy, and wall thickness is difficult to assess if the bowel is not distended.

■ Therefore, **orally administered contrast**, frequently given in temporally divided doses to allow earlier contrast to reach the colon while later contrast opacifies the stomach, **is routinely utilized for most abdominal CT scans** except those performed for **trauma**, the *stone search study*, and studies specifically directed towards evaluating vascular structures like the **aorta**.
  • Oral contrast used for CT examinations is either a dilute solution containing barium or iodinated contrast.

➡ There are **several important findings** common to any part of the bowel, which are key to the diagnosis of bowel abnormalities by CT.

■ **Thickening of the bowel** wall. The normal **small bowel** lumen does not exceed about 2.5 cm in diameter, and the wall is usually **no thicker than 3 mm. The colonic wall does not exceed 3 mm** with the lumen distended.
■ **Submucosal edema or hemorrhage.** Submucosal infiltration produces varying degrees of *thumbprinting*, nodular indentations into the bowel lumen representing focal areas of submucosal infiltration by edema, hemorrhage, inflammatory cells, tumor (lymphoma), or amyloid.
■ **Hazy or strandlike infiltration of the surrounding fat.** Extension of inflammatory reaction outside of the bowel into the adjacent fat is a sentinel finding that heralds associated disease (Fig. 18-10).
■ **Extraluminal contrast or extraluminal air.** Indicates the presence of a bowel perforation (Fig. 18-11).

Small Bowel: Crohn Disease

■ Crohn disease is a **chronic, relapsing, granulomatous inflammation of the small bowel and colon** resulting in ulceration, obstruction and fistula formation. Crohn disease

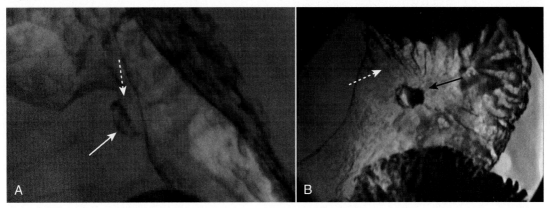

Figure 18-6 Benign lesser curvature gastric ulcer. A, Seen in profile is a large collection of barium that protrudes beyond the expected contour of the normal body of the stomach along the lesser curvature representing a gastric ulcer (*solid white arrow*). This ulcer collection was present on multiple views (an important characteristic of an ulcer called *persistence*). The mound of edematous tissue that surrounds the ulcer (*dotted white arrow*) is called an **ulcer collar. B,** Seen *en face,* there are numerous gastric folds (*dotted white arrow*) that all radiate to the ulcer margin and a central collection (*solid black arrow*) representing the ulcer itself. This was a benign gastric ulcer.

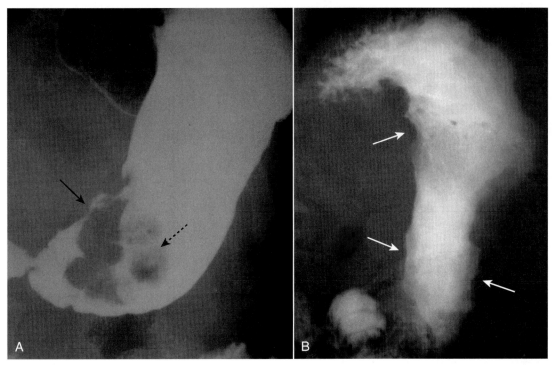

Figure 18-7 Carcinomas of the stomach. A, There is a large, polypoid filling defect in the antrum of the stomach that displaces the barium around it (*solid black arrow*). Contained within the mass and seen *en face* is an irregularly shaped collection of barium that represents an ulceration in the mass (*dotted black arrow*). This was an adenocarcinoma of the stomach. **B,** The entire body of the stomach displays a lack of distensibility, losing the normal ballooning outward that every portion of the GI tract demonstrates when filled with enough barium or air. Instead, the walls of the stomach are concave inward (*solid white arrows*) and **rigid,** a sign of malignancy. This stomach would display the same appearance on all images. This is the typical appearance for **linitis plastica,** caused by an infiltrating adenocarcinoma of the stomach.

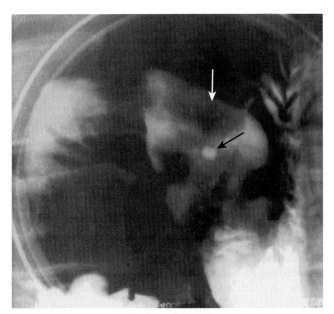

Figure 18-8 Acute duodenal ulcer. Contained within the duodenal bulb on its anterior wall is a collection of barium (*solid black arrow*), shown to be persistent on a number of other images, surrounded by a zone of edema (*solid white arrow*) that displaces the barium from around the ulcer. This collection is characteristic of an acute duodenal ulcer. When duodenal ulcers heal, they are likely to do so with scarring that deforms the normal triangular contour of the bulb.

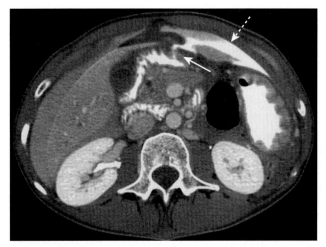

Figure 18-9 Perforated duodenal ulcer. Axial CT scan of the upper abdomen done with oral and intravenous contrast shows a leak of oral contrast from the duodenum (*solid white arrow*) into the peritoneal cavity (*dotted white arrow*). Obstruction, perforation, and hemorrhage are common complications of ulcer disease. The patient had a perforated duodenal ulcer repaired at surgery.

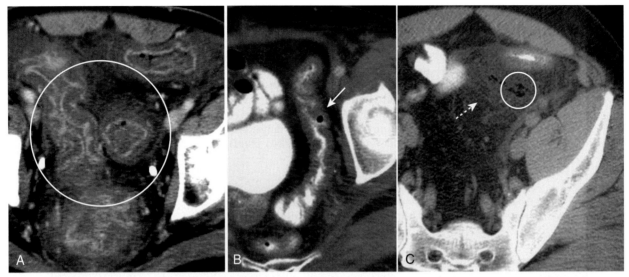

Figure 18-10 Key findings on CT of the GI tract. Findings applicable to any part of the bowel and key to the diagnosis of bowel abnormalities on CT. **A,** There is thickening and enhancement of the wall of the bowel (*circle*). When distended, as these loops of large bowel are, the bowel wall is normally very thin. **B,** There is submucosal infiltration of the wall (thumbprinting) (*solid white arrow*). In this case of ischemic colitis, it most likely represents edema with some hemorrhage. **C,** Infiltration of the surrounding fat is seen (*dotted white arrow*), a sentinel finding that usually heralds adjacent inflammation. There is also extraluminal air (*circle*), a sign of bowel perforation.

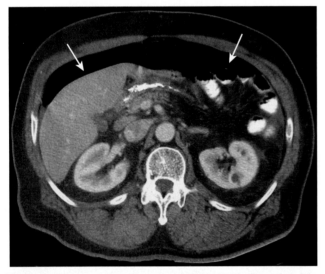

Figure 18-11 Free air from bowel perforation. With the patient lying supine for this CT scan, free intraperitoneal air (*solid white arrows*) rises to the highest part of the abdomen beneath the anterior abdominal wall. Most cases of free intraperitoneal air (**pneumoperitoneum**) are due to perforations from gastric and duodenal ulcers.

typically **involves the ileum and right colon,** presents with *skip areas* (abnormal bowel interposed between normal bowel), is prone to **fistula formation,** and has a **propensity for recurring** following surgical resection and reanastamosis in whatever loop of bowel becomes the new terminal ileum.

■ Crohn disease may be imaged either with a barium **small bowel follow-through** (series) or **CT of the abdomen and pelvis.**

➡ Imaging findings in Crohn disease include **narrowing, irregularity, and ulceration of the terminal ileum** frequently with proximal small bowel dilatation; **separation of the loops of bowel** due to fatty infiltration of the mesentery surrounding the ileum, making the affected loop(s)

stand apart from the surrounding loops of small bowel (**proud loop**); the *string sign*—narrowing of the terminal ileum into a near slitlike opening by spasm and fibrosis; and **fistulae**—especially between the ileum and colon but also to the skin, vagina, and urinary bladder (Fig. 18-12).

Large Bowel

■ The intraluminal surface of the colon is most often studied with optical or virtual colonoscopy or double contrast barium enema examination. Structures outside of the colon are usually studied by CT examination of the abdomen and pelvis with oral or rectal contrast.

Diverticulosis

■ **Colonic diverticula,** like most diverticula of the GI tract, represent herniation of the mucosa and submucosa through a defect in the muscular layer (*false diverticula*).

➡ They occur more frequently with increasing age and may be due, at least in part, to increase in intraluminal pressure and weakening of the colonic wall. They are **usually multiple (*diverticulosis*),** are almost always **asymptomatic** (about 90% of the time) but **can become inflamed or bleed. Diverticulosis is the most common cause of massive lower GI bleeding.** When they bleed, the **right-sided** diverticula seem to bleed more than those on the left.

■ They occur most often in the sigmoid colon and are readily **identified on either barium enema or CT examination as small spikes or smoothly contoured collections of air or contrast attached to the colon** (Fig. 18-13).

Diverticulitis

■ Diverticula can become inflamed and perforate (*diverticulitis*), most often secondary to mechanical irritation or

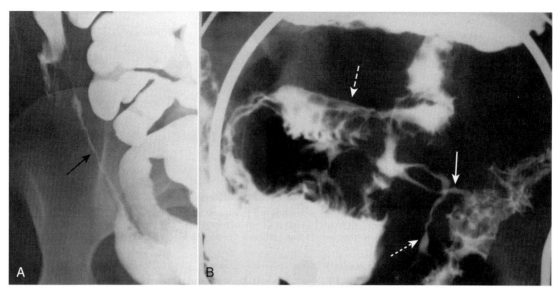

Figure 18-12 Crohn disease. A, The terminal ileum (*solid black arrow*) is markedly narrowed (***string sign***) and stands apart from other loops of small bowel (***proud loop***). **B,** A close-up image of the right lower quadrant from a small bowel follow-through study in another patient shows multiple streaks of barium (*solid* and *dotted white arrows*) representing multiple enteric fistulae originating from an abnormal loop of small bowel (*dashed white arrow*) and connecting with each other and the large bowel. Fistula formation is a common complication of this disease.

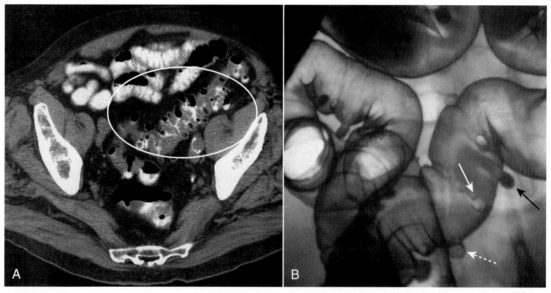

Figure 18-13 Diverticulosis. A, In this CT scan of the pelvis, diverticula contain air and appear as small, usually round outpouchings, especially in the region of the sigmoid colon (*white oval*). **B,** There are numerous outpouchings containing barium seen in the sigmoid colon of this air-contrast barium enema examination. Some diverticula are filled with barium (*solid black arrow*), while others contain air and are outlined with barium (*dotted white arrow*). Where a diverticulum is seen *en face,* it produces a circular density (*solid white arrow*), which can mimic the appearance of a polyp.

obstruction. **CT is the modality of choice** for the **diagnosis of diverticulitis** since the pericolonic soft tissues can be visualized using CT, which is impossible with either barium enema or optical endoscopy.

CT findings of diverticulitis start with the **presence of diverticula** and include **thickening** of the adjacent colonic wall (>4 mm); **pericolonic inflammation**—hazy areas of increased attenuation or streaky, disorganized linear and amorphous densities in the pericolonic fat; **abscess formation**—multiple small bubbles of air or pockets of fluid contained within a pericolonic soft tissue, masslike density; and **perforation of the colon**—extraluminal air or contrast either around the site of the perforation or, less likely, free in the peritoneal cavity (Fig. 18-14).

Colonic Polyps

- The **incidence of polyps increases with age** and the **incidence of malignancy increases with the size** of the polyp. Patients with polyposis syndromes, in which multiple adenomatous polyps are present, have a much higher risk of developing a colonic malignancy.

Most colonic polyps are **hyperplastic polyps** that have **no malignant potential. Adenomatous polyps** carry a low **potential for malignancy that increases with the size of the polyp** so that those **>1.5 cm in size** have about a **10% chance of being malignant.** Therefore, early detection and removal of adenomatous polyps will decrease the chances of malignant transformation.

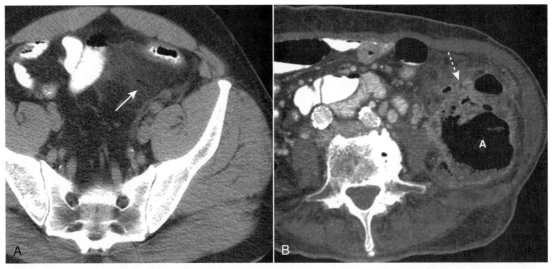

Figure 18-14 Diverticulitis, CT. A, Infiltration of the pericolonic fat is demonstrated by a hazy increase in attenuation (*solid white arrow*) of the normal fat. Focal infiltration of fat is a common characteristic of inflammatory disease. **B,** There is a large abscess cavity (*A*) in the left lower quadrant in this close-up of a CT scan of the lower abdomen. There are adjacent small bubbles of gas that are not contained within the bowel and infiltration of the normal fat (*dotted white arrow*). These findings are secondary to a confined perforation with abscess formation from diverticulitis.

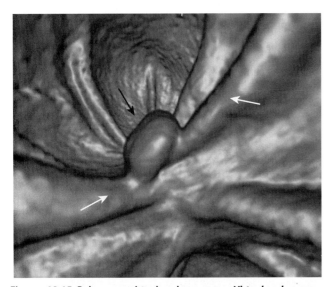

Figure 18-15 Polyp on virtual colonoscopy. *Virtual colonoscopy* utilizes CT scanning of the abdomen to allow for the three-dimensional reconstruction of the appearance of the inside of the bowel without the use of an endoscope. A polyp in the descending colon (*solid black arrow*) is seen as a distinct mass, while the normal haustral folds (*solid white arrows*) are ridgelike structures present throughout the large bowel.

- Colonic polyps can be visualized using barium enema examination, CT (virtual colonoscopy), or optical colonoscopy.
- *Virtual colonoscopy* is a technique made possible by newer, faster CT and MRI scanners and complex computer algorithms that allow for the three-dimensional reconstruction of the appearance of the inside of the bowel lumen including time-of-flight (motion) displays without the use of an endoscope. Virtual colonoscopy also allows for visualization of the other abdominal structures outside of the colon (Fig. 18-15).
- Polyps may be **sessile** (attach directly to the wall) or **pedunculated** (attach to the wall by a stalk) (Fig. 18-16). A polyp **may contain numerous fronds** that produce an irregular, wormlike surface with numerous crypts that may

contain barium (***villous polyp***). Villous polyps tend to be larger and have more of a malignant potential than other adenomatous polyps (Fig. 18-17).
- Occasionally, a polyp may serve as a ***lead point*** for an ***intussusception***, in which the polyp drags and prolapses one part of the bowel into the lumen of the bowel immediately ahead of it. The bowel proximal to the intussusception is usually obstructed and dilated. Intussusception may produce a characteristic ***coiled-spring*** appearance on barium enema or CT (Fig. 18-18).

Colonic Carcinoma

Colon cancer is the **most common cancer of the GI tract**. Most colon cancers occur in the **rectosigmoid** region and take years to develop. **Risk factors** include adenomatous polyps, ulcerative colitis and Crohn disease, polyposis syndromes, family history of colonic polyps or colon cancer, and prior pelvic irradiation.

- The imaging findings of carcinoma of the colon include the presence of a persistent, large, polypoid filling defect; annular constriction of the colonic lumen producing an **apple core lesion** (Fig. 18-19); and **frank or microperforation**—infiltration of the pericolonic fat with streaky or hazy densities of increased attenuation with or without the presence of extraluminal air.
- Other findings of carcinoma of the colon can include large bowel obstruction—either antegrade obstruction or retrograde obstruction demonstrated by the inability of rectally administered barium to pass the point of the colon cancer (Fig. 18-20) and **metastases**, especially to the liver and the lungs.

Colitis

- Colitis is **inflammation of the large bowel.** There are numerous **causes** of colitis, including infectious, ulcerative and granulomatous, ischemic, radiation-induced, and

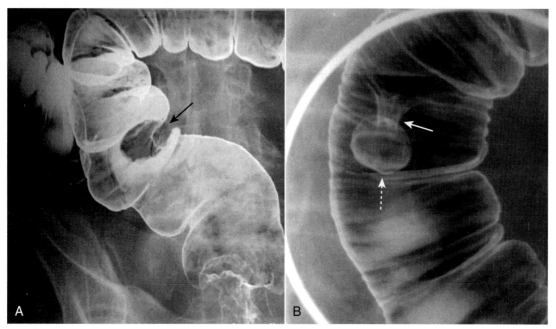

Figure 18-16 Sessile and pedunculated polyps of the colon. Polyps can be recognized as persistent filling defects in the colon; barium is displaced by the polyp. **A,** There is a *sessile* filling defect in the pool of barium along the left lateral wall of the sigmoid colon (*solid black arrow*). The size of the lesion should raise concern for malignancy. **B,** In another patient with a filling defect in the sigmoid colon etched by barium (*dotted white arrow*), the polyp is seen to be attached to the wall of the colon by a stalk (*solid white arrow*). Polyps on a stalk are called *pedunculated polyps.*

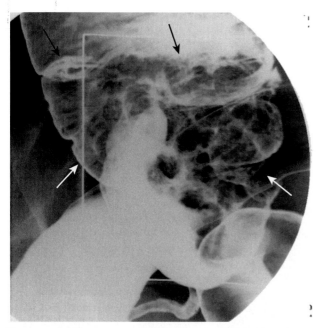

Figure 18-17 Villous tumor of cecum. There is a large, polypoid mass in the cecum (outlined by both *black* and *white solid arrows*). Contained within the mass is an interlacing network of white lines representing barium that is trapped within the interstices of the frondlike projections from this tumor. This is a characteristic appearance for a villous adenomatous tumor.

antibiotic-associated etiologies. Because many forms of colitis appear similar radiographically, clinical history is of paramount importance.

CT findings of colitis include segmental **thickening** of the bowel wall, irregular narrowing of the bowel lumen due to edema (i.e., *thumbprinting*) (Fig. 18-21), **and infiltration** of the surrounding fat.

- **Mesenteric ischemia** produces colitis due to diminished blood flow from either occlusion of vessels **(thrombus)** or from **slow flow**, as in congestive heart failure, and may differ in appearance from some of the other colitides by its lack of bowel wall enhancement with IV contrast (see Fig. 14-12). There may also be intramural or portal venous gas present (see Fig. 15-15B).

Appendicitis

- Pathophysiologically, the development of appendicitis is invariably preceded by obstruction of the appendiceal lumen. CT is now the modality of choice in diagnosing appendicitis. Appendicitis is also diagnosed using ultrasound and MRI.
- An **appendicolith is a calcified concretion found in the appendix** of about 15% of all people. It will manifest, especially on CT, as a calcification in the lumen of the appendix. The combination of **abdominal pain** and the **presence of an appendicolith** is associated with **appendicitis about 90% of the time** and indicates a higher probability for **perforation.**

The key CT findings of acute appendicitis are identification of a **dilated appendix** (> 6 mm) which does **not** fill with oral contrast; **periappendiceal inflammation—** which is evidenced by streaky, disorganized linear high-attenuation densities in the surrounding fat (Fig. 18-22A); and **increased contrast enhancement of the wall of the appendix** due to inflammation.

- **Perforation** occurs in up to 30% of cases and is **recognized by small quantities of periappendiceal extraluminal air or a periappendiceal abscess.** Since obstruction of the appendiceal lumen is a prerequisite for

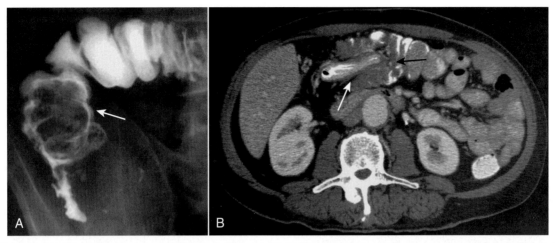

Figure 18-18 Intussusception, barium enema, and CT scan. A, When one loop of bowel prolapses inside the loop immediately distal to it, the resultant obstruction produces a ***coiled-spring*** appearance on barium enema examination as two loops of bowel are superimposed on one another (*solid white arrow*). **B,** In another patient with an intussusception, a loop of large bowel (*solid white arrow*) is seen prolapsing into the loop distal to it (*solid black arrow*) producing a filling defect and obstructing the lumen.

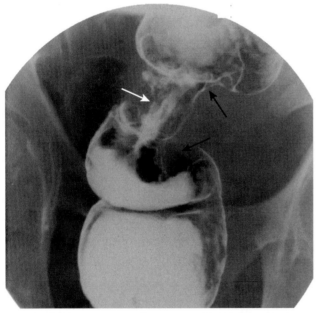

Figure 18-19 Annular constricting carcinoma of the rectum. This is a characteristic ***apple-core*** lesion of the rectum caused by circumferential growth of a colonic carcinoma. The margins of the lesion (*solid black arrows*) demonstrate what is called an ***overhanging edge*** where tumor tissue projects into and overhangs the normal lumen, typical of this type of lesion. The "core" of the "apple" (*solid white arrow*) is composed of tumor tissue—all of the normal colonic mucosa has been replaced. Identification of such a lesion is pathognomonic for carcinoma.

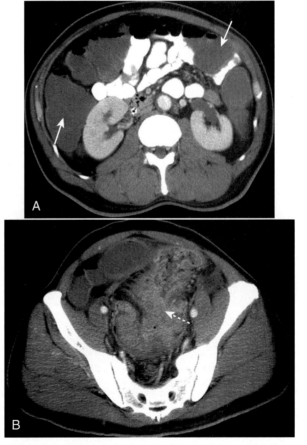

Figure 18-20 Large bowel obstruction, CT. Two CT images from the same patient demonstrate **(A)** dilated and fluid-filled loops of large bowel (*solid white arrows*). In **(B),** a large soft-tissue mass in the sigmoid (*dotted white arrow*) represents the patient's obstructing carcinoma of the sigmoid colon.

appendicitis, the presence of free intraperitoneal air should point to another diagnosis (Fig. 18-22B).

- The use of ultrasound in appendicitis will be discussed in Chapter 19.
- The **appendix** of this book (not to be surgically removed) lists the **studies of first choice** for many **different clinical scenarios** relating to **abdominal pain.**

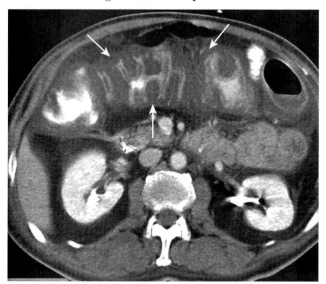

Figure 18-21 Colitis. The colon demonstrates ***thumbprinting*** (*solid white arrows*) and a pattern that is called the ***accordion sign.*** This patient had *C. difficile* colitis, formerly called pseudomembranous colitis, and now known to be caused almost exclusively by toxins produced by *Clostridium difficile.* It frequently follows antibiotic therapy. The diagnosis is usually made clinically by visualization of the pseudomembrane on endoscopy. The accordion sign represents contrast that is trapped between enlarged folds and indicates the presence of marked edema or inflammation, but it is not specific for *C. difficile* colitis.

PANCREAS

Pancreatitis

- The two **most common causes of pancreatitis** are **alcoholism** and **gallstones**. Inflammation of pancreatic tissue leading to disruption of the ducts and spillage of pancreatic juices occurs readily because of the lack of a capsule surrounding the pancreas.

> Pancreatitis is a **clinical diagnosis**, with CT serving to document either a **cause** (e.g., gallstones) or **complication** (e.g., pseudocyst formation).

- Recognizing acute pancreatitis on CT:
  - **Enlargement** of all or part of the pancreas (normal measurements for the pancreas are 3 cm for the head; 2.5 cm for the body, and 2 cm for the tail) (Fig. 18-23).
  - **Peripancreatic stranding** or **fluid collections.**
  - **Low-attenuation** lesions in the pancreas from **necrosis.** Areas of nonviable pancreas; usually develop **early** in the course of the disease; requires IV contrast administration and is important in predicting prognosis.
  - **Pseudocyst formation.** Fibrous tissue encapsulates a walled-off collection of pancreatic juices released from the inflamed pancreas. The **wall of a pseudocyst is usually visible by CT** and **may contrast-enhance** (Fig. 18-24).
- Chronic pancreatitis
  - Chronic pancreatitis is a continuous and irreversible disease of the pancreas most often secondary to **alcohol abuse** leading to **fibrosis, atrophy of the gland, ductal dilatation,** and frequently **diabetes.**

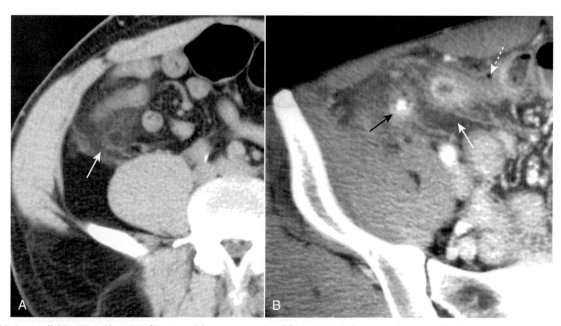

Figure 18-22 Appendicitis, CT. A, There is infiltration of the periappendiceal fat in the right lower quadrant manifest by the increased attenuation in the mesenteric fat (*solid white arrow*). Focal infiltration of fat is a common characteristic of inflammatory diseases and helps in their localization. **B,** Contained within the lumen of the appendix is a small calcification (*solid black arrow*) or ***appendicolith.*** There is inflammatory infiltration of the surrounding fat producing high attenuation (*solid white arrow*). A very small amount of air is present outside of the appendiceal lumen from a confined perforation (*dotted white arrow*). An appendicolith can be found in about one-fourth of the cases of acute appendicitis. The combination of an appendicolith and acute appendicitis is a strong predictor of a perforated appendix.

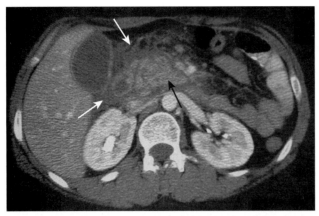

Figure 18-23 Acute pancreatitis. The body of the pancreas is enlarged (*solid black arrow*). There is infiltration of the peripancreatic fat (*solid white arrows*). These findings are consistent with acute pancreatitis in the proper clinical setting. This patient had a markedly elevated amylase and lipase.

 The **hallmarks** of the disease are **multiple, amorphous calcifications** that form within the **dilated ducts** of the atrophied gland (see Fig. 16-11).

Pancreatic Adenocarcinoma

- Risk factors for pancreatic adenocarcinoma include **alcoholism, cigarette smoking, chronic pancreatitis,** and **diabetes.** Pancreatic adenocarcinoma has an **exceedingly poor prognosis:** most tumors are unresectable and incurable at the time of diagnosis. **Most of the time** (75%), the tumor is located in the **head** of the pancreas; about 10% occur in the body, and 5% in the tail. About half of the patients present with **jaundice;** most of the time, **there is associated pain.**
- **Ultrasound is the study of choice in the initial workup of the jaundiced patient** (see Chapter 19).

 Recognizing pancreatic adenocarcinoma on CT:

- **Focal pancreatic mass,** usually **hypodense** to the remainder the gland (Fig. 18-25).
- **Ductal dilatation,** usually involving **both the pancreatic and biliary ducts.** The normal **pancreatic duct** measures **less than 4 mm** in the head and tapers to the tail; the **common duct** should be **less than 7 mm** in diameter.
- Other findings of pancreatic carcinoma include spread to contiguous organs, enlarged lymph nodes, and ascites.

HEPATOBILIARY ABNORMALITIES

Liver: General Considerations

- CT evaluation of **liver masses** is usually done with a **combination** of scans obtained **before and after intravenous contrast** injection. **Postcontrast** scans are obtained in **two phases:** one is done quickly (**hepatic-arterial phase**) and a second is done about a minute later (**portal-venous phase**), the combination helping to best define and characterize liver masses. This combination of three separate scans done **without contrast** and then during the **arterial**

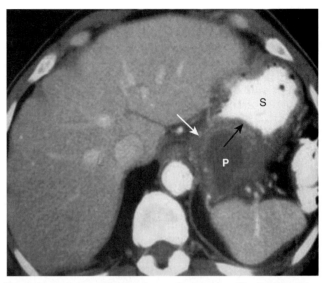

Figure 18-24 Pancreatic pseudocyst. Pseudocysts (*P*) of the pancreas occur when fibrous tissue encapsulates a walled-off collection of pancreatic juices released from the inflamed pancreas. Pseudocysts may have an enhancing wall (*solid white arrow*). The cyst is indenting a loop of adjacent bowel, in this case the posterior wall of the stomach (*S*). The indentation on a loop of bowel by an extrinsic mass is called a ***pad sign*** (*solid black arrow*).

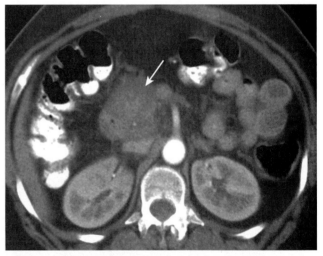

Figure 18-25 Pancreatic adenocarcinoma. The head of the pancreas is enlarged by a mass (*solid white arrow*). Normally, the head of the pancreas should roughly be the same size as the width of the lumbar vertebral body visible on the same cut. Most pancreatic adenocarcinomas are located in the head (75%), and jaundice is a common presenting sign.

phase followed by the **venous phase** is called a *triple-phase scan* (Fig. 18-26).
- **MRI** is increasingly utilized as the modality of choice in the evaluation of both focal and diffuse liver disease. MRI can often definitively characterize hepatic lesions described as indeterminate on CT scan as cysts, benign hepatic neoplasms such as hemangioma and focal nodular hyperplasia, hepatocellular carcinoma, and metastatic disease. It is **particularly useful in the evaluation of small (1 cm or less) lesions** compared to CT.
- For routine MRI imaging of the liver, an intravenous contrast agent called ***gadolinium*** is typically administered, and multiple postgadolinium enhanced images are obtained. Gadolinium will be discussed in Chapter 20.

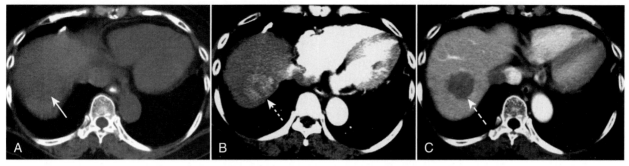

Figure 18-26 **Triple-phase CT scan of the liver, hepatocellular carcinoma.** Evaluation of liver masses is usually done with a combination of scans including an unenhanced scan **(A)** and then two postcontrast scans: one obtained quickly (hepatic-arterial phase) **(B)** and a second (portal-venous phase) slightly delayed **(C)**. The combination of three scans is called a triple-phase scan. This case shows the typical findings of a focal hepatocellular carcinoma. Most are low density (hypodense) or the same density as normal liver (isodense) without contrast (*solid white arrow* in **A**), enhance on the arterial phase with IV contrast (hyperdense) (*dotted white arrow* in **B**) and then return to hypodense or isodense on the venous phase (*dashed white arrow* in **C**).

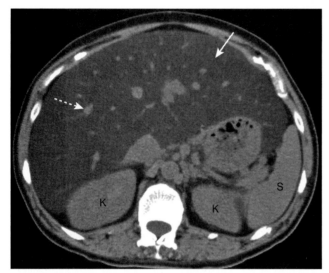

Figure 18-27 **Diffuse fatty liver (hepatic steatosis).** Normally, on noncontrast CT scans, the liver is always denser than or equal to the density of the spleen. In this patient with diffuse fatty infiltration of the liver, the spleen (*S*) is denser than the liver (*solid white arrow*). Notice how the vessels stand out in the fatty liver (*dotted white arrow*). (*K* = kidneys.)

Fatty Infiltration

Fatty infiltration (also known as *hepatic steatosis*) of the liver is a **very common** abnormality in which there is fat accumulation in the hepatocytes in such diseases as alcoholism, obesity, diabetes, hepatitis, or cirrhosis. Most patients with a fatty liver are **asymptomatic**. The **fatty infiltration** may be **diffuse** or **focal**, and focal lesions may be **solitary** or **multiple**.

- When diffuse, the **liver is usually slightly enlarged.** The **blood vessels stand out prominently** but are usually **neither obstructed nor displaced.**
- Normally, on noncontrast CT scans, the liver is always **denser than or equal to the density of the spleen. With fatty infiltration of the liver, the spleen is denser than the liver** without intravenous contrast (Fig. 18-27).

Focal fatty infiltration can produce an appearance that **mimics tumor,** but fatty infiltration usually produces **no mass effect** and has the ability to **appear and disappear** in a matter of weeks, quite unlike tumor masses.

- **MRI is the most accurate modality in the evaluation of a fatty liver,** using a phenomenon called *chemical shift imaging* to detect the presence of microscopic, intracellular lipid present in such a liver. Chemical shift relates to the way that lipid and water protons behave in the magnetic field (Fig. 18-28).

Cirrhosis

- Cirrhosis is a chronic, irreversible disease of the liver which features destruction of normal liver cells and diffuse fibrosis and appears to be the final common pathway of many abnormalities including **hepatitis B and C, alcoholism, nonalcoholic fatty infiltration of the liver,** and miscellaneous diseases like **hemochromatosis** and **Wilson disease.** Complications of cirrhosis include **portal hypertension, ascites, renal dysfunction, hepatocellular carcinoma, hepatic failure,** and **death.**

Recognizing cirrhosis of the liver on CT:

- **Early** in the disease, the liver may demonstrate **diffuse fatty infiltration.** As the disease progresses, the liver **contour becomes lobulated.** The **liver shrinks in volume** with the **right lobe** characteristically becoming **smaller** while the **caudate lobe and left lobe become disproportionately larger,** especially in alcoholic cirrhosis (Fig. 18-29).
- There is a **mottled, inhomogeneous** appearance to the liver parenchyma following intravenous contrast enhancement due to a mixture of regenerating nodules, focal fatty infiltration, and fibrosis.
- **Portal hypertension** may develop which can lead to **dilated vessels** around the stomach, splenic hilum, and esophagus representing **varices.**
- **Splenomegaly** may develop.

Ascites may be present. Sometimes it can be difficult to differentiate between ascites and pleural effusion on CT examinations (Box 18-1, Fig. 18-30).

Space-Occupying Lesions of the Liver

- One of the primary aims of imaging studies, no matter what part of the body is being studied, is to accurately

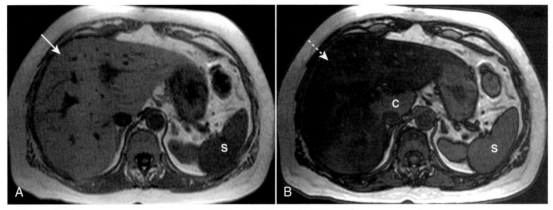

Figure 18-28 Fatty liver, MRI. Using a phenomenon called **chemical shift imaging** to detect the presence of microscopic, intracellular lipid present in a fatty liver, MRI is the most accurate imaging modality in identifying a fatty liver. Chemical shift relates to the way that lipid and water protons behave in the magnetic field. **A,** The liver (*solid white arrow*) appears normal, brighter than the spleen (*S*). **B,** This is called an **opposed-phase image,** and it demonstrates marked signal loss (signal dropout) throughout the liver (*dotted white arrow*), indicating a fatty liver. Most of the liver is now darker than the spleen (*S*), except for the caudate lobe (*C*), which is normal.

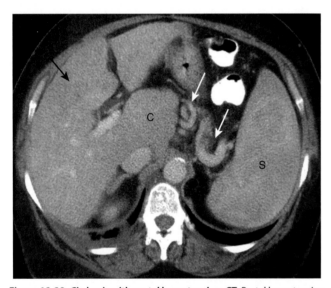

Figure 18-29 Cirrhosis with portal hypertension, CT. Portal hypertension can lead to dilated vessels around the stomach, splenic hilum (*solid white arrows*), and esophagus representing varices. Splenomegaly may develop (*S*). There is characteristic enlargement of the caudate lobe (*C*) relative to the right lobe of the liver (*solid black arrow*), especially in alcoholic cirrhosis.

Box 18-1 Differentiating Ascites from Pleural Effusion

Patients may have a combination of ascites and pleural effusion for a number of reasons, including cirrhosis, ovarian tumors, metastatic disease, hypoproteinemia, and congestive heart failure.

Differentiating between ascitic fluid and pleural fluid at the lung base on CT examinations may be difficult because both may appear posterior to the liver.

Ascitic fluid will appear **anterior to the hemidiaphragm** in the axial plane (see Fig. 18-30A).

Pleural effusion will be located **posterior to the hemidiaphragm.**

Ascitic fluid **will not spread to the "bare" area of the liver posteriorly** where there is no peritoneal lining.

Therefore, **fluid that appears posterior to the bare area is pleural in location** (see Fig. 18-30B).

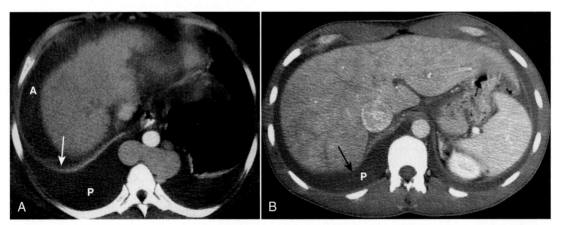

Figure 18-30 Differentiating pleural effusion from ascites. A, Patients may have a combination of ascites (*A*) and pleural effusions (*P*) for a number of reasons, cirrhosis being one of them. Ascitic fluid will appear anterior to the hemidiaphragm (*solid white arrow*) in the axial plane. Pleural effusion will be located posterior to the hemidiaphragm. **B,** Ascites will never completely encircle the liver because of the "bare area" (*solid black arrow*), not covered by peritoneum. Fluid posterior to the bare area must be in the pleural space (*P*).

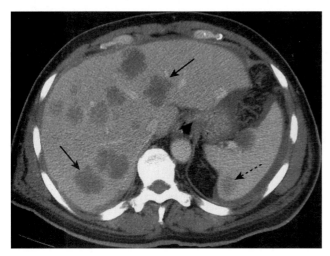

Figure 18-31 Metastases to the liver and spleen. Metastases usually appear as multiple, low-attenuation masses (*solid black arrows*). There are also low-attenuation lesions in the spleen (*dotted black arrow*). The patient had a primary adenocarcinoma of the colon.

differentiate between benign and malignant processes using techniques that do not place the patient in danger or subject the patient to unnecessary pain. This is the central goal in evaluating liver masses as well.

- CT studies are best at demonstrating liver masses when performed **both with and without contrast** because either study alone may fail to reveal an *isodense* mass, i.e., one that has the identical attenuation as the surrounding normal tissue.
- **MRI is useful in characterizing liver masses**, particularly small lesions 1 cm or less.

Metastases

Metastases are the **most common malignant hepatic masses**. While **most are multiple**, metastases also represent the **most common cause** of a **solitary malignant mass** in the liver.

- **Most liver metastases originate in the gastrointestinal tract,** particularly the **colon,** and almost all reach the liver via the bloodstream. Other primary sites of metastatic spread to the liver include stomach, pancreas, esophagus, lung, melanoma, and breast.
- **Recognizing liver metastases on CT and MRI:**
  - Metastases are usually **multiple, low-attenuation masses** (Fig. 18-31). **Larger metastases** may demonstrate areas of necrosis that can be recognized as mottled areas of low attenuation within the mass. **Mucin-producing carcinomas,** such as might originate in the stomach, colon, or ovary, can **calcify** both the primary tumor and the metastases (see Fig. 16-14).
  - **MRI** is **as sensitive** as CT in detecting liver metastases but is usually used in a **problem-solving role**. In general, MRI is more expensive than CT scanning and may suffer from more motion artifact than CT.

Hepatocellular Carcinoma (Hepatoma)

- Hepatocellular carcinoma is the most **common primary malignancy** of the liver. Virtually all arise in livers with

preexisting abnormalities such as **cirrhosis** or **hepatitis**. **Most are solitary**, but up to one out of five can be multiple, mimicking metastases. **Vascular invasion is common**, particularly of the portal system.

- **Recognizing hepatocellular carcinoma (HCC) on CT and MRI:**
  - There are **three patterns** of presentation for hepatocellular carcinoma: **solitary mass**, large **multiple nodules**, **diffuse infiltration** throughout a segment, lobe or the entire liver (see Fig. 18-26).
  - On CT, most HCCs are **low density (hypodense)** or the same density as normal liver **(isodense) without contrast**, enhance on the **arterial phase** with IV contrast **(hyperdense)** and then return to **hypodense** or **isodense** on the **venous phase** (Fig. 18-32).
  - Low attenuation areas from **necrosis** are common. **Calcification** occurs relatively frequently.
  - **MRI** can demonstrate certain features that are fairly specific for **hepatocellular carcinoma**, as well as detect intrahepatic metastases and venous invasion. Unlike benign lesions like hemangiomas of the liver which tend to retain intravenously-administered gadolinium contrast, hepatocellular carcinomas **show washout** of the contrast material.

Cavernous Hemangiomas

Cavernous hemangiomas are the **most common primary liver tumor** and **second in frequency to metastases for localized liver masses**. They are more common in **women**, are usually **solitary** and are almost always **asymptomatic**. They are complex structures composed of multiple, large vascular channels lined by a single layer of endothelial cells.

- **Recognizing cavernous hemangiomas of the liver on CT and MRI:**
  - **Cavernous hemangiomas are usually hypodense lesions on unenhanced CT scans**; they have a characteristic nodular enhancement **from the periphery** inward following injection of intravenous contrast and **become isodense** in the venous phase.
  - Contrast tends to be **retained** within the numerous vascular spaces of the lesion so that they characteristically appear **denser than the rest of the liver on delayed** (10 minute) **scans** (Fig. 18-33).
  - **MRI is frequently the preferred modality** in the evaluation of hemangiomas, as it is **more sensitive** than a nuclear medicine tagged red blood cell scan and more specific than a multiphase CT scan.
  - Similar to CT, **hemangiomas on MRI** usually have a characteristic nodular enhancement from the periphery inward following injection of intravenous contrast. Contrast tends to be retained within the numerous vascular spaces of hemangiomas so that they characteristically appear brighter than the rest of the liver on delayed (10 minute) scans (Fig. 18-34).

Hepatic Cysts

- Believed to be **congenital** in origin, they are easily identified as **sharply marginated**, spherical lesions of **low**

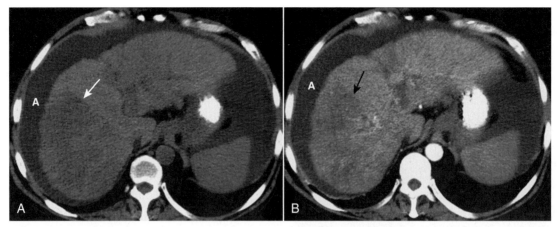

Figure 18-32 Diffuse hepatocellular carcinoma of the liver, CT. There are three patterns of appearance for hepatocellular carcinoma: solitary mass (see Fig. 18-26), multiple nodules and diffuse infiltration throughout a segment, lobe (as in this case), or the entire liver. **A,** A typical low-attenuation lesion is seen in the right lobe of the liver on the nonenhanced scan (*solid white arrow*). **B,** The arterial phase demonstrates patchy enhancement (*solid black arrow*) indicating the probability of tumor necrosis in the low-attenuation areas. There is ascites present (*A*). The overall volume of the liver is decreased, and the contour is lobulated from underlying cirrhosis.

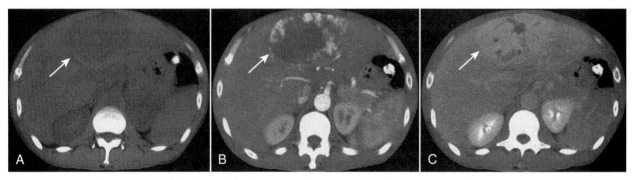

Figure 18-33 Cavernous hemangioma of the liver, triple-phase CT study. (A) Cavernous hemangiomas (*solid white arrow* on all images) are usually hypodense lesions on unenhanced scans. They characteristically enhance from the periphery inward following injection of intravenous contrast during the arterial phase **(B)** and eventually become isodense. Contrast then tends to be retained within the numerous vascular spaces of the lesion so that it characteristically appears denser than the rest of the liver on delayed scans **(C).**

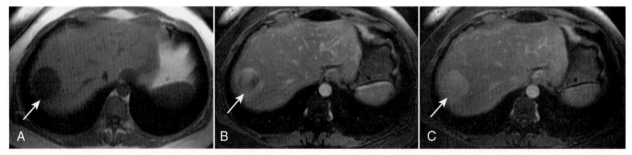

Figure 18-34 Cavernous hemangioma of the liver, MRI. (A) This image (an axial T1-weighted image) demonstrates a well-circumscribed, slightly lobular dark mass in the right hepatic lobe (*solid white arrow* in all images). **(B)** Subsequent images following the administration of intravenous contrast (gadolinium) show peripheral-to-central enhancement, until the entire mass homogeneously enhances on a delayed 10-minute image **(C).** The combination of this enhancement pattern and the signal characteristics of the lesion allows an unequivocal diagnosis of hemangioma.

attenuation (fluid density) compared to the remainder of the liver, on both unenhanced and enhanced CT scans. MRI is much better than CT at characterizing cysts. They are usually **solitary** and are **homogeneous** in density (Fig. 18-35).

Biliary System: Magnetic Resonance Cholangiopancreatography (MRCP)

- MRCP (magnetic resonance cholangiopancreatography) is a **noninvasive** way to image the biliary tree **without**

requiring injection of contrast material. MRCP utilizes MRI imaging sequences that make fluid-filled structures like the bile ducts, pancreatic ducts and gallbladder extremely bright, and everything else dark. Patients are imaged during a single-breath hold.

- MRCP is excellent at depicting **biliary or ductal strictures, ductal dilatation, stones in the bile ducts (choledocholithiasis), gallstones, adenomyomatosis of the gallbladder, choledochal cysts, and pancreas divisum**.
- If there is a concern for malignancy (such as pancreatic adenocarcinoma or cholangiocarcinoma) as the cause of

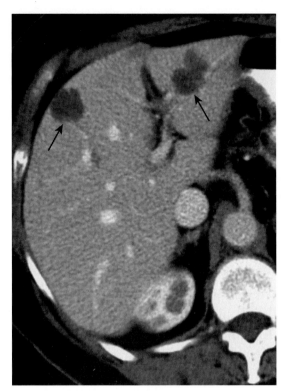

Figure 18-35 Hepatic cysts, CT. Believed to be congenital in origin, hepatic cysts are easily identified as sharply marginated, spherical lesions of low attenuation (fluid density), compared to the remainder of the liver on both unenhanced and enhanced scans (*solid black arrows*). They are homogeneous in density.

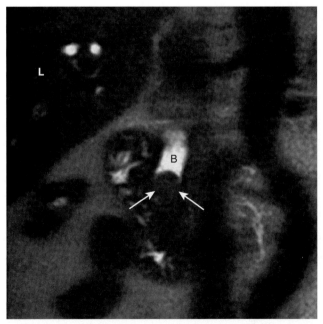

Figure 18-36 Choledocholithiasis and biliary ductal dilatation on magnetic resonance cholangiopancreatography (MRCP). This is a coronal close-up of the right upper quadrant utilizing MR imaging. There is a large obstructing gallstone (*solid white arrows*) in the distal common bile duct (*B*), which is dilated to 13 mm. Because of the signal characteristics of bile, an MRCP can be done without the need for the injection of contrast. (*L* = liver.)

pancreaticobiliary ductal dilatation, then additional pulse sequences following the administration of gadolinium can be obtained. Contrast administration allows better detection of malignancy (Fig. 18-36).

URINARY TRACT

Kidneys: General Considerations

- The kidneys are retroperitoneal organs, encircled by varying amounts of fat and enclosed within a fibrous capsule. So long as they are functioning properly, the **kidneys are the route** through which intravenously injected, iodinated **contrast and gadolinium-based MRI contrast agents are excreted from the body**.
- Following injection of iodinated contrast agents, the kidneys should therefore **enhance**. If the kidneys are not functioning properly, iodinated contrast is excreted though alternative pathways (bile, bowel), a process called *vicarious excretion* of contrast.
- Ultrasound is utilized in the characterization of renal masses, particularly in assessing their cystic or solid nature and involvement of the collecting system or surrounding vessels.

Space-Occupying Lesions

Renal Cysts

- Simple renal cysts are a **very common** finding on CT and US scans of the abdomen occurring in more than half of the population over 55 years of age.
- Simple cysts are **benign, fluid-filled** structures which are frequently **multiple** and **bilateral**. On CT scans, they tend to have a **sharp margin** where they meet the normal renal parenchyma. They have density measurements (Hounsfield numbers) of **water density** (−10 to +20). They **do not contrast-enhance** (Fig. 18-37A).
- On **ultrasound examinations**, simple cysts are **echo-free** (anechoic) masses with **strong through transmission** of the ultrasound signal; they have **sharp borders** where they meet the renal parenchyma and **round or oval shapes**. Thickening of the wall or dense internal echoes raise suspicion for a malignant lesion (Fig. 18-37B).

Renal Cell Carcinoma (Hypernephroma)

- Renal cell carcinoma is the **most common primary renal malignancy in adults**. Solid masses in the kidneys of adults are usually renal cell carcinomas. They have a propensity for **extending into the renal veins**, into the **inferior vena cava** and producing **nodules in the lung**.
- When they metastasize to bone, they are **purely lytic** and **often expansile**.

➡ Recognizing renal cell carcinoma on CT:

- A dedicated CT scan for renal cell carcinoma usually consists of images obtained before and after intravenous contrast administration.
- Ranging from **completely solid** to **completely cystic**, renal cell carcinomas are **usually solid lesions which may**

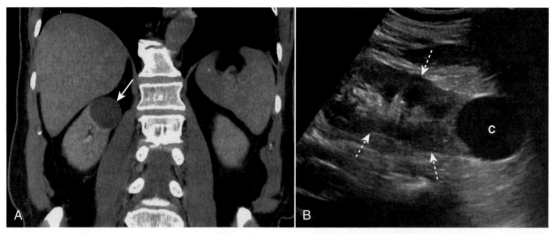

Figure 18-37 Renal cysts, CT urogram and US. A, This is an image from a CT urogram that demonstrates a low-attenuation mass (*solid white arrow*) in the upper pole of the right kidney, which is homogeneous in density and sharply marginated. These findings are characteristic of a simple cyst. **B,** A sagittal ultrasound of the kidney (*dotted white arrows*) demonstrates an anechoic mass (*C*) with features consistent with a simple cyst of the lower pole.

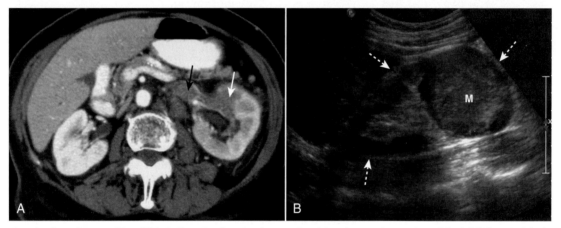

Figure 18-38 Renal cell carcinomas CT and US. A, There is a low-density mass involving the anterior portion of the left kidney (*solid white arrow*). The tumor is seen to extend directly into the left renal vein (*solid black arrow*), a propensity for renal cell carcinomas. **B,** Sagittal ultrasound on another patient with renal cell carcinoma shows an echogenic mass (*M*) occupying the mid portion of the kidney (*dotted white arrows*).

contain **low-attenuation areas of necrosis**. Even though renal cell carcinomas **enhance with intravenous contrast**, they still tend to remain **lower in density than the surrounding normal kidney**.

- **Renal vein invasion occurs in up to one in three cases** and may produce filling defects in the lumen of the renal veins (Fig. 18-38A).
- On **ultrasound**, smaller renal cell carcinomas are **usually hyperechoic**; as the lesion increases in size and undergoes necrosis it may be hypoechoic. Its wall, however, should be thicker and more irregular than a simple cyst (Fig. 18-38B).
- The primary role of **MRI of the kidneys** is in the evaluation of **small masses** less than 1.5 cm or in any renal mass characterized as indeterminate for malignancy by either CT or US.

PELVIS

General Considerations

- **Ultrasound is the study of first choice in evaluation of suspected abnormalities of the female pelvis** (see Chapter 19).
- **MRI** (see Chapter 20) has assumed an increasingly important role in defining the anatomy of the uterus and ovaries

and in clarifying questions about patients in whom US findings are confusing. MRI is also used in staging and surgical planning.

- MRI can be particularly useful in evaluating ovarian dermoid cysts, endometriosis, hydrosalpinges (fluid-filled fallopian tubes), and in determining whether an ovarian cystic lesion is simple (benign) or contains a solid component (often malignant).

URINARY BLADDER

Bladder Tumors

- Most malignant bladder tumors are **transitional cell tumors**. Transitional tumors may occur simultaneously anywhere along the uroepithelium from the bladder to the ureter to the kidney. The **primary tumor** appears as **focal thickening of the bladder wall** or may produce a **filling defect in the contrast-filled bladder** (Fig. 18-39).

Adenopathy

- Lymphoma can involve any part of the GI or GU tract. While thoracic lymphoma is almost always due to Hodgkin

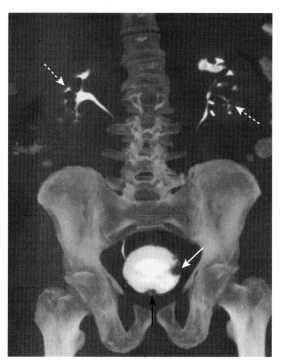

Figure 18-39 Transitional cell carcinoma of the bladder, CT urogram. There is a filling defect in the left lateral wall of the contrast-filled bladder (*solid white arrow*) representing a tumor. The defect at the base of the bladder (*solid black arrow*) is caused by the prostate gland. The calyceal collecting systems (*dotted white arrows*) are normal.

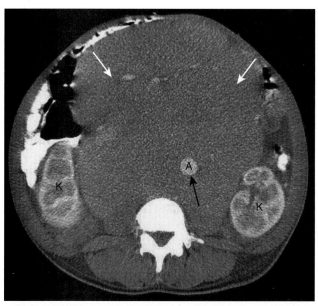

Figure 18-40 Massive lymphadenopathy, lymphoma. There is massive abdominal lymphadenopathy occupying most of the abdomen (*solid white arrows*) and displacing the kidneys (*K*) laterally and the aorta (*A*) anteriorly far from its normal location next to the spine (*solid black arrow*). The patient had non-Hodgkin lymphoma.

disease, **the stomach is the most common extranodal site of gastrointestinal non-Hodgkin lymphoma.**

■ Extranodal involvement and noncontiguous spread to other organs or nodes are features of non-Hodgkin lymphoma.

 Recognizing the CT findings of lymphoma:

■ **Multiple enlarged lymph nodes.** Pelvic lymph nodes are considered pathologically enlarged if they exceed 1 cm in their shortest dimension.
■ **Conglomerate masses of coalesced nodes.** Bulky tumor masses that can encase and obstruct vessels.
■ Lymphadenopathy will classically **displace the aorta and/or vena cava anteriorly** (Fig. 18-40).
■ Other malignancies can produce abdominal or pelvic adenopathy besides lymphoma. Even benign disease like sarcoid can produce abdominal adenopathy.

· ·

WEBLINK

Registered users may obtain more information on Recognizing Gastrointestinal, Hepatic, and Urinary Tract Abnormalities on StudentConsult.com.

🏠 TAKE-HOME POINTS

Recognizing Gastrointestinal, Hepatic, and Urinary Tract Abnormalities

CT, ultrasound, and MRI have essentially replaced conventional radiography and, in some instances, barium studies for the evaluation of the GI tract.

Esophageal diverticula occur in the neck (Zenker), around the carina (traction) and just above the diaphragm (epiphrenic); only the Zenker diverticulum tends to produce symptoms.

Esophageal carcinoma has a poor prognosis with an increasing incidence of adenocarcinomas forming in Barrett esophagus, a condition in which GERD plays a major role in stimulating metaplasia of the squamous to columnar epithelium.

Esophageal carcinomas appear in one or more forms, including an annular-constricting lesion, a polypoid mass, and a superficial, infiltrating type lesion.

Hiatal hernias are a common abnormality that may be associated with GERD, although GERD can occur even in the absence of a demonstrable hernia; they are usually of the sliding variety in which the EG junction lies above the diaphragm.

The radiologic findings of *gastric ulcer* include a persistent collection of barium that extends outward from the lumen beyond the normal contours of the stomach, usually along the lesser curvature or posterior wall in the region of the body or antrum; the ulcer may have radiating folds which extend to the ulcer margin and a surrounding margin of edema.

The key finding in *gastric carcinoma* is a mass that protrudes into the lumen and produces a filling defect, displacing barium; gastric carcinomas may be associated with rigidity of the wall, nondistensibility of the lumen, and irregular ulceration or thickening of the gastric folds (>1 cm), especially localized to one area of the stomach.

The radiologic findings of *duodenal ulcers* include a persistent collection of contrast, more often seen *en face* with surrounding spasm and edema. Healing of duodenal ulcers produces scarring and deformity of the bulb.

Any imaging evaluation of the bowel should ideally be carried out with the bowel distended with air or contrast because collapsed and unopacified loops of bowel can introduce artifactual errors of diagnosis.

Key abnormal findings of bowel disease on CT are thickening of the bowel wall, submucosal edema or hemorrhage, hazy infiltration of fat, and extraluminal air or contrast.

Crohn disease is a chronic, relapsing, granulomatous inflammation of the small bowel and colon, usually involving the terminal ileum, resulting in ulceration, obstruction, and fistula formation; it may have skip areas, is prone to fistula formation, and has a propensity for recurring following surgical removal of an involved segment.

Colonic *diverticulosis* increases in incidence with increasing age, most often involves the sigmoid colon, and is almost always asymptomatic, although it can lead to diverticulitis or massive GI bleeding, especially from right-sided diverticula.

CT is the study of choice for imaging *diverticulitis*; the findings include pericolonic inflammation, thickening of the adjacent colonic wall (>4 mm), abscess formation and confined perforation of the colon.

Most *colonic polyps* are hyperplastic and have no malignant potential; adenomatous polyps carry a malignant potential that is related, in part, to their size. Colonic polyps can be visualized using barium enema examination, CT (virtual colonoscopy), or optical colonoscopy.

Imaging signs of colonic polyps include a persistent filling defect in the colon with or without a stalk; some larger, villous adenomatous polyps have a higher malignant potential and may contain barium within the interstices of their fronds.

The imaging findings of *colonic carcinoma* are a persistent, large, polypoid or annular constricting filling defect of the colon which may have frank or micro-perforation or large bowel obstruction and metastases, especially to the liver and the lungs.

Colitis of any etiology can cause thickening of the bowel wall, narrowing of the lumen, and infiltration of the surrounding fat.

CT is the study of choice in diagnosing *appendicitis*. Findings include a dilated appendix (>6 mm) that does not fill with oral contrast, periappendiceal inflammation, increased enhancement of the wall of the appendix with intravenous contrast, and sometimes identification of an appendicolith (fecolith).

The two most common causes of *pancreatitis* are gallstones and alcoholism; pancreatitis is a clinical diagnosis, with CT serving to document a cause or a complication of the disease; CT findings include enlargement of the pancreas, peripancreatic stranding, pancreatic necrosis, and pseudocyst formation.

Pancreatic adenocarcinoma has a very unfavorable prognosis, occurs most often in the pancreatic head, and usually manifests as a focal hypodense mass, which may be associated with dilatation of the pancreatic and/or biliary ducts.

Fatty infiltration of the liver is very common and can produce focal or diffuse areas of decreased attenuation that characteristically do not displace or obstruct the hepatic vessels; the liver appears less dense than the spleen.

In its later stages, *cirrhosis* produces a small liver (especially the right lobe) with a lobulated contour, inhomogeneous appearance of the parenchyma, prominent left and caudate lobes, splenomegaly, varices, and ascites.

Evaluation of liver masses is frequently done utilizing a *triple-phase scan* that includes a precontrast scan and two postcontrast scans, one in the hepatic-arterial phase and then another in the portal venous phase.

Metastases are the most common malignant hepatic masses; metastases mostly originate in the GI tract and appear as multiple, low-density masses that may necrose as they become larger.

Hepatocellular carcinoma is the most common primary hepatic malignancy; these lesions are usually solitary and typically enhance with IV contrast on CT.

Cavernous hemangiomas are usually solitary, more common in females, and typically produce no symptoms; they have a characteristic centripetal pattern of enhancement and frequently retain contrast longer than the remainder of the liver.

MRCP (magnetic resonance cholangiopancreatography) is a noninvasive way to image the biliary tree without requiring injection of contrast material; it can be used to demonstrate biliary strictures, gallstones, and congenital anomalies.

Renal cysts are a very common finding, are frequently multiple and bilateral, do not enhance, and typically have sharp margins where they meet the normal renal parenchyma. On US, simple cysts are well-defined anechoic masses.

Renal cell carcinoma is the most common primary renal malignancy and shows a propensity for extension into the renal vein and for metastasizing to lung and bone; on CT, it is usually a solid mass that enhances with IV contrast but remains less dense than the normal kidney. On US, renal cell carcinomas are frequently echogenic masses.

Ultrasound is the imaging study of first choice in evaluating the female pelvis.

Abdominal and pelvic adenopathy may be caused by lymphoma, other malignancies, or benign diseases like sarcoid; multiple enlarged nodes or conglomerate masses of nodes may be seen on CT.

Chapter 19

Ultrasonography: Understanding the Principles and Recognizing Normal and Abnormal Findings

- *Ultrasound (US)* occupies an acoustical frequency that is hundreds of times greater than humans can hear. *Ultrasonography* is the medical imaging modality that utilizes that acoustical energy to localize and characterize human tissues.

HOW IT WORKS

- The creation of a sonographic image (*sonogram*) depends on three major components: the production of a high frequency sound wave, the reception of a reflected wave or echo, and the conversion of that echo into the actual image.
- The sound wave is produced by a *probe* that contains one of more *transducers,* which send out extremely short bursts of acoustical energy at a given frequency.
  - For most imaging, the probe is placed **externally on the skin surface** and moved by the sonographer who sweeps the probe back and forth over the area to be scanned while viewing the images obtained in real time on a monitor. In order to produce the best contact between the probe and the skin, a coupling gel is applied to the skin surface first.
  - On occasion, more detailed images can be obtained by inserting the probe into the body, such as is done with *transvaginal, transrectal,* and *transesophageal* sonography.
- Like all sound waves, the pulses produced by the transducer travel at different speeds depending on the **density** of the medium through which they are traveling.
- Where the wave strikes an **interface** between tissues of **differing densities,** some of the sound will be **transmitted forward** while some will be **reflected back** to the transducer.

How much sound is transmitted versus how much is reflected is a property of the tissues that make up the interface and is called the *acoustical impedance.* Large **differences** in acoustical impedance will result in **greater sound reflection; small differences** will result in **greater transmission.**

- If the pulse encounters **fluid,** most of the acoustical energy is **transmitted.** If the pulse encounters **gas or bone,** so much of the acoustical energy is **reflected** back that it is usually not possible to define deeper structures.
- When the echo arrives back at the transducer (a matter of microseconds), it is converted from sound into electrical pulses that are then sent to the scanner itself.

- Using an on-board computer, the scanner determines the length of **time** it took for the echo to be received, the **frequency** of the reflected echo, and the magnitude or **amplitude** of the signal. With this information, a sonographic image of the scanned body part can be generated by the computer and recorded digitally, on film, or sometimes on videotape.
- A tissue that reflects many echoes is said to be **echogenic (hyperechoic)** and is usually depicted as **bright or white** on the sonogram; a tissue that has few or no echoes is said to be **sonolucent (hypoechoic or anechoic)** and is usually depicted as being **dark or black.**

Images can be produced in any plane by adjusting the direction of the probe. By convention, two **common imaging planes** utilized are those **along the long axis** of the body or body part being scanned, called the **sagittal or longitudinal plane,** or **perpendicular to the long axis** of the body or body part being scanned, called the **transverse plane.**

- Also by convention, sonographic images are viewed with the patient's **head** to your **left** and the patient's **feet** toward your **right; anterior** is **up** and **posterior** is **down.**
- There are several types of ultrasound used in medical imaging. They are described in Table 19-1.

DOPPLER ULTRASONOGRAPHY

- You are probably familiar with the common examples of a passing train whistle or police siren as illustrations of the *Doppler effect,* which generally states that sound changes in frequency as the object producing the sound approaches or recedes from your ear.
- Sonography makes use of the Doppler effect to determine if an object, usually blood, is **moving toward** or **away** from the transducer and at what **velocity** it is moving.
  - The transducer sends out a signal of known frequency; the frequency of the echo returned is compared to the known frequency of the original signal.
  - If the returned echo has a **lower frequency** than the original, then the object is **moving away** from the transducer. If the returned echo has a **higher frequency** than the original, then the object is **moving toward** the transducer.

The **direction of flow** of blood is represented sonographically by the colors **red and blue.** By convention, **red indicates flow toward** and **blue indicates flow away** from the transducer.

TABLE 19-1 TYPES OF ULTRASOUND

A-Mode	Simplest; spikes along a line represent the signal amplitude at a certain depth; used mainly in ophthalmology.
B-Mode	Mode most often used in diagnostic imaging; each echo is depicted as a dot and the sonogram is made up of thousands of these dots; can depict real-time motion.
M-Mode	Used to show moving structures such as blood flow or motion of the heart valves.
Doppler	Uses the Doppler effect to assess blood flow; used for vascular ultrasound. *Pulsed Doppler* devices emit short bursts of energy that allow for an accurate localization of the echo source and has replaced continuous wave Doppler.
Duplex ultrasonography	Utilized in vascular studies; refers to the simultaneous use of both gray-scale or color Doppler to visualize the structure of and flow within a vessel and spectral waveform Doppler to quantitate flow.

TABLE 19-2 ADVANTAGES AND DISADVANTAGES OF ULTRASONOGRAPHY

Advantages	Disadvantages
No ionizing radiation	Difficulty penetrating through bone
No known long-term side effects	Gas-filled structures reduce its utility
"Real-time" images	Obese patients may be difficult to penetrate
Produces little or no patient discomfort	Dependent on the skills of the operator scanning
Small, portable, inexpensive, ubiquitous	

ADVERSE EFFECTS AND SAFETY ISSUES

- The procedure is **well tolerated**. Scans can be obtained quickly, done at the bedside if necessary, and, for the most part, require no patient preparation other than eating no food before abdominal studies (Table 19-2).
- Ultrasound has the short-term potential to cause **minor elevation of heat** in the area being scanned, though not at levels used in diagnosis.

> There are **no known long-term side effects** that have been scientifically demonstrated from the use of medical ultrasound in humans. Nevertheless, like all medical procedures, it should be utilized only when medically necessary. The U.S. Food and Drug Administration warns against the use of ultrasound during pregnancy to produce "keepsake photos or videos."

MEDICAL USES OF ULTRASONOGRAPHY

- **Ultrasound is widely used in medical imaging.** It is usually **the study of first choice** in imaging the female pelvis and in pediatric patients, in differentiating cystic versus solid lesions in all patients, in noninvasive vascular imaging, imaging of the fetus and placenta during pregnancy, and in real-time, image-guided fluid aspiration and biopsies.

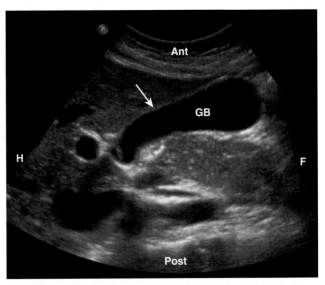

Figure 19-1 Normal gallbladder, sagittal view. The gallbladder (*GB*) is normally filled with bile and is sonolucent. The wall of the gallbladder is less than 3 mm in size and slightly echogenic (*solid white arrow*). By convention on a sagittal view, the patient's head is to your left (*H*), feet to your right (*F*), anterior is up (*Ant*), and posterior is down (*Post*).

- Other common uses are evaluation of cystic versus solid breast masses, thyroid nodules, tendons, and in assessing the brain, hips, and spine in newborns. Ultrasound is used everywhere from intraoperative scanning in the surgical suite to the medical unit in the battlefield and in locations as remote as the South Pole.
- We will look at several common abnormalities in which ultrasound plays a primary imaging role.

BILIARY SYSTEM

- **Ultrasound is the study of first choice for abnormalities of the biliary system.** Patients who present with the relatively common complaint of right upper quadrant pain usually undergo an ultrasound examination first. CT may be helpful in cases with difficult or unusual anatomy, for detecting masses, or in determining the extent of disease already diagnosed, but **CT is less sensitive than ultrasound in detecting gallstones.**

Normal Ultrasound Anatomy

- The **gallbladder** is an elliptical sac that lies inferior and medial to the right lobe of the liver. Although different layers of its wall have different echogenic properties, the gallbladder overall consists of a fluid-filled **sonolucent lumen** surrounded by an **echogenic wall.** In the fasting patient, the gallbladder is about **4 × 10 cm in size** and the **wall is normally no thicker than 3 mm** (Fig. 19-1).

Gallstones and Acute Cholecystitis

- **Cholelithiasis** is estimated to affect more than 20 million Americans. In almost all cases, acute cholecystitis starts with a gallstone **impacted in the neck of the gallbladder or cystic duct.** The presence of gallstones does not, by itself, mean that the patient's pain is from the gallbladder

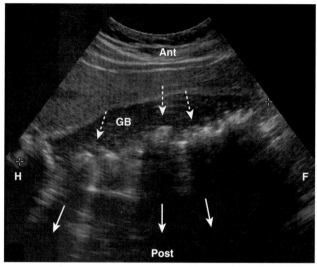

Figure 19-2 Cholelithiasis, sagittal view. There are numerous echogenic stones (*dotted white arrows*) in the gallbladder (*GB*). The stones cast acoustical shadows as they reflect most of the sound waves (*solid white arrows*).

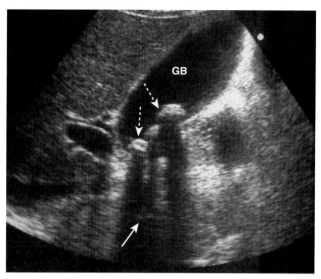

Figure 19-3 Acoustical shadowing. There is a band of reduced echoes (*solid white arrow*) behind echogenic gallstones (*dotted white arrows*) that reflect most, but not all, of the sound waves. The presence of acoustical shadowing can have diagnostic value in identifying the presence of calculi in the gallbladder (*GB*).

because asymptomatic gallstones are common. Cholecystitis can also occur less commonly in the absence of stones (*acalculous cholecystitis*).

■ **Gallstones usually fall to the most dependent part of gallbladder,** which will depend on the patient's position at the time of the scan. This helps to differentiate gallstones from polyps or tumors, which may be attached to a nondependent surface. Gallstones are characteristically **echogenic** and produce *acoustical shadowing* because they reflect most of the signal (Fig. 19-2).

Acoustical shadowing describes a band of reduced echoes behind an echo-dense object (e.g., a gallstone) that reflects most, but not all, of the sound waves. While acoustical shadowing reduces the diagnostic effectiveness of ultrasound through such tissues as bone and bowel gas, its presence can have diagnostic value in identifying the presence of calculi, such as in the gallbladder and kidney (Fig. 19-3).

Biliary sludge can be found in the lumen of the gallbladder and is an aggregation that may contain cholesterol crystals, bilirubin, and glycoproteins. It is often associated with biliary stasis. While it may be echogenic, **sludge does not produce acoustical shadowing like gallstones** (Fig. 19-4).

■ **Signs of acute cholecystitis on ultrasound:**
  • The presence of gallstones, possibly impacted in the neck of the gallbladder or cystic duct.
  • Thickening of the gallbladder wall (>3 mm) (Fig. 19-5A).
  • **Pericholecystic fluid** (fluid around the gallbladder) (Fig. 19-5B).
  • A positive *Murphy sign* (pain that is elicited by compression of the gallbladder with the ultrasound probe).
■ In the presence of gallstones and gallbladder wall thickening, ultrasound has a positive predictive value for acute cholecystitis as high as 94%.

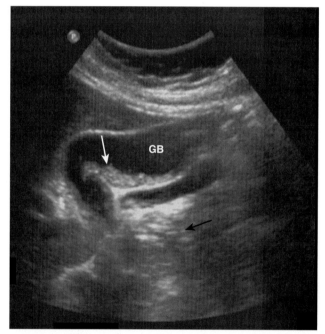

Figure 19-4 Sludge in the gallbladder. Sludge (*solid white arrow*) in the gallbladder (*GB*) is associated with biliary stasis. While it may be echogenic, sludge does not produce acoustical shadowing like gallstones (the absence of shadowing is shown by *solid black arrow*).

■ Radionuclide scans (**HIDA scans**) **are also used in the diagnosis of acute cholecystitis.**
  • Hepatoiminodiacetic acid (the "HIDA" in HIDA scan) is tagged with a radioactive tracer (Technetium Tc 99m), injected intravenously and imaged with a special camera after it has been excreted by the liver into the bile and emptied into the small intestine.
  • In patients with **obstruction of the cystic duct,** the tracer will not appear in the **gallbladder.** In patients with **obstruction of the common bile duct,** the tracer **will not appear in the small intestine.** Either finding usually is caused by an obstructing gallstone (Fig. 19-6).

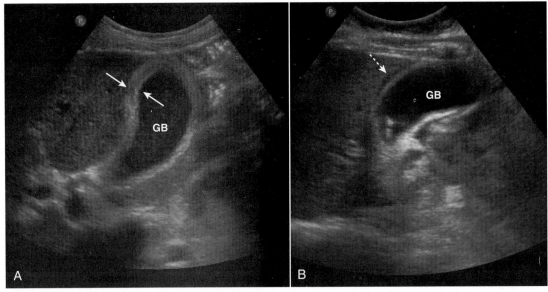

Figure 19-5 Acute cholecystitis, sagittal views, two patients. A, Thickening of gallbladder (*GB*) wall. The wall should be 3 mm or less. This wall is markedly thickened at 6 mm (*solid white arrows*). **B,** There is an echo-free crescent (*dotted white arrow*) surrounding a thickened gallbladder (*GB*) wall representing pericholecystic fluid. The patient had a positive sonographic Murphy sign.

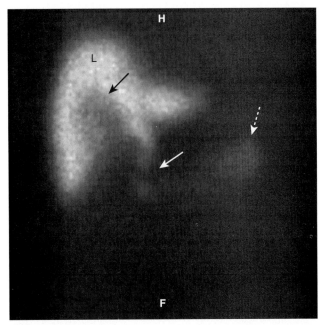

Figure 19-6 HIDA scan in cystic duct obstruction. HIDA, a radioactive labeled isotope, concentrates in the liver (*L*) and is then excreted into the biliary ducts. On this delayed image, the common bile duct (*solid white arrow*) and small bowel (*dotted white arrow*) fill normally because the common bile duct is patent. The cystic duct and gallbladder do not fill because the cystic is obstructed, by a stone in this case. There is a tracer-free (photopenic) area in the gallbladder fossa because the nuclide cannot fill the gallbladder lumen (*solid black arrow*).

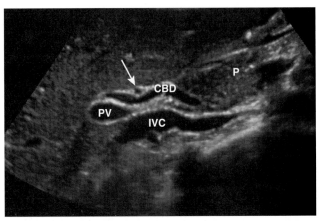

Figure 19-7 Normal common bile duct, portal vein, and hepatic artery, sagittal view. The common bile duct (*CBD*) measures 3 mm (normal <6 mm). The *solid white arrow* points to the hepatic artery, seen on end. The portal vein (*PV*) is posterior to the common duct, and the inferior vena cava (*IVC*) is seen posterior to the portal vein. The pancreas (*P*) is anterior to the CBD.

Bile Ducts

■ Ultrasound plays a key role in evaluation of the intrahepatic and extrahepatic bile ducts and pancreatic duct. The intrahepatic biliary radicals drain into the left and right hepatic ducts, which join to form the common hepatic duct (CHD). Where the cystic duct from the gallbladder joins the CHD is the origin of the common bile duct (CBD), which drains either within or adjacent to the head of the pancreas via the ampulla of Vater into the second portion of the duodenum. **The CBD lies anterior to the portal vein and lateral to the hepatic artery in the porta hepatis** (Fig. 19-7).

➤ The CHD and proximal CBD can be visualized normally on virtually all ultrasound studies of the right upper quadrant. **The CHD measures no more than 4 mm** (inner wall to inner wall) and the **CBD measures no more than 6 mm** in diameter. The **pancreatic duct measures <2 mm.**

■ Normal intrahepatic bile ducts are not visible. When the CBD is obstructed, the **extrahepatic ducts dilate before the intrahepatic ducts.** Over time, both the intrahepatic and extrahepatic ducts will be dilated (Fig. 19-8).

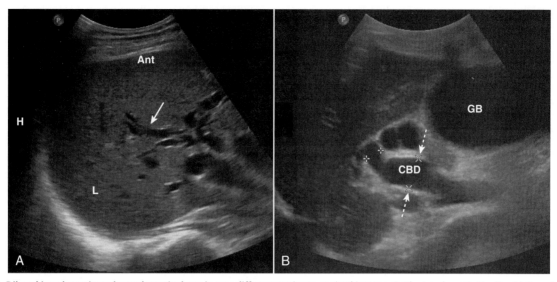

Figure 19-8 Dilated intrahepatic and extrahepatic ducts in two different patients, sagittal images. A, The intrahepatic (*L* = liver) biliary ducts are normally not visible by ultrasound. In this case, they are dilated (*solid white arrow*) from obstruction by a pancreatic carcinoma (not shown). **B,** The *CBD* is dilated at 15 mm (*dotted white arrows*) and the gallbladder (*GB*) is distended from an obstructing stone (not shown).

- **Causes of bile duct obstruction** include gallstones, pancreatic carcinoma, strictures, sclerosing cholangitis, cholangiocarcinoma, and metastatic disease.

URINARY TRACT

Normal Ultrasound Anatomy

- The kidneys normally measure **9-12 cm in length, 4-5 cm in width, and are 3-4 cm thick.** The **renal sinus** is home to the renal pelvis and the major branches of the renal artery and vein. Because the renal sinus contains fat, it normally appears **brightly echogenic. The calyces are normally not visible. The medullary pyramids are hypoechoic.** The renal parenchyma has **uniformly low echogenicity,** which is **usually less** than that of the adjacent **liver and spleen** (Fig. 19-9).
- Renal masses are discussed in Chapter 18.

Hydronephrosis

- **Hydronephrosis** is defined as dilatation of the renal pelvis and calyces.
- In patients experiencing renal colic, ultrasound is used primarily to **evaluate for the presence of hydronephrosis** since the ureters are difficult to visualize with US. The *stone search* itself is almost always carried out by CT scanning (see Chapter 16).
- The typical appearance of obstructive uropathy is a **dilated calyceal system.** The echogenic **renal sinus** contains a **dilated, fluid-filled, and therefore anechoic renal pelvis.** The ureter may be dilated to the level of the obstructing stone. Severe hydronephrosis may distort the appearance of the kidney (Fig. 19-10).

Medical Renal Disease

- **Medical renal disease** refers to a host of diseases that primarily affect the **renal parenchyma.** They include such

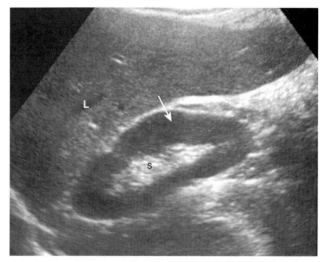

Figure 19-9 Normal right kidney, sagittal view. The renal sinus (*S*) is home to the renal pelvis and the major branches of the renal artery and vein. Because the renal sinus contains fat, it normally appears brightly echogenic. The normal renal pelvis is not visible in the renal sinus. The renal parenchyma (*solid white arrow*) has uniformly low echogenicity and is usually less echogenic than the adjacent liver (*L*) or spleen.

diseases as glomerulonephritis, diseases that cause nephrotic syndrome, and renal involvement in collagen vascular diseases.

- In the early stages of medical renal disease, the kidneys may appear normal. Later, changes in the echo architecture occur but these are usually nonspecific as to the actual etiology. The **renal parenchyma becomes more echogenic (brighter) than the liver and spleen,** the reverse of the normal echo pattern. **Renal size** is also an important reflection of the chronicity of a disease, the renal parenchyma almost always **decreasing in size with chronic disease.** A biopsy may be performed to determine the etiology of the disease (Fig. 19-11).

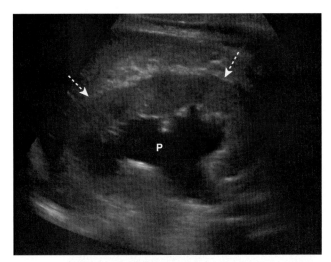

Figure 19-10 Hydronephrosis, sagittal view, right kidney. The renal sinus now contains a markedly dilated, fluid-filled and anechoic renal pelvis (*P*) in this patient with hydronephrosis. The renal parenchyma remains normal in size and echogenicity (*dotted white arrows*). The patient had an obstructing stone at the ureteropelvic junction.

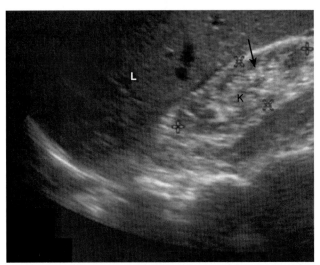

Figure 19-11 Chronic medical renal disease, sagittal view. The right kidney (*K*) is small, measuring 6 × 3 cm between cursor marks. The renal parenchyma (*solid black arrow*) is more echogenic (brighter) than the adjacent liver (*L*), the reverse of the normal echo pattern. This patient had chronic glomerulonephritis from long-standing diabetes.

ABDOMINAL AORTIC ANEURYSMS

- An aneurysm is defined as a localized dilation of an artery by at least **50% over its normal size.** Most aortic aneurysms occur in the abdominal aorta **inferior to the origin of the renal arteries** and **frequently extend into one or both iliac arteries.**
  - Most aortic aneurysms are either **fusiform** in shape or produce **uniform dilatation** of the entire vessel.

 The abdominal aorta normally measures no more than 3 cm in diameter (outer wall to outer wall).

- The **size of an aneurysm** is directly **related to its risk of rupture.** For aneurysms **less than 4 cm** in diameter, there is **less than a 10%** chance of rupture, but for aneurysms

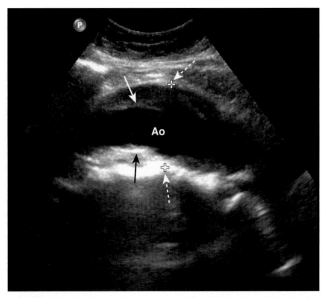

Figure 19-12 Abdominal aortic aneurysm, sagittal view. There is fusiform dilatation of the abdominal aorta (*Ao*) measuring 4.9 cm between marks (*dotted white arrows*). Hypoechoic thrombus is seen in the aneurysm (*solid black and white arrows*). Ultrasonography is the screening study of choice when an asymptomatic, pulsatile abdominal mass is palpated. For aneurysms 4-5 cm in diameter, the risk of rupture increases to almost 25%.

4-5 cm in diameter, the risk of rupture increases to **almost 25%.**
- **Recognizing an abdominal aortic aneurysm**
  - **Ultrasonography is the screening study of choice** when an asymptomatic, pulsatile abdominal mass is palpated.
  - Because it is moving, blood within the lumen of the aorta will appear anechoic; thrombus in the wall of the aneurysm will appear echogenic (Fig. 19-12).
  - Unenhanced CT has the advantage of depicting the absolute size of the aneurysm, but **in order to define the extent of mural thrombus and the presence of dissection, intravenous contrast must be used.**
    - **Mural thrombus** can be recognized as a **filling defect** in the contrast-filled aneurysm (Fig. 19-13).
  - Rupture of an aneurysm can be inferred if **soft tissue encircles the aorta** (although other lesions can produce this finding) and is definite if **extravasation is identified** on a contrast-enhanced CT scan (see Fig. 19-13).

FEMALE PELVIC ORGANS

- **Ultrasonography is the imaging study of choice in evaluating a pelvic mass or pelvic pain in the female.** Leiomyomas confined to the myometrium are the most common tumors of the uterus. Endometrial carcinomas are usually confined to the uterus at the time of discovery. The most common mass in the ovary is a functional cyst. Generally, uterine masses are solid and ovarian masses are cystic.

Normal Ultrasound Anatomy of the Uterus

- The uterus is made up of a thick muscular layer (**myometrium**) and a mucous surface (**endometrium**). It is divided into a **body**, with **cornu** to receive the fallopian tubes, and

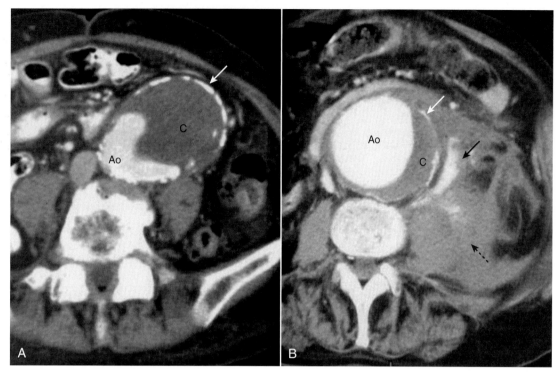

Figure 19-13 Abdominal aortic aneurysms on CT: mural thrombus and rupture. A, The aorta is enlarged. Contrast is present in the lumen (*Ao*) along with a large clot (*C*). Calcification is seen in the wall of the aorta (*solid white arrow*). The aneurysm is almost in contact with the anterior abdominal wall. **B,** This aneurysm, in another patient, has ruptured. Contrast is seen in the lumen (*Ao*) along with a crescentic clot (*C*), and there is calcification present in the wall (*solid white arrow*), just as in the previous case. The major finding here is active extravasation of contrast-containing blood outside of the aorta (*solid black arrow*) producing a large retroperitoneal hematoma (*dotted black arrow*).

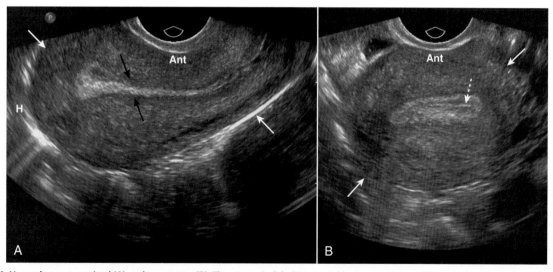

Figure 19-14 Normal uterus, sagittal (A) and transverse (B). The uterus (*solid white arrows*) has a pear shape with maximum dimensions of approximately 8 cm in length, 5 cm in width, and 4 cm in AP dimension. **A,** The endometrium lines the uterine cavity and is measured in the sagittal view (*solid black arrows*). **B,** The collapsed uterine cavity is within the center of the endometrium and is visualized as a thin, echogenic line (*dotted white arrow*).

the **cervix.** Anterior to the uterus is the peritoneal space called the **anterior cul-de-sac.** The **posterior cul-de-sac** is also called the **rectouterine recess.**

- The uterus is usually **anteverted** (axis of the cervix relative to the vagina) and **anteflexed** (position of the uterine body relative to the cervix). In the adult, the uterus has a **pear shape** with maximum dimensions of approximately **8 cm in length, 5 cm in width, and 4 cm in AP dimension**. The size of the normal uterus increases with multiparity; with aging, the uterus regresses in size (Fig. 19-14).

- The normal **endometrial cavity** forms a **thin echogenic stripe or line** between the opposing surfaces of the endometrium. By convention it is measured as a double thickness on a sagittal view of the mid-uterus. The appearance of both the endometrium and the ovaries varies depending on the phase of the menstrual cycle.

  The standard **transabdominal** (through the abdominal wall) study of the uterus is done with a **full urinary bladder.** The full bladder provides an **acoustical window** to

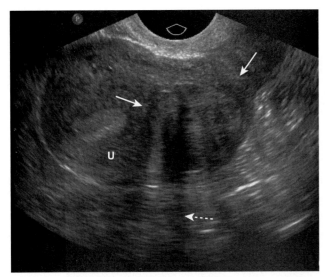

Figure 19-15 Leiomyoma of the uterus, sagittal view. There is a heterogeneously hypoechoic mass (*solid white arrows*) in the uterus (*U*). Uterine leiomyomas may display some areas that contain many echoes and others that demonstrate few echoes. They frequently absorb enough sound to produce acoustical shadowing (*dotted white arrow*). Where they are necrotic, they may be cystic. If they contain calcium, the calcium will produce acoustical shadowing.

the uterus by pushing bowel loops out of the pelvis and also helps to delineate the bladder itself.

- **Transvaginal** studies are done with higher frequency probes and thus provide **better resolution** images and are done with the **bladder empty.** Transabdominal and transvaginal studies are considered complementary techniques.
- **Sonohysterography** is a procedure in which saline is instilled in the uterine cavity in conjunction with images obtained using transvaginal ultrasound. It provides excellent visualization of the uterine cavity and fallopian tubes and can be used to detect small uterine polyps, submucosal myomas, and adhesions.

Uterine Leiomyomas (Fibroids)

- Leiomyomas are **benign smooth muscle tumors** of the uterus that occur in up to 50% of women over the age of 30. Although most women with fibroids are **asymptomatic,** fibroids can cause **pain, infertility, menorrhagia,** and urinary or bowel symptoms if they grow large enough.
- **Ultrasound (transabdominal and transvaginal) is the imaging study of choice** in evaluating uterine fibroids. MRI is used mainly to evaluate complicated cases or in surgical planning. Fibroids are also frequently visualized on CT scans of the pelvis, usually performed for other reasons.
- **Recognizing uterine leiomyomas on US**
  - Uterine leiomyomas are **heterogeneously hypoechoic, solid masses,** meaning they may display some areas that contain many echoes and others that demonstrate few echoes. They frequently absorb enough sound to produce **acoustical shadowing.** Where they are **necrotic,** they may be anechoic. If they **contain calcium,** the calcium will produce **acoustical shadowing** (Fig. 19-15).
- **Recognizing uterine leiomyomas on CT**
  - Characteristically, they are **lobulated soft tissue masses** that **frequently calcify** with **amorphous or popcorn**

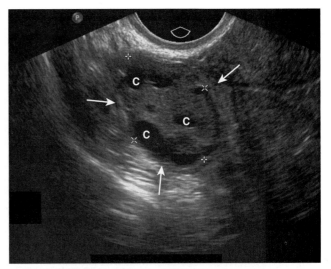

Figure 19-16 Normal right ovary, sagittal view. In premenopausal women, the ovaries are approximately 2 × 3 × 4 cm in size (*solid white arrows*), usually containing small cystic follicles (*C*) as shown here.

calcification. When they grow large, they frequently **undergo central necrosis** which manifests as **low attenuation** areas (see Fig. 16-12B).
- The **myometrium** is very vascular and **markedly enhances** on contrast-enhanced CT scans of the pelvis. The viable portions of uterine myomata also enhance dramatically following injection of intravenous contrast.

Normal Ultrasound Anatomy of the Ovaries

- Ultrasound is the **imaging study of choice** for evaluating the ovaries.
- **Normal ovarian anatomy and physiology**
  - In premenopausal women, the ovaries are approximately **2 × 3 × 4 cm in size,** frequently containing cystic follicles. The ovaries atrophy after menopause (Fig. 19-16).
  - The normal ovary changes in appearance not only with age but also with the phase of each menstrual cycle. Under normal hormonal stimulation, one egg-containing follicle becomes dominant and attains a size of about 2.5 cm at the time of ovulation (Fig. 19-17).

  If one of the nondominant follicles fills with fluid and does not rupture, a **follicular cyst** is formed. Follicular cysts are **unilateral, usually asymptomatic,** and usually **involute** during the next menstrual cycle or two. If they persist or enlarge, they are pathologic.

- A *corpus luteum* is the structure that forms after expulsion of an egg from the dominant ovarian follicle. If the corpus luteum fills with fluid, a **corpus luteal cyst** will develop. Though **less common** than follicular cysts, corpus luteal cysts are **more symptomatic (pain) and can be larger.** Still, most usually **involute** in 6-8 weeks.

Ovarian Cysts

- **Follicular cysts** and **corpus luteum cysts** are called **functional cysts** of the ovary because they occur as a result of the hormonal stimuli associated with ovulation.

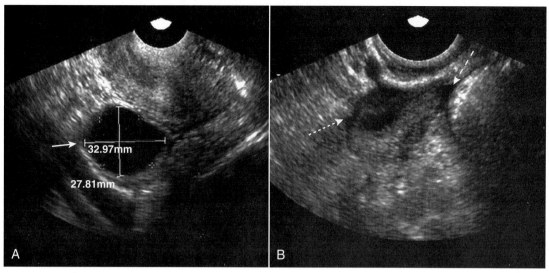

Figure 19-17 Dominant follicle ruptures during scan. Under normal hormonal stimulation, one egg-containing follicle becomes dominant and attains a size of about 2.5 cm at the time of ovulation. **A,** The dominant follicle is 3.3 × 2.8 cm at the start of the study (*solid white arrow*). **B,** A few minutes later, during the study, the follicle ruptures (ovulation occurs) and the follicle shrinks dramatically in size (*dotted white arrow*). A small, physiologic amount of free fluid appears in the peritoneal cavity (*dashed white arrow*).

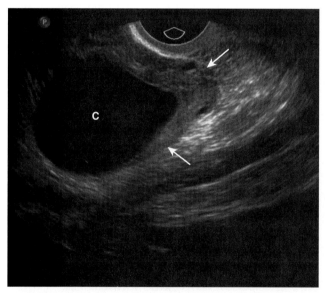

Figure 19-18 Simple ovarian cyst, sagittal view. Contained within the left ovary (*solid white arrows*) is a well-defined, thin-walled, anechoic structure representing a simple ovarian cyst (*C*). Ovarian cysts may contain echogenic material if hemorrhage occurs into the cyst.

■ Both are characteristically **well-defined, thin-walled, anechoic structures with homogeneous internal fluid density.** They may contain echogenic material if hemorrhage occurs into the cyst (Fig. 19-18).

■ **Nonfunctional cysts** of the ovary include **dermoid cysts, endometriomas, and polycystic ovaries.**

• **Dermoid cysts** are **mature teratomas** composed of cells from all three germ layers—ectoderm, mesoderm, and endoderm—although the ectodermal elements (hair, bone) predominate. They are most commonly found in women of reproductive age and are bilateral in up to 25% of cases (Fig. 19-19).

• **Endometriomas,** part of the disease *endometriosis,* are cystic ovarian lesions, sometimes called *"chocolate cysts"* because they are filled with brownish-red blood. Endometriomas can become large and multilocular.

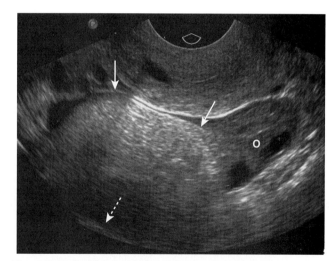

Figure 19-19 Ovarian dermoid cyst. There is a large, solid echogenic mass (*solid white arrows*) in the right ovary (*O*) with acoustical shadowing (*dotted white arrow*). Dermoid cysts of the ovary are most commonly found in women of reproductive age and are bilateral in up to 25% of cases.

• **Polycystic ovarian disease** is an endocrine abnormality that allows for numerous ovarian follicles (>12 per ovary) to develop in various stages of hormonal growth and atresia. When associated with oligomenorrhea, hirsutism, and obesity, it is called *Stein-Leventhal syndrome* (Fig. 19-20).

Ovarian Tumors

■ Most ovarian tumors arise from the **surface epithelium** that covers the ovary, **serous tumors** being more **common** (*serous cystadenomas, adenocarcinomas*) than **mucinous** tumors (*mucinous cystadenomas, adenocarcinomas*). Most serous **tumors,** and the overwhelming number of mucinous tumors, are **benign.**

 On ultrasound, primary tumors of the ovary are **usually cystic in nature.** Keys to differentiating ovarian cysts

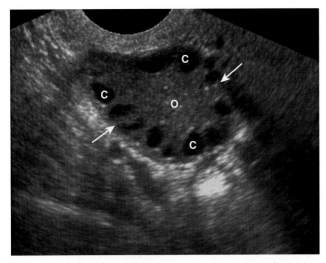

Figure 19-20 Polycystic ovarian disease. Polycystic ovarian disease is an endocrine abnormality that allows for numerous ovarian follicles (>12 per ovary) to develop in various stages of hormonal growth and atresia. This ovary (*O*) is enlarged (*solid white arrows*) and contains multiple peripheral cysts, some of which are labeled (*C*). When associated with oligomenorrhea, hirsutism, and obesity, polycystic ovarian disease is called ***Stein-Leventhal syndrome.***

from tumors include **thick and irregular walls** and **internal septations** seen in tumors (Fig. 19-21).

- The primary route of spread for ovarian cancer is throughout the **peritoneal cavity.** *Omental cake* is the term that applies to metastatic implants in the omentum and on the peritoneal surface frequently producing an elongated nodular mass. **Ascites** usually indicates peritoneal spread.

Pelvic Inflammatory Disease

- Pelvic inflammatory disease (PID) is a term used to describe a **group of infectious diseases affecting the uterus, fallopian tubes, and ovaries.** Most cases of PID **begin as a transient endometritis** and ascend to infection of the tubes and ovaries. Patients can have pain, vaginal discharge, adnexal tenderness and elevated white blood cell counts. Complications include **infertility, chronic pain, or ectopic pregnancy.**
- **Recognizing PID on ultrasound**
  - **Enlarged ovaries** with multiple cysts and periovarian inflammation
  - Fluid-filled and dilated fallopian tube (***pyosalpinx***) (Fig. 19-22A)

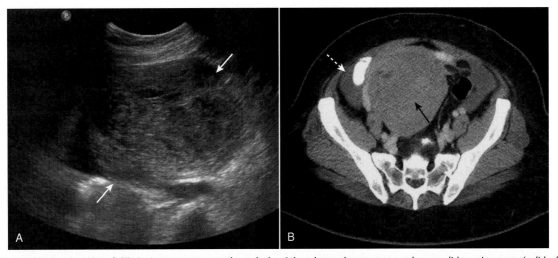

Figure 19-21 Ovarian tumor, US and CT. A, A transverse scan through the right adnexa demonstrates a large, solid ovarian mass (*solid white arrows*). **B,** CT on the same patient shows a large heterogeneous mass arising from the right adnexa (*solid black arrow*). A small amount of ascites is seen (*dotted white arrow*). This patient had a fibroma of the ovary, a tumor sometimes associated with ascites and pleural effusion (**Meig syndrome).**

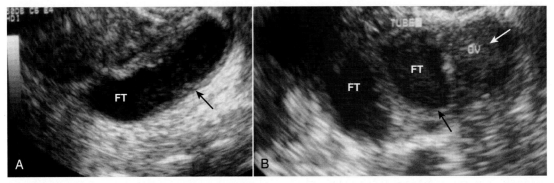

Figure 19-22 Pelvic inflammatory disease, sagittal and transverse views, US. A, A fluid-filled and dilated fallopian tube (*FT*) containing pus and debris (*solid black arrow*) representing a pyosalpinx is demonstrated. **B,** Due to progressive inflammation, there is fusion of a dilated and tortuous fallopian tube (*solid black arrow, FT*) and the adjacent ovary (*solid white arrow, OV*) producing a **tubo-ovarian complex.**

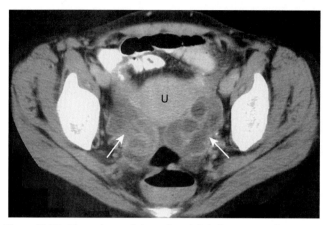

Figure 19-23 Bilateral pyosalpinges in pelvic inflammatory disease, CT. There are dilated, serpiginous, and fluid-filled tubular structures bilaterally (*solid white arrows*) representing pyosalpingitis of both fallopian tubes on this scan of the pelvis in a young female with pelvic inflammatory disease. (*U* = uterus.)

- Fusion of the dilated fallopian tube and ovary (***tubo-ovarian complex***) (Fig. 19-22B)
- Multiloculated mass with septations (***tubo-ovarian abscess***)
- CT can be used for cases of complicated PID or those in whom the history may not suggest that diagnosis.
- Recognizing **PID on CT** requires the use of intravenous contrast material. Findings include:
  - **Haziness of pelvic fat**
  - **Thickened tubes**—may be folded upon themselves and appear as a fluid-filled multicystic mass (Fig. 19-23)
  - **Enlarged uterus** with increased endometrial enhancement and fluid and enlarged ovaries that enhance with contrast
  - **Pyosalpinx and tubo-ovarian abscess**—adnexal mass with focal areas of hypodensity
  - **Pelvic ascites**

Ascites

Ascites is the **abnormal accumulation of fluid in the peritoneal cavity.** In the recumbent position, ascitic fluid flows up the **right paracolic gutter** to the right **subphrenic space** so ascites is generally easier to detect by ultrasound in the right upper quadrant between the liver and the diaphragm.

- Ascitic fluid that is a **transudate** is primarily **sonolucent.** Fluid collections that are **exudates** or contain hemorrhage or pus may contain **echoes** (Fig. 19-24).
- Ultrasound is frequently used to identify the best **location** to perform a **paracentesis** to remove ascitic fluid. The ultrasonographer may place a mark on the patient's skin indicating the best portal from which to withdraw fluid while avoiding any visceral organ.

APPENDICITIS

- The normal appendix may not be visualized on ultrasound. The diameter of the appendix is usually **less than 6 mm.**

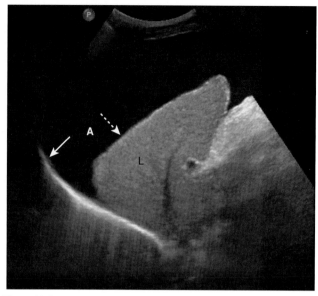

Figure 19-24 Ascites, sagittal US. Ascitic fluid flows up the right paracolic gutter to the right subphrenic space so ascites (*A*) is generally easier to detect by ultrasound in the right upper quadrant between the liver (*L*) and the diaphragm (*solid white arrow*). The liver is contracted and has a nodular margin (*dotted white arrow*), both features of cirrhosis. If the fluid is a transudate, as in this case of ascites due to cirrhosis, the fluid will be anechoic. Exudates will produce internal echoes.

When visible, the **normal appendix compresses** when pressure is applied with the transducer.
- The pathophysiology of acute appendicitis begins with obstruction of the appendiceal lumen followed by progressive distension of the obstructed appendix until perforation occurs and a periappendiceal abscess forms.

In **acute appendicitis,** the appendix may be recognized on ultrasound as a blind-ending, aperistaltic tube with a **diameter of 6 mm or more.** The appendix is **noncompressible** (using a technique called ***graded compression***). It may be **tender when palpated** with the probe. In about a third of the cases of appendicitis, a **fecalith** will be present (Fig. 19-25).

PREGNANCY

- Ultrasound has provided a **safe and reliable** means of visualizing the fetus in utero and the ability to do so repeatedly during the course of a pregnancy, if necessary. The overwhelming majority of mothers in North America and Western Europe undergo at least one ultrasound evaluation sometime during pregnancy.
- Even before pregnancy, ultrasound can be used for assessing the time of ovulation to aid in the process of successful fertilization.
- The uses of ultrasound during pregnancy are outlined in Box 19-1.
- The goals of sonography during pregnancy may differ depending on the timing of the scan. During the **first trimester,** goals are to exclude an ectopic pregnancy, estimate the age of the pregnancy, determine fetal viability, and determine if there are multiple fetuses present. During the **second and third trimesters,** goals may include estimates

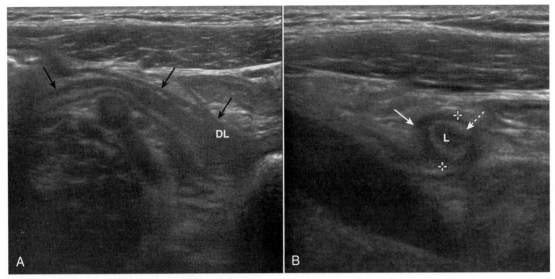

Figure 19-25 Acute appendicitis, sagittal and transverse views. A, There is a blind-ending tubular structure (*solid black arrows*) that has a thick wall and a distended lumen (*DL*) representing an inflamed and distended appendix. **B,** In this transverse view, the appendix (*solid white arrow*) measures 7 mm between marks (normal <6 mm). The lumen (*L*) contains fluid, and there is an echogenic ring that represents the mucosa (*dotted white arrow*) surrounding it. The appendix may be tender when palpated with the probe.

Box 19-1 Uses of Ultrasound During Pregnancy
Fetal presence and gestational age
Fetal abnormalities and viability
The presence of multiple pregnancies
Placental localization
Amniotic fluid volume
Intrauterine growth retardation
In helping guide invasive studies like amniocentesis, chorionic villus sampling, and intrauterine transfusions

of amniotic fluid volume, detection of fetal anomalies, determination of placental and fetal positioning, or guidance for invasive studies to determine the likelihood of fetal viability in the event of a premature birth.

■ A discussion of all of the ultrasound findings during pregnancy is beyond the scope of this text. We'll look at three important uses of ultrasound.

Ectopic Pregnancy

■ Most ectopic pregnancies are **tubal in location** and occur near the **fimbriated (ovarian) end**. The classical clinical findings of **pain, abnormal vaginal bleeding, and a palpable adnexal mass** are seen in only about half of cases. The incidence of ectopic pregnancies is increasing, most likely because of increasing risk factors, but the mortality rate has declined, in part because of their early diagnosis by ultrasound.

➡ Using transvaginal scanning, **ultrasound is best at identifying the presence** of a **normal, intrauterine pregnancy**; ultrasound does less well at directly visualizing an ectopic pregnancy.

■ If a **gestational sac** (the earliest sonographic finding in pregnancy, appearing at about 4-5 weeks gestational age),

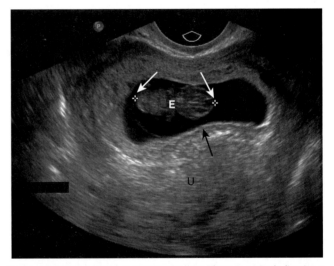

Figure 19-26 Early intrauterine pregnancy. There is a single live intrauterine pregnancy (*solid white arrows*) contained within the gestational sac (*solid black arrow*) inside the uterus (*U*). Using a measurement called the crown-rump length, (between the *white arrows*) the embryo (*E*) was estimated at 9 weeks of age. Sonographic gestational age begins on the first day of the last normal menstrual cycle because, for most individuals, that is a more certain date than the actual date of ovulation.

yolk sac (first structure to be seen normally in gestational sac), or **viable fetus** is identified **in the uterine cavity**, an **ectopic pregnancy** is effectively **excluded**. Endovaginal examinations are usually performed to find the gestational sac (Fig. 19-26).

⚠ While it is possible to have **simultaneous** intrauterine and extrauterine pregnancies, such *heterotopic pregnancies* are **extremely rare**, other than in fertility patients, so that identification of an intrauterine pregnancy effectively excludes an ectopic pregnancy.

■ Conversely, the demonstration of a **live embryo outside of the uterus is diagnostic of an ectopic pregnancy.** This is

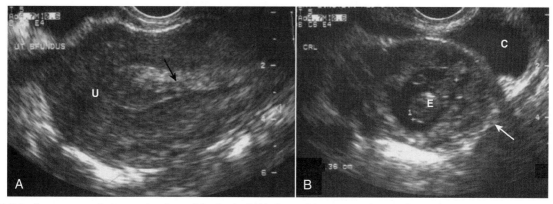

Figure 19-27 **Ectopic pregnancy. A,** A normal endometrial stripe (*solid black arrow*) is present with no evidence of a pregnancy in the uterus (*U*). **B,** There is an adnexal mass (*solid white arrow*) containing an embryo (*E*). There is fluid in the cul-de-sac (*C*). The demonstration of an embryo outside of the uterus is diagnostic of an ectopic pregnancy.

not a common occurrence with most ectopic pregnancies (Fig. 19-27).

■ Most often, an ectopic location is diagnosed by a combination of findings that includes the demonstrated **absence of an identifiable intrauterine pregnancy** while the quantitative **serum human chorionic gonadotropin hormone (β-HCG)** rises above the discriminatory level, at which point a normal intrauterine pregnancy **should almost always be identified.** If those two criteria are met, **an ectopic pregnancy is presumed present.**

■ The **beta (β) subunit of HCG** is specific for the hormone produced by placental tissue shortly after the implantation of a fertilized ovum in the uterus. The levels of HCG roughly double every 2-3 days in a normal pregnancy. At a β-HCG level of around **1,500 milli-international units per milliliter (mIU/mL), a normal intrauterine pregnancy should be visible** with transvaginal ultrasound.

⚠ Serial β-HCG determinations may help in differentiating an ectopic pregnancy from an *early abortion,* both of which may display similar sonographic findings. Patients with an early abortion will display **falling β-HCG levels** on serial serum studies, while **ectopic pregnancies will rise,** though usually **more slowly** than normal intrauterine pregnancies.

■ An ectopic pregnancy is also presumed present when there are **large amounts of free fluid (blood) inside the abdominal cavity.** Small amounts of free fluid can occur from other causes, such as spontaneous abortion, ruptured ovarian cysts, and normal ovulation.

■ Ectopic pregnancies are **managed** either surgically (usually laparoscopic surgery) or medically with an abortifacient such as methotrexate. Some spontaneously resolve.

Fetal Abnormalities

■ Ultrasound is used extensively to monitor normal fetal growth and development.

■ Certain fetal anomalies can be recognized by ultrasound in utero that are known to be universally fatal after birth, such as anencephaly or complete ectopia cordis. The accurate interpretation of sonograms by someone trained and accredited in obstetric ultrasound is critical in detecting such anomalies.

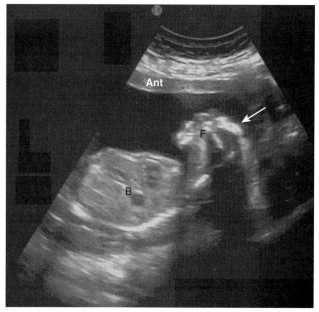

Figure 19-28 **Anencephaly, sagittal view.** There is a single live intrauterine pregnancy. The body (*B*) and face (*F*) are present, but the cranium and all of the cerebrum and cerebellum are absent (*solid white arrow*). Anencephaly involves a failure of closure of the neural tube during the 3rd-4th weeks of development. It virtually always leads to fetal demise, stillbirth, or neonatal death.

■ Many fetal anomalies may be diagnosed by ultrasound in utero. Among them:
  • **Central nervous system abnormalities:** Hydrocephalus, abnormalities of the prosencephalon, agenesis of the corpus callosum, intrauterine infections, cysts, meningomyelocele, anencephaly (Fig. 19-28)
  • **Skeletal anomalies:** Dwarfism, skeletal dysplasias, achondroplasia, osteogenesis imperfecta, asphyxiating thoracic dysplasia, limb anomalies
  • **Gastrointestinal abnormalities:** Esophageal atresia and tracheoesophageal fistula, duodenal atresia, small and large bowel obstruction, abdominal wall defects, congenital diaphragmatic hernias, choledochal cyst
  • **Genitourinary tract abnormalities:** Renal agenesis, congenital ureteropelvic junction and ureterovesicle junction obstruction, bladder outlet obstruction, multicystic dysplastic kidney, polycystic kidney disease

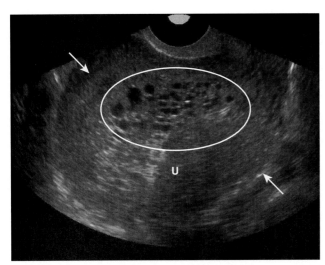

Figure 19-29 Molar pregnancy, sagittal view. The uterus (*U*) is enlarged and filled with echogenic tissue (*solid white arrows*). There are innumerable, relatively uniform-sized cystic spaces that represent hydropic villi (*oval*) in this complete molar pregnancy. In a complete molar pregnancy, there is no fetus.

- **Cardiac anomalies:** Hypoplastic left heart syndrome, tricuspid atresia, endocardial cushion defects, Ebstein anomaly, tetralogy of Fallot, transposition of the great vessels, coarctation of the aorta, cardiac arrhythmias
- In detecting fetal anomalies, ultrasound has played a major role in obstetrical management of pregnancy. Ultrasound's role should increase as more reliable markers for chromosome abnormalities that can be quickly assessed without prolonged waiting periods become more available.

Molar Pregnancy

- **Molar pregnancy** is the most common of a group of disorders of the placenta that also includes **invasive mole** and **choriocarcinoma.** Pathologically, molar pregnancies feature **cystic (grapelike or hydatidiform) degeneration of chorionic villi** and **proliferation of the placental trophoblast.**
- A molar pregnancy is suggested by **uterine size that is disproportionately large** for the dates of gestation, **β-HCG levels in excess of 100,000 mIU/mL** (normal pregnancies are less than 60,000 mIU/mL), vomiting, vaginal bleeding, and toxemia.
- **Sonographic findings of molar pregnancy:**
  - **Enlarged uterus** filled with echogenic tissue that enlarges the endometrial cavity
  - **Innumerable,** uniform-sized **cystic spaces** that represent hydropic villi (Fig. 19-29)
  - **Enlarged and cyst-filled ovaries**
  - In a *complete molar pregnancy,* there is no fetus.
- Therapy is uterine evacuation. About 20% of those with complete molar pregnancies may harbor persistent trophoblastic tissue, so follow-up is carried out with serial HCG determinations.

VASCULAR ULTRASOUND

- Vascular ultrasound studies combine morphologic images of the vessels with the simultaneous recording of the

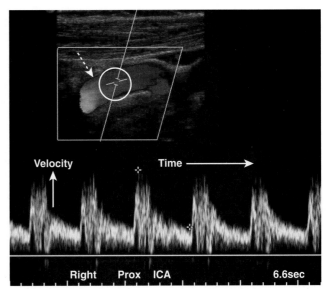

Figure 19-30 Normal proximal right internal carotid artery, duplex sonogram. The upper display (*dotted white arrow*) depicts flow in the artery (the original displayed the flow in color). Within the *white circle* is the Doppler sampler volume, the measurements for which are shown on the lower graphical display, called the **Doppler spectral waveform**. The x axis represents time; the height of the waveforms represents the velocity of blood flow within the Doppler sampler volume. The velocity normally increases with each systole and decreases with each diastole.

velocity of flow displayed by the **Doppler spectral waveform.**

- The combination of the two is called **Duplex sonography,** and its use helps assure that the sample being measured accurately represents the area of interest.

The **Doppler spectral waveform** is a graphic representation of the **velocity of flow over time** within a focused area. It is depicted along an x (time) and y (velocity) axis. Flow toward the transducer is displayed above the baseline; flow away below the baseline. Different arteries have distinctive spectral waveforms depending, in part, on whether there is normally a high or low resistance to flow within them.

- **Color flow Doppler imaging** adds the dimension of superimposing moving blood (shown in color) over a gray-scale image of the anatomic structure enabling a more rapid identification of potential abnormalities. The Doppler spectral waveform quantitates the flow.
- **Carotid ultrasonography** has become the study of choice for the noninvasive assessment of extracranial atherosclerotic disease. Extracranial carotid occlusive disease accounts for more than one half of strokes. Carotid ultrasound is also used to evaluate bruits, as preoperative screening prior to other major vascular surgery and to assess the patency of the vessel after endarterectomy (Fig. 19-30).

Carotid stenosis begins to cause elevations in the velocity of flow when there is greater than 50% narrowing of the lumen. Significant stenosis alters the Doppler waveform **proximal, at,** and **distal** to the **point of stenosis.**

- Ultrasound is used to assess the **thickness of the vessel wall** (it gets thicker with atherosclerosis), the **presence and**

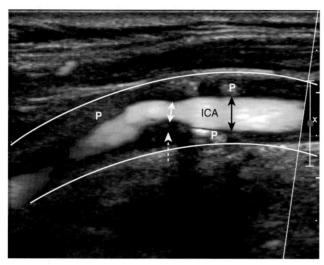

Figure 19-31 Stenotic right internal carotid artery, sagittal view. The *white lines* indicate the normal location of the wall of the right internal carotid artery (*ICA*). The lumen is narrowed (*double black arrows*) due the presence of plaque (*P*) throughout the wall. At the site of the *dotted white arrow*, the lumen narrows to less than 50% of its normal diameter (*double white arrow*) from thicker plaque.

nature of plaque, and analysis of the Doppler spectral waveform.

- Any vessel in the body of large enough size which is accessible to the ultrasound transducer can be studied. Besides the carotid arteries, the jugular veins, vertebral artery, renal arteries, and peripheral arteries are commonly studied. CT-angiography may also be used for vascular studies, but it requires ionizing radiation and intravenous contrast.

- **Arterial flow in the extremities** produces a **high resistance waveform** due to the downstream high resistance of the arterial bed. With significant arterial disease, there is a **focal increase** in the velocity of flow at the point of stenosis. A normal high resistance flow becomes low resistance when the scan sample is distal to the point of obstruction (Fig. 19-31).

DEEP VEIN THROMBOSIS

- The majority of patients with deep venous thrombosis are **asymptomatic.** The most serious complication of deep vein thrombosis (DVT) is pulmonary embolism.

- The highest yield sonographic examination for DVT using US occurs in the **symptomatic** patient who has symptoms **above the knee.** US has a much lower sensitivity in asymptomatic patients.

- The ultrasound examination for deep venous thrombosis is performed by examining the leg along the course of certain anatomical landmarks: the common femoral vein, proximal deep femoral vein, greater saphenous vein, and the popliteal vein.

Sonographic evaluation for DVT of the leg is mainly based on the principle that **normal venous structures will easily be compressed and completely collapsed** by the transducer, whereas veins harboring thrombi will not compress. Sonographic evaluation also seeks to visualize the echogenic thrombus itself (Fig. 19-32).

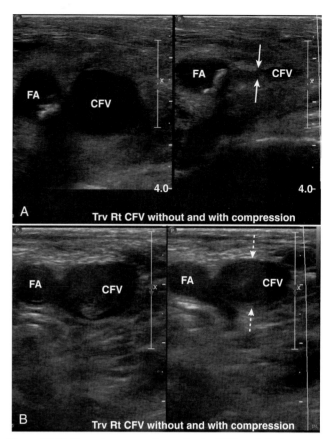

Figure 19-32 Normal common femoral vein (CFV) and deep venous thrombosis (DVT). Normal veins will compress and collapse by pressure from the transducer, whereas veins harboring thrombi will not compress. Arteries will also not collapse. These are paired images done both without and with compression of the CFV in two different patients. **A,** In this normal patient, the *CFV* collapses normally with compression (*solid white arrows*). The femoral artery, as expected, (*FA*) does not. **B,** In this patient with a DVT, the CFV does not collapse with compression (*dotted white arrows*) implying the presence of a clot contained within it.

WEBLINK

Registered users may obtain more information on Ultrasonography: Understanding the Principles and Recognizing Normal and Abnormal Findings on StudentConsult.com.

TAKE-HOME POINTS

Ultrasonography: Understanding the Principles and Recognizing Normal and Abnormal Findings

Creation of a sonographic image (sonogram) depends on three major components: the production of a high frequency sound wave, the reception of a reflected wave or echo, and the conversion of that echo into the actual image.

A tissue that reflects many echoes is said to be **echogenic (hyperechoic)** and is usually depicted as bright or white on the sonogram; a tissue that has few or no echoes is said to be **sonolucent (hypoechoic or anechoic)** and is usually depicted as being dark or black.

Sonography makes use of the Doppler effect to determine if an object, usually blood, is moving toward or away from the transducer and at what velocity it is moving.

There are no known long-term side effects that have been scientifically demonstrated from the use of medical ultrasound in humans.

Gallstones are characteristically echogenic and produce acoustical shadowing because they reflect most of the signal.

Biliary sludge can be found in the lumen of the gallbladder and is often associated with biliary stasis. While it may be echogenic, sludge does not produce acoustical shadowing like gallstones.

The typical appearance of *obstructive uropathy* is a dilated calyceal system. The normally echogenic renal sinus contains a dilated, fluid-filled, and anechoic renal pelvis.

In *medical renal disease*, the renal parenchyma becomes more echogenic (brighter) than the liver and spleen, the reverse of the normal echo pattern.

Ultrasonography is the screening study of choice when an asymptomatic, pulsatile abdominal mass is palpated. The normal abdominal aorta measures <3 cm in diameter.

Leiomyomas confined to the myometrium are the most common tumors of the uterus. The most common mass in the ovary is a functional cyst. Generally, uterine masses are solid and ovarian masses are cystic.

Follicular cysts and corpus luteum cysts are called functional cysts of the ovary. Follicular cysts are more common. Functional cysts are characteristically well-defined, thin-walled, anechoic structures with homogeneous internal fluid density. They may contain echogenic material if hemorrhage occurs into the cyst.

Nonfunctional cysts of the ovary include dermoid cysts, endometriomas, and polycystic ovaries.

Tumors of the ovaries most often arise from the surface covering and are either serous or mucinous. Most serous tumors and the overwhelming number of mucinous tumors are benign.

Pelvic inflammatory disease (PID) is a term used to describe a group of infectious diseases affecting the uterus, fallopian tubes, and ovaries, most beginning as a transient endometritis.

In the recumbent position, ascitic fluid flows up the right paracolic gutter to the right subphrenic space so *ascites* is generally easier to detect by ultrasound in the right upper quadrant between the liver and the diaphragm.

In *acute appendicitis*, the appendix may be a blind-ending, aperistaltic tube with a diameter of 6 mm or more. It is noncompressible and may be tender when palpated with the probe. In about a third of the cases of appendicitis, a fecalith will be present.

Ultrasound has provided a safe and reliable means of visualizing the fetus in utero and the ability to do so repeatedly during the course of a pregnancy, if necessary.

Most *ectopic pregnancies* are tubal in location and occur near the fimbriated (ovarian) end. An ectopic pregnancy can be effectively *excluded* if an intrauterine pregnancy is present and *included* if an extrauterine pregnancy is seen. Most often, an ectopic pregnancy is diagnosed by a combination of absence of an identifiable intrauterine pregnancy while the β-HCG rises above a certain level.

A *molar pregnancy* is suggested by a uterine size that is disproportionately large for the dates of gestation and β-HCG levels in excess of 100,000 mIU/mL (normal pregnancies are less than 60,000 mIU/mL).

Vascular ultrasound studies combine morphologic images of the vessels with the simultaneous recording of the velocity of flow displayed by the Doppler spectral waveform. *Carotid stenosis* begins to cause changes in the velocity of flow when there is greater than 50% narrowing of the lumen.

Sonographic evaluation for *DVT* of the leg is mainly based on the principle that normal venous structures will be easily compressed and collapsed by the transducer, whereas veins harboring thrombi will not compress. Sonographic evaluation also seeks to visualize the echogenic thrombus itself.

Chapter 20

Magnetic Resonance Imaging: Understanding the Principles and Recognizing the Basics

DANIEL J. KOWAL

HOW MRI WORKS

- Magnetic resonance imaging (MRI) involves the use of a very strong magnetic field to manipulate the electromagnetic activity of atomic nuclei in a way that releases energy in the form of radiofrequency signals, which are recorded by the scanner's receiving coils and then computer-processed to form an image.
  - Our bodies are composed of atoms, each of which has a nucleus made up of protons and neutrons. The only exception, but an important one, is the hydrogen nucleus, which is made up of only one proton.
  - *Proton* and *hydrogen nucleus* are interchangeable terms.
  - Although MRI could be used to evaluate many different nuclei, **clinical MRI scanners are based on hydrogen nuclei** due to their abundance in the human body. The body is mostly composed of water molecules, which have an abundance of hydrogen nuclei.
  - Nuclei (like the hydrogen nucleus) that have an **odd number** of **protons or neutrons** will have a **net magnetic moment** and behave like mini-bar magnets, which is what MRI requires to make an image.
- Each proton has a **positive electrical charge**, and because protons also have a spin, this charge is **constantly moving.**
  - You might remember that a **moving electrical charge is also an electrical current**, and because an electrical current **induces a magnetic field**, each proton has its own small magnetic field (or *magnetic moment*).
- Normally, protons in the body spin randomly.
- When a patient enters an MRI scanner, though, the mini-magnet protons all align with the more powerful external magnetic field of the MRI magnet.
  - Most of these protons will point **parallel to the field** and others point **antiparallel** to the field, but they will all align with the external magnetic field of the MRI.
  - The **sum of all magnetic moments** is called the *net magnetization vector.* **Any tissue** placed in a large magnetic field **will have a net magnetization vector.**
- Protons don't like to be couch potatoes, so they *precess* (wobble like a spinning top) along the magnetic field lines of the MRI.
- We'll return to our little protons in a (magnetic) moment.

HARDWARE THAT MAKES UP AN MRI SCANNER

Main Magnet

- The main magnet in an MR scanner is usually a *superconducting magnet.*
- Superconducting magnets contain a conducting coil that is cooled down to **superconducting temperature** in order to carry the current (4° K or −269° Celsius).

At temperatures that low (close to absolute zero), **resistance to the flow of electricity in the conductor practically disappears.**

- Therefore, an electric current sent once through this ultra-cold conducting material **will continuously flow and create a permanent magnetic field. The magnet in an MRI scanner is always "on."**
- To reach temperatures this low, *cryogens* such as liquid helium and nitrogen are utilized.
- If the temperature increases above these superconducting temperatures, a *quench* occurs, and there is suddenly resistance to flow of electricity. The energy stored in the magnetic coils then becomes converted to heat. A quench can be initiated manually if there is an emergent need to turn off the MRI magnet, but it is extremely expensive to turn the magnet back on after a quench.
- Most scanners today have a **magnetic field strength** between **0.5 and 3 Tesla.**
  - **One tesla (T) = 10,000 gauss (G).**
    - No, tesla does not refer to the 1980s hair metal band, but to Nikola Tesla, the father of alternating current.
  - To provide a reference for how strong this magnetic field is, **the earth's magnetic field is only 50 microTesla.**
  - The MRI scanner's external magnetic field is so strong it can pull a metallic oxygen tank into the scanner like a missile.
  - **Open MRI scanners,** those that do not completely encircle the patient in the scanning circle, have **lower field strengths** of 0.1-1.0 T.
  - In general, **higher field strength magnets have better spatial resolution,** but **lower field strength magnets**

have better tissue contrast and are less expensive to install and operate.

Coils

- An important part of the MRI scanner are the **coils** placed within the magnet. These coils are responsible for either transmitting the **radiofrequency (RF) pulses (transmitter coils)** that excite the protons, or receiving the signal (or **echo**) given off by these excited protons (**receiver coils**).
- Types of coils
  - Volume coils
    - These coils surround the part of the body to be imaged, and are **permanently part of the scanner.** They act as the transmitters of the RF pulse (transmitter coils) and can also act as receiver coils.
  - Surface coils
    - These coils are placed directly on the area to be imaged and thus have different shapes, depending on the body part.
    - These coils are **good for superficial structures,** but are poor for deep structures because the detected signal intensity falls rapidly with increased distance from the coil.
    - Unlike volume coils, these coils only act as receiver coils and receive the signal of the excited nuclei, with the RF pulse transmitted by the volume coil.
  - **Gradient coils**

These coils generate additional linear, electromagnetic fields that vary the magnetic field and are important because they help **relate the signal to an exact location and tissue,** and make slice selection and spatial information possible. These coils are the source of the repetitive, machine-gunlike **banging noise** characteristic of MRI, and are **essential for creating** images.

- There are **three sets of gradient coils** corresponding to the three dimensions in space: x, y, and z orientations (i.e., the axial, coronal, and sagittal orientations). It is **these gradient coils that help the MRI scanner detect from which tissue the signal is coming.**

Computer

- A computer dedicated to the MRI scanner processes the radiofrequency signals received by the receiver coils and generates an image.
- The **imaging parameters** set at the MRI console determine how different images will be **weighted,** and ultimately how different tissues will look.

WHAT HAPPENS ONCE SCANNING BEGINS

- When the patient is placed in the scanner magnet, the **transmitter coils** send a short (measured in milliseconds) electromagnetic pulse called a **radiofrequency (RF) pulse.**
  - The spinning protons in the patient **align** with the external magnetic field of the magnet.
  - This RF pulse is sent at a particular frequency that can change the orientation of the protons, **flipping their net**

magnetization vector and **displacing them from their original alignment in the external field.**
- There are two important, different magnetization vector components that play a role in this process: **longitudinal magnetization (parallel to the magnetic field)** and **transverse magnetization (perpendicular to the magnetic field).**
- When the **RF pulse is turned off,** the displaced protons **relax and realign** with the main magnetic field, and energy subsequently released in the form of radiofrequency signals (the echo) is detected by the receiver coils.

The times it takes for this recovery and decay to occur and the echo to be generated are called *T1* and *T2.*

- **T1 and T2 are both time constants,** and it is the values of the T1 and T2 relaxation times that allow different tissues to be identified.
  - T1 is called the **longitudinal relaxation time.**
  - T2 is called the **transversal relaxation time.**
- **T1 relaxation (or recovery)** is the time it takes for the tissue to recover to its longitudinal state, the time before the RF pulse was administered.
- **T2 relaxation (or decay)** is the time it takes for the tissue to regain its transverse orientation, before the RF pulse was administered.
- **In summary,** as soon as the RF pulse stops, relaxation begins (transversal magnetization disappears, and longitudinal magnetization reappears) and the spinning nuclei release energy which is subsequently picked up by the receiver coil and ultimately used to produce an image.

PULSE SEQUENCES

- **Pulse sequences** consist of a set of **imaging parameters** determined in advance by protocols for specific diseases and body parts and then preselected by the MRI technologist at the computer at the time of the study to send a set of instructions to the RF generator and gradient amplifiers.
  - **Pulse sequences** will determine the way different tissues will appear.
  - The orientation of the image (axial, coronal, or sagittal) is also predefined as part of the pulse sequence.
  - Each pulse sequence can take as little as 20 seconds to as long as 15 minutes to complete.
  - **A particular imaging protocol** (e.g., a routine MRI brain protocol) **consists of a series of multiple pulse sequences.** Depending on the number and the time for each pulse sequence, MRI studies can last from a few minutes to over an hour.
- There are **two main pulse sequences: spin echo (SE) and gradient recalled echo (GRE).**
  - Both of these sequences will produce an echo (the radiofrequency signal returning from the protons in the tissue being scanned), and the signal from this echo is used to create an MRI image. **All of the other pulse sequences used in MRI scanning are based on these two sequences.**

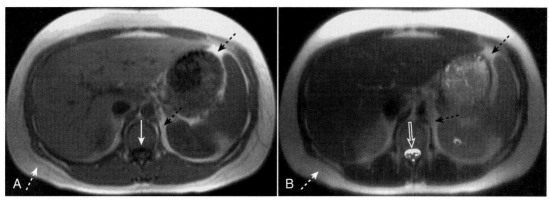

Figure 20-1 **Normal T1-weighted and T2-weighted axial images of the abdomen.** Because cerebrospinal fluid is similar to water in density, it appears dark on the T1-weighted image **(A)** (*solid white arrow*), and bright on the T2-weighted image **(B)** (*open white arrow*). Subcutaneous fat (*dotted white arrows*) and intraabdominal fat (*dotted black arrows*) are bright on both T1-weighted and T2-weighted images.

- **TR and TE**
  - These parameters are set by the MRI operator at the console prior to scanning.
  - Changing the TR and TE will alter how the image is **"weighted."**
  - **TR** is the **repetition time between two RF pulses,** and it influences the amount of *T1 weighting.*
    - Pulse sequences which feature a **short TR** (meaning a short amount of time between the RF pulses) will create what is called a **T1-weighted image.**
  - **TE** is the **echo time between a pulse and its resultant echo,** and it influences the amount of *T2 weighting.*
    - Pulse sequences which feature a **long TE** (meaning a long amount of time between the RF pulse and the echo) will create what is called a **T2-weighted image.**

HOW CAN YOU IDENTIFY A T1-WEIGHTED OR T2-WEIGHTED IMAGE?

- Different tissues have different T1 and T2 values (relaxation and recovery time constants), which is why fat, muscle, and bone, for example, will appear differently not only from each other but also with different pulse sequences.

 Tissues that have a short T1 will be bright.

- Tissues with a long T2 will be bright.
- "Bright" translates into "whiter" or having "increased signal intensity" on MRI scans. "Dark" translates into "blacker" or having "decreased signal intensity" on MRI.
- A key point is that **water will be dark on T1-weighted images and bright on T2-weighted images. Water is T1-dark and T2-bright.**
  - A **bright** way to remember this fact is that the number "2" is both in H_2O (water) and T2-weighted image.
  - Therefore, when you are looking at any MR image, **first try to find something you know is fluid (water),** such as the CSF in the ventricles and spinal canal or **urine** in the bladder, for example.
  - **If the fluid is dark, then you are probably looking at a T1-weighted sequence** (Fig. 20-1A).
  - **If this fluid is bright, then chances are you are looking at a T2-weighted image** (Fig. 20-1B).

 Certain tissues and structures **are typically bright on T1-weighted images.**

- **Fat:** subcutaneous and intraabdominal fat, fat within yellow bone marrow, fat-containing tumors (see Fig. 20-1A)
- **Hemorrhage:** although this varies depending on the age of the hemorrhage (Fig. 20-2)
- **Proteinaceous fluid:** proteinaceous fluid in renal or hepatic cysts, cystic neoplasms (Fig. 20-3)
  - However, a simple cyst containing water will be dark on T1 (and bright on T2), because remember that water is T1-dark (Fig. 20-4)
- **Melanin,** e.g., melanoma (Fig. 20-5)
- **Gadolinium and other paramagnetic substances (manganese, copper)**
- Certain tissues and structures **are typically bright on T2-weighted images.**
  - **Fat:** subcutaneous and intraabdominal fat, fat within yellow bone marrow, fat-containing tumors (see Fig. 20-1B)
  - **Water, edema,** (Figs. 20-6 and 20-7) **inflammation, infection, cysts** (see Fig. 20-4)
  - **Hemorrhage:** although this varies depending on the age of the hemorrhage (see Fig. 20-2).
- Notice that **both fat and hemorrhage can be T1-bright and T2-bright.**
- **Suppression**
  - A useful feature of MRI is the ability to **cancel out** or **suppress** the signal from certain tissues, thus making that tissue look **dark** on the image, and making other structures and pathology more conspicuous.
  - **A tissue that is often suppressed is fat.**
  - **Fat** is normally bright on T1-weighted images, but **will be dark on T1-fat suppressed images** (Fig. 20-8).
  - This feature is useful when attempting to identify fat-containing lesions such as **ovarian dermoid cysts, adrenal myelolipomas,** and **liposarcomas** (Fig. 20-9), as they will appear to change from bright on the nonfat suppressed images to dark on the fat-suppressed images.
  - Fat suppression is **also useful** for evaluation of tissues **after the administration of gadolinium contrast.**
- There are many other pulse sequences besides T1-weighted and T2-weighted images that typically comprise a particular MRI scan protocol, such as *diffusion-weighted images*

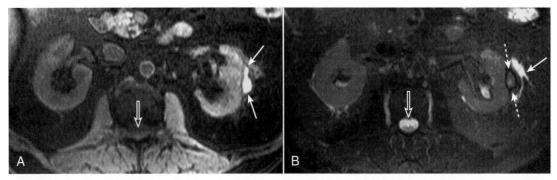

Figure 20-2 Subcapsular hematoma of the kidney. A, Axial T1-weighted fat-suppressed image demonstrates a bright subcapsular hematoma (*solid white arrows*) involving the left kidney laterally. We can tell that this is a T1-weighted image because cerebrospinal fluid (CSF) in the spinal canal is dark (*open white arrow*). **B,** Axial T2-weighted, fat-suppressed image again demonstrates a slightly bright left subcapsular hematoma with a dark rim of hemosiderin (*dotted white arrows*) indicating surrounding older blood. There is a small amount of adjacent left perinephric fluid (*solid white arrow*). The bright signal of the CSF helps us to recognize this image as a T2-weighted image (*open white arrow*).

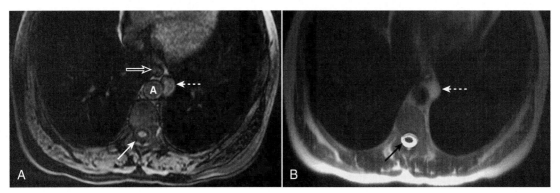

Figure 20-3 Proteinaceous enteric cyst. A, Axial T1-weighted fat-suppressed image demonstrates a left-sided, mediastinal bright mass (*dotted white arrow*) adjacent to the esophagus (*open white arrow*) and aorta (*A*). Notice that this mass is brighter than the CSF in the spinal canal (*solid white arrow*). **B,** Axial T2-weighted image shows that the mass is T2 bright (*dotted white arrow*), but not as bright as the CSF in the spinal canal (*solid black arrow*). Contrast-enhanced images (not shown) demonstrated no enhancement. At surgery, this mass was found to represent a benign enteric cyst containing proteinaceous (as opposed to purely simple) fluid.

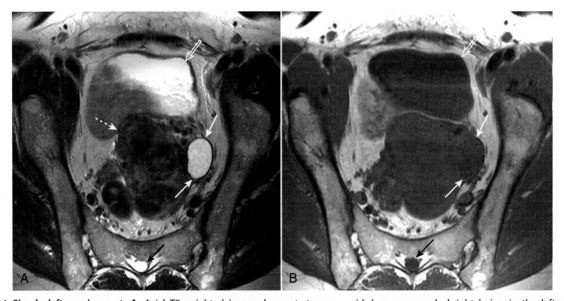

Figure 20-4 Simple left ovarian cyst. A, Axial T2-weighted image demonstrates an ovoid, homogeneously bright lesion in the left ovary (*solid white arrows*) adjacent to a fibroid uterus (*dotted white arrows*). Note that urine in the bladder (*open white arrow*) and CSF in the spinal canal (*solid black arrow*) are both bright, which helps us identify this image as a T2-weighted image. **B,** Axial T1-weighted image shows that this left ovarian lesion is dark (*solid white arrows*) and therefore consistent with simple fluid. Urine in the bladder (*open white arrow*) and CSF in the spinal canal (*closed black arrow*) are also dark.

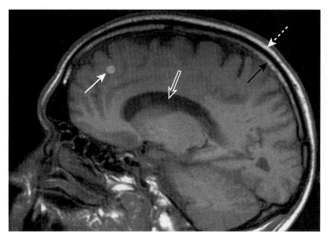

Figure 20-5 Metastatic melanoma. Sagittal T1-weighted image of the brain demonstrates a bright mass (*solid white arrow*) in the frontal lobe representing metastatic melanoma. Notice that both the yellow bone marrow within the skull (*solid black arrow*) and the overlying subcutaneous fat (*dotted white arrow*) are bright. We can tell that this is a T1-weighted image because the CSF in the lateral ventricles is dark (*open white arrow*).

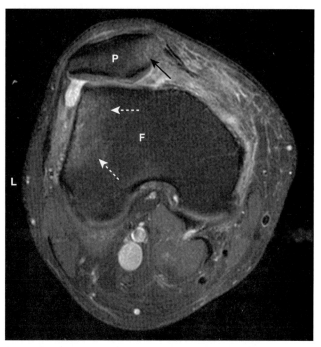

Figure 20-7 Bone marrow edema due to transient patellar dislocation. Axial proton-density, fat-saturated image (a T2-like sequence) demonstrates bright bone marrow edema involving the lateral (*L*) femoral (*F*) condyle (*dotted white arrows*) and medial aspect of the patella (*P*) (*solid black arrow*). This edema is due to recent lateral patellar dislocation with contusion as it struck the femur.

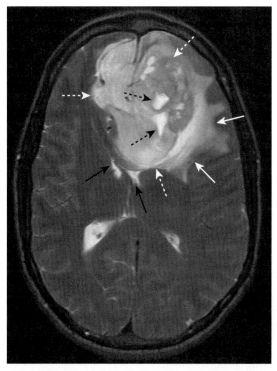

Figure 20-6 Glioblastoma multiforme with surrounding edema. Axial T2-weighted image demonstrates bright vasogenic type edema (*solid white arrows*) surrounding a large, lobulated frontal lobe mass (*dotted white arrows*) representing glioblastoma multiforme, an aggressive brain tumor. There are a few bright areas of cystic degeneration (*dotted black arrows*) within this mass. The frontal horns of the lateral ventricles are compressed (*solid black arrows*).

(*DWI*), ***proton density-weighted images,*** and an entire alphabet soup of catchy acronyms like ***STIR*** and ***MRA/TOF.***

MRI CONTRAST: GENERAL CONSIDERATIONS

- **Gadolinium** is the most common intravenous contrast agent used in clinical MRI imaging.

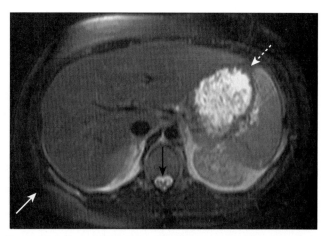

Figure 20-8 Normal T2-weighted fat-suppressed axial image of the abdomen. We can tell that this is a T2-weighted image because the CSF in the spinal canal is bright (*solid black arrow*). Also, it is a fat-suppressed image because the subcutaneous (*solid white arrow*) and intraabdominal (*dotted white arrow*) fat are dark. Fat is normally bright on a T2-weighted image without fat suppression.

- It is a rare-earth, heavy metal ion that is chelated to different compounds to form MRI contrast agents. When chelated to an acid known as DTPA (Gd-DTPA), it forms *gadopentetate dimeglumine*, also known as the commonly used contrast agent *Magnevist®*.
- Gadolinium-based contrast agents are **used in the same fashion that iodinated contrast media is used in CT.** They can be injected intravascularly or intraarticularly.
- After intravenous injection, Gd-DTPA enters the blood pool, enhances organ parenchyma, and then is excreted by the kidneys via glomerular filtration.

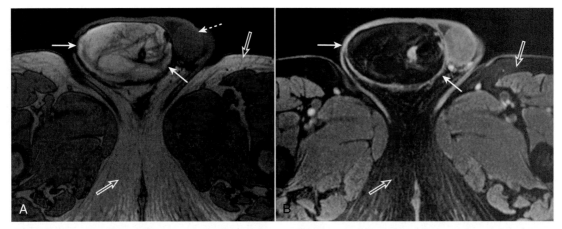

Figure 20-9 Fat in a liposarcoma of the right spermatic cord. A, Axial T1-weighted image of the scrotum demonstrates a bright, heterogeneous right scrotal mass (*solid white arrows*). The left testis is unremarkable (*dotted white arrow*), and the right testis is not visualized. Note that subcutaneous fat is normally bright (*open white arrows*). **B,** Axial T1-weighted, fat-suppressed, gadolinium-enhanced image demonstrates that the bright signal in the right scrotal mass is now dark, consistent with fat (*solid white arrows*). The subcutaneous fat of the thighs is also dark (*open white arrows*). This was an unusual malignancy of the spermatic cord derived from fat cells.

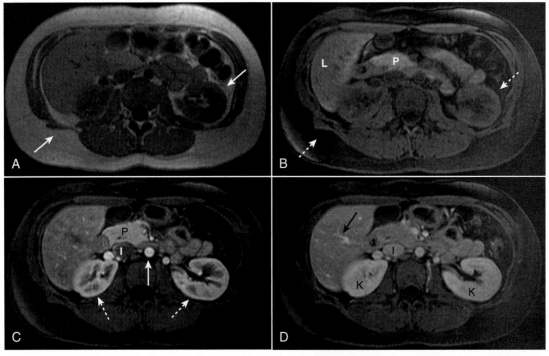

Figure 20-10 Fat suppression and normal enhancement of the abdomen following the administration of intravenous gadolinium. A, T1-weighted image of a normal abdomen demonstrates normal bright subcutaneous and intraabdominal fat (*solid white arrows*). **B,** T1-weighted, fat-suppressed image shows that the signal from the fat has been suppressed (*dotted white arrows*) and is now dark. Intraabdominal organs such as the pancreas (*P*) and liver (*L*) now appear brighter relative to the adjacent suppressed fat. **C,** T1-weighted, fat-suppressed, early phase post-gadolinium image shows the normal enhancement of the aorta (*solid white arrow*) which enhances earlier than the inferior vena cava (*I*). The kidneys demonstrate normal corticomedullary phase enhancement (*dotted white arrows*), and the pancreas (*P*) enhances maximally during this phase. **D,** T1-weighted, fat-suppressed, later phase post-gadolinium image shows that the hepatic veins (*solid black arrow*) and inferior vena cava (*I*) are now well enhanced. The kidneys (*K*) now demonstrate normal homogeneous enhancement, the optimal phase to detect renal masses.

- Other special types of gadolinium-based contrast agents have a component of biliary excretion.

➤ **Gadolinium's effect is to shorten the T1 relaxation times** of hydrogen nuclei (and to a lesser extent also shorten T2).

■ **T1 shortening will cause a brighter signal on T1-weighted images,** and it is for this reason that **images obtained after**

gadolinium administration are usually T1-weighted to take advantage of this effect.

■ Fat is bright on T1 even before the administration of gadolinium. In order to increase detection of contrast enhancement in fat, the precontrast and postcontrast images are typically fat-suppressed (meaning darkened) to enhance the effect of the gadolinium (Fig. 20-10).

■ Structures that become **bright on postgadolinium images are typically vascular** (such as tumors) (Fig. 20-11)

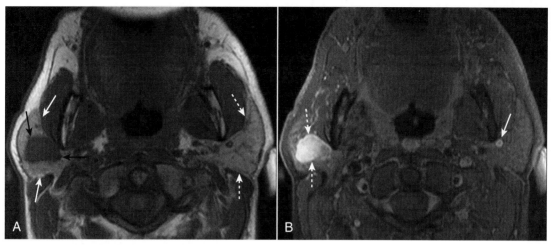

Figure 20-11 Right parotid pleomorphic adenoma. A, Axial T1-weighted image of the neck demonstrates a dark, ovoid mass with a slightly lobular contour (*solid black arrows*) located within the right parotid gland (*solid white arrows*). The left parotid gland is unremarkable (*dotted white arrows*). **B,** Axial T1-weighted, fat-suppressed, post-gadolinium enhanced image demonstrates that the right parotid mass is very bright due to intense enhancement (*dotted white arrows*). Surgical resection of this mass yielded a pleomorphic adenoma, the most common benign tumor of the parotid gland. A clue that this image is a gadolinium-enhanced image is the presence of bright, enhancing vascular structures such as the left retromandibular vein (*solid white arrow*).

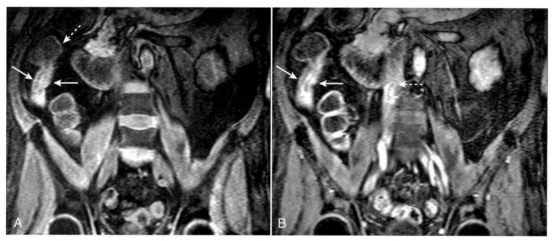

Figure 20-12 Active inflammation in Crohn disease. A, Coronal T1-weighted fat-suppressed image from an MR enterography examination demonstrates thickening of the wall of the distal terminal ileum (*solid white arrows*). The adjacent cecum is normal (*dotted white arrow*). **B,** Coronal T1-weighted, fat-suppressed, gadolinium-enhanced image demonstrates marked enhancement of the wall of the terminal ileum (*solid white arrows*) indicating that this wall thickening represents active inflammatory narrowing of the lumen. Gadolinium is also seen within the inferior vena cava (*dotted white arrow*), a finding that helps us determine that this is an enhanced image.

and **inflammation** (Fig. 20-12), and are described as **enhancing.**

MRI SAFETY ISSUES

General Considerations

- **No harmful biological effects** have been demonstrated from exposure to **static magnetic fields below 10 T.** The maximum clinical MR field strength is well below that value, currently at 3.0 T.

Claustrophobia

- Patients can occasionally suffer such extreme claustrophobia in the small confines of the MR scanner that **they will be unable to begin or complete** the study. Pretreatment with sedation may help in the appropriate clinical situation.

- Alternatively, the patient can be scanned in an **open magnet,** which is not as confining. The trade-off, however, is that open magnets in general have lower magnetic field strengths and poorer spatial resolution.

Ferromagnetic Objects

- Any ferromagnetic object inside the patient **can be moved** by the magnetic field of the MR scanner and could damage adjacent tissues. Such internal ferromagnetic objects also hold the potential to be **heated and cause burns** to surrounding tissues.

⮕ **Ferromagnetic objects in a location where motion of the object may be harmful to the patient represent an absolute contraindication to MR imaging.** These objects include medically inserted items such as cerebral aneurysm repair clips, vascular clips, and surgical staples.

Many vascular clips and staples are now manufactured to be MRI-compatible.

- Some **foreign bodies, such as bullets, shrapnel, and metal in the eyes** (as can be seen in metal workers) can also be ferromagnetic.
  - Patients who may have a history of possible metallic foreign bodies in the eyes must have conventional orbital radiographs before undergoing an MRI and, if metal is present, an alternative means of imaging should be utilized.
  - If a patient who has metallic foreign bodies in the eyes undergoes an MRI, motion of these foreign bodies could cause blindness.
- Ferromagnetic objects outside of the patient such as **oxygen tanks, scissors, scalpels,** and **metallic tools,** also pose a risk to the patient as **they could become airborne** once they enter the magnetic field and for this reason are strictly forbidden in the MRI scanning room. **Nonferromagnetic equipment ("MR-safe equipment") is now available,** and is used for MRI-guided procedures such as biopsies.

Mechanical or Electrical Devices

MRI **cannot** be performed in patients who have **pacemakers, pain stimulator implants, insulin pumps, other implantable drug infusion pumps, and cochlear implants.**

- The presence of a pacemaker or implantable cardiac defibrillator represents an **absolute contraindication to MR imaging** because the device may be deactivated by the magnetic field, and there may also be heating induced in the leads that could injure the endocardium.

Pregnant Patients

- Although there are no known biological risks associated with MR imaging in adults, the effects of MRI on the fetus are not definitely known (Fig. 20-13).

Because only limited data exists and because the fetus is more susceptible to injury in the first trimester of pregnancy, **pregnancy is considered by some to be an absolute contraindication to MR imaging** due to theoretical harmful effects to the fetus.

- The American College of Radiology, however, states that pregnant patients **can** undergo MRI scans at any stage of pregnancy if it is decided that the risk-benefit ratio to the patient weighs in favor of performing the study.

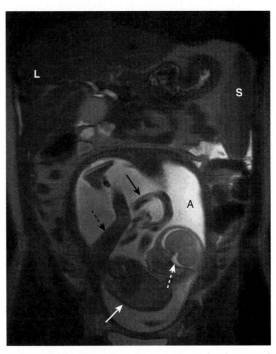

Figure 20-13 **MRI in pregnancy.** Coronal T2-weighted image demonstrates an intrauterine pregnancy. The maternal liver (*L*) and spleen (*S*) are partially imaged. The bright amniotic fluid (*A*) and fetal CSF (*dotted white arrow*) help us to recognize this image as a T2-weighted image. The fetal body (*solid white arrow*) and leg (*dotted black arrow*) can be seen clearly. The umbilical cord (*solid black arrow*) is partially visualized.

TABLE 20-1 USES OF MRI

System	Organ	Diseases
Musculoskeletal	Evaluate bone marrow menisci, tendons, muscles	Meniscal tears; ligamentous and tendon injuries; contusions
	Bones	Occult or stress fractures
	Osteomyelitis	High negative predictive value if normal
	Spine (Chapter 24)	Disk disease and marrow infiltration; differentiating scarring from prior surgery from new disease
Neurologic	Brain (Chapter 25)	Ideal for studying brain, especially posterior fossa; tumor, infarction; multiple sclerosis
	Peripheral nerves	Impingement; injury
GI	Liver (Chapter 18)	Characterize liver lesions; detect small lesions; cysts, hemangiomas; hepatocellular carcinoma; focal nodular hyperplasia; hemochromatosis; fatty infiltration
	Biliary system (Chapter 18)	Magnetic resonance cholangiopancreatography for strictures, ductal dilatation
	Small and large bowel	MR enterography; appendicitis in pregnant females
Endocrine/ reproductive	Adrenal glands	Adenomas; adrenal hemorrhage
	Female pelvis	Anatomy of uterus and ovaries; leiomyomas; adenomyosis; ovarian dermoid cysts; endometriosis; hydrosalpinx
	Male pelvis	Staging of rectal, bladder, and prostate carcinoma
GU	Kidneys	Renal masses; cysts versus masses

- MRI should probably not be performed **electively** in early term pregnancy due to this unknown risk to the fetus.
- **Gadolinium is not recommended in pregnant patients,** as gadolinium crosses the placenta, is subsequently excreted by the fetal kidneys, and has unknown effects on the fetus.

Nephrogenic Systemic Fibrosis

- In patients with renal insufficiency, gadolinium-based contrast agents have been associated with a rare, painful, debilitating, and sometimes fatal disease called **nephrogenic systemic fibrosis (NSF).**
- NSF produces fibrosis of skin, eyes, joints, and internal organs resembling scleroderma.
- Patients with **preexisting renal dysfunction,** especially those on dialysis, are at the **greatest risk.**
  - **Caution** is exercised **when administering gadolinium** to patients who have **moderate renal disease** (estimated glomerular filtration rate [eGFR] between 30-60 mL/min/1.73m^2). Gadolinium is typically avoided in patients with severe renal disease (eGFR < 30).
- There is currently no evidence to suggest that patients with normal renal function are at risk of developing NSF, and contrast-enhanced MRI imaging remains extremely safe in the vast majority of patients.

DIAGNOSTIC APPLICATIONS OF MRI

- Some of the many clinical uses of MRI are outlined in Table 20-1. The chapters in which some of the diseases are discussed in greater detail are indicated.

WEBLINK

Registered users may obtain more information on Magnetic Resonance Imaging: Understanding the Principles and Recognizing the Basics on StudentConsult.com.

TAKE-HOME POINTS

MRI: Understanding the Principles and Recognizing the Basics

MRI uses a very strong magnetic field to influence the electromagnetic activity of hydrogen nuclei, also called protons.

Protons each have a charge and possess a spin. The constant movement of protons generates a small magnetic field causing the proton to behave like a mini-magnet. When the protons are placed in the much more powerful magnetic field of the MRI scanner, they all align with this external magnetic field.

A radiofrequency (RF) pulse, transmitted by a transmitter coil, displaces the protons from their original alignment with the external magnetic field of the scanner.

When the RF pulse is turned off, the displaced protons relax and realign with the main magnetic field,

producing a radiofrequency signal (the echo) as they do so. Receiver coils receive this signal (or echo) given off by the excited protons. A computer reconstructs the information from the echo to generate an image.

The main magnet in an MRI scanner is usually a superconducting magnet that is cooled to extremely low temperatures in order to carry the electrical current.

There are three major types of coils within the MRI scanner: volume, surface, and gradient coils.

Pulse sequences consist of a set of imaging parameters that determine the way a particular tissue will appear. The two main pulse sequences that all MRI pulse sequences are based on are called spin echo (SE) and gradient recalled echo (GRE).

T1 and T2 are both time constants. T1 is called the longitudinal relaxation time, and T2 is called the transversal relaxation time.

TR is the repetition time between two RF pulses. A short TR creates a T1-weighted image.

TE is the echo time between a pulse and its resultant echo. A long TE creates a T2-weighted image.

On T1-weighted images, fat, hemorrhage, proteinaceous fluid, melanin, and gadolinium are typically bright (white).

On T2-weighted images, fat, water, edema, inflammation, infection, cysts, and hemorrhage are typically bright.

In summary, fat is T1-bright and T2-bright. Water is T1-dark and T2-bright.

Suppression is a feature of MRI that will cancel out or eliminate signal from certain tissues and is most often used for fat. Although normally T1-bright, fat will be dark on T1-weighted fat suppressed images. Fat suppression is particularly useful for tissue characterization after administration of gadolinium.

Gadolinium is the most common intravenous contrast agent used in clinical MR imaging, and its effect is to shorten the T1 relaxation time of hydrogen nuclei yielding a brighter signal. Vascular structures such as tumors and areas of inflammation enhance after gadolinium administration and become more conspicuous.

Ferromagnetic objects must be kept outside of the MRI scanning room as they could become airborne when exposed to the magnetic field. Patients who may have metallic foreign bodies in their eyes must first have conventional orbital radiographs to see if metal is present.

In pregnancy, MRI is preferred in the second and third trimester, and gadolinium is contraindicated.

Nephrogenic systemic fibrosis is a debilitating fibrotic disease that can occur in patients with renal insufficiency who receive intravenous gadolinium-based contrast agents. Therefore, gadolinium is typically avoided in patients with severe renal disease.

Chapter 21

Recognizing Abnormalities of Bone Density

NORMAL BONE ANATOMY

Conventional Radiography

- On conventional radiographs, bones consist of a dense *cortex* of **compact bone**, which completely envelopes a less dense *medullary cavity* containing **cancellous bone** arranged as *trabeculae*, separated primarily by blood vessels, hematopoietic cells, and fat. The proportions of cortical versus trabecular bone vary in different skeletal sites and even at different locations in the same bone, i.e., the **cortex is naturally thicker in some places than in others.**
- When viewed in **tangent** on conventional radiographs, the **cortex** produces a **smooth white shell** of varying thickness that appears as a dense white band along the outer margins of the bone.
- The **medullary cavity** on conventional radiographs appears as a core of less dense, **grayish material inside the cortical shell, interlaced with a fine network of bony trabecular markings.** The *corticomedullary junction* is the edge between the inner margin of the cortex and the medullary cavity (Fig. 21-1).
- It is important to remember that **the cortex completely surrounds the entire bone** but on conventional radiographs is best seen where it is viewed in profile, i.e., where the x-ray beam passes tangentially to the bone.
- Almost all **examinations of bone start with conventional radiographs** obtained with at least **two views exposed at a 90° angle to each other** (called *orthogonal views*) so as to localize abnormalities better and to visualize as much of the circumference of the bone as possible.
    - Still, **conventional radiographs cannot visualize the entire circumference of a tubular bone** and **they are not particularly sensitive for demonstrating musculoskeletal soft tissue abnormalities** other than soft tissue swelling.

CT and MRI

- CT and MRI are able to demonstrate the entire circumference and internal matrix of bone, including, especially with MRI, surrounding soft tissues not visible on conventional radiographs. This is accomplished by computer-aided reformatting and a superior ability to display more subtle differences in tissue densities (Fig. 21-2).
- In addition to bony trabeculae, the marrow cavity contains *red and yellow bone marrow*. The **red marrow** produces the precursors of blood cells. **Yellow marrow** contains fat. The composition of marrow is different for different bones of the body and changes during life to become less

hematopoietically active with age so that, around age 30, most of the appendicular skeleton contains only yellow marrow while most of the red marrow resides in the axial skeleton. Unlike conventional radiography, **MRI is an excellent means of studying** the components of marrow, a fact that makes MRI so useful in the study of **marrow pathology.**
- Whereas the cortex is the part of the bone most easily visualized on conventional radiographs, **cortical bone has a very low signal intensity on conventional MRI** sequences.

THE EFFECT OF BONE PHYSIOLOGY ON BONE ANATOMY

- Bones reflect the general metabolic status of the individual. Their composition requires a **protein-containing, collagenous matrix (*osteoid*)** upon which **bone mineral**, principally *calcium phosphate*, is transformed into cartilage and bone.
- Bones are continuously undergoing remodeling processes that include **resorption of old or diseased bone by osteoclasts** and **formation of new bone by osteoblasts.** While osteoblasts are responsible for bone matrix production, osteoclasts resorb both the matrix and mineral.
- Both osteoclastic and osteoblastic activity depend on the presence of a viable blood supply to bring those cells to the bone
- **Bones** also **respond to mechanical forces**—for example, the contractions of muscles and tendons, the process of bearing weight, constant use, or prolonged disuse—that help to form or maintain the shape as well as the content of each bone.
- In this chapter, we arbitrarily divide abnormalities of bone density into two major categories based primarily on their appearance on conventional radiographs—those that produce a pattern of either **increased** or **decreased** bone density and then subdivide those two patterns by **extent of disease: focal** versus **diffuse** (or **generalized**) changes (Table 21-1).
- If **MRI** were used as the basis for categorization, bone (marrow) disorders could be divided into four other categories:
    - **Reconversion** refers to the reversal of the normal conversion of marrow cells so that red marrow repopulates bone from which it had been replaced by yellow marrow. Chronic anemias such as sickle cell disease are examples of this category.
    - **Marrow replacement** such as by metastatic cells, multiple myeloma, or leukemia.

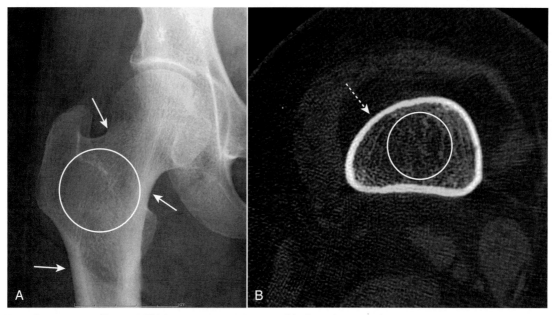

Figure 21-1 Normal appearance of bone. A, This is an anteroposterior view of the hip. When viewed in tangent, the cortex is seen as a white line, varying in thickness in different parts of the bone (*solid white arrows*). In the medullary cavity, cancellous bone is seen to contain an interlacing network of trabeculae (*white circle*). **B,** An axial CT scan through the proximal femur. The entire 360° circumference of the cortex (*dotted white arrow*) is seen surrounding the less-dense medullary cavity containing both bony trabeculae and fat (*white circle*). The image is optimized to display bone so that the muscles and subcutaneous fat are less well seen.

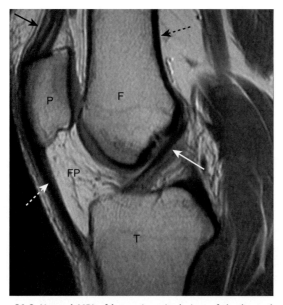

Figure 21-2 Normal MRI of knee. A sagittal view of the knee demonstrates the superior display of the internal matrix of bone and the surrounding soft tissues. There is fatty marrow in the distal femur (*F*), proximal tibia (*T*), and patella (*P*). The quadriceps (*solid black arrow*) and patellar (*dotted white arrow*) tendons are shown. The anterior cruciate ligament (*solid white arrow*) is visible. There is bright signal fat in the infrapatellar fat pad (*FP*). Notice how the cortex of bone has a very weak signal (*dotted black arrow*).

- **Myeloid depletion** involves the loss of red marrow by such agents as radiation, chemotherapy, or aplastic anemias.
- **Myelofibrosis** involves the replacement of marrow by fibrous tissue such as might result from chemotherapy or radiation treatments.
- Fractures and dislocations, arthritis, and spinal diseases are discussed in subsequent chapters.

TABLE 21-1 CHANGES IN BONE DENSITY

Density	Extent	Examples Used in this Chapter
Increased Density ↑	Diffuse	Diffuse osteoblastic metastases Osteopetrosis (rare)
	Focal	Localized osteoblastic metastases Avascular necrosis of bone Paget disease
Decreased Density ↓	Diffuse	Osteoporosis Hyperparathyroidism Rickets and osteomalacia
	Focal	Localized osteolytic metastases Multiple myeloma Osteomyelitis

RECOGNIZING A GENERALIZED INCREASE IN BONE DENSITY

- On conventional radiographs and CT, there will be an **overall whiteness (sclerosis)** to all or most of the bones.
- This leads to a **diffuse loss of visualization of the normal network of bony trabeculae in the medullary cavity** because of replacement of the normal intertrabecular fatty marrow by bone-producing elements.
- There is also a **loss of visualization of the normal corticomedullary junction** because of the abnormally increased density of the medullary cavity relative to the cortex (Fig. 21-3).
- Examples of diseases that cause a diffuse increase in bone density are shown in Box 21-1.

Carcinoma of the Prostate

- Diffuse, blood-borne, metastatic disease from *carcinoma of the prostate* is the **prototype for generalized increase in**

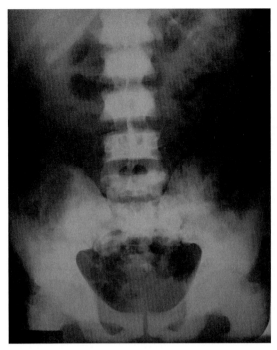

Figure 21-3 Diffuse metastatic disease from carcinoma of the prostate. The bones are diffusely sclerotic. You can no longer see the normal trabeculae or the junction between the medullary cavity and the cortex as the medullary cavities have been filled in with osteoblastic metastatic disease that obscures these normal boundaries and increases the overall bone density. Contrast this picture with that of Paget disease of the pelvis (see Fig. 21-12).

Box 21-1 **Diffuse Increase in Bone Density**
Carcinoma of the prostate (which can also cause a focal increase in bone density)
Osteopetrosis

bone density. Osteoblastic activity occurs **beyond the control** of normal physiologic constraints.

- Metastatic disease to bone **occurs in over 80% of autopsied patients with carcinoma of the prostate. Multiple bone metastases** from carcinoma of the prostate occur much **more frequently** than do **solitary bone lesions.**

- With diffuse bone metastases, a so-called *superscan* may be seen on radionuclide bone scan. The superscan demonstrates high radiotracer uptake throughout the skeleton, with poor or absent renal excretion of the radiotracer (Fig. 21-4).

Osteopetrosis

- *Osteopetrosis* (also called *marble bone disease* for obvious reasons) is a **rare** hereditary **defect in osteoclastic activity** that ultimately results in an **increase in bone density** affecting the entire skeleton (Fig. 21-5).

- Although the bones are increased in density, they are **mechanically inferior** to normal bone and are more prone to **pathologic fractures.**

- In the **infantile form** of this disease, the defective osseous material can replace **normal bone marrow** leading to **anemia, thrombocytopenia, and leukopenia** (*pancytopenia*).

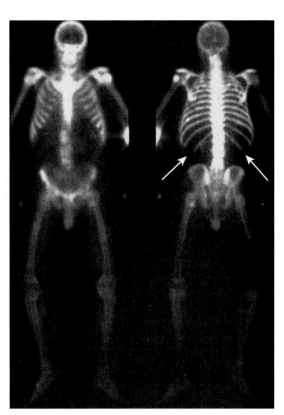

Figure 21-4 Radionuclide bone superscan. Anterior and posterior views of the axial and appendicular skeleton show the increased distribution of bone radiotracer uptake throughout the skeleton. This is the picture of the so-called **superscan** produced by osteoblastic metastatic disease involving every bone leading to high uptake throughout the skeleton, with poor or absent renal excretion of the radiotracer (*solid white arrows* point to the absence of excretion by the kidneys).

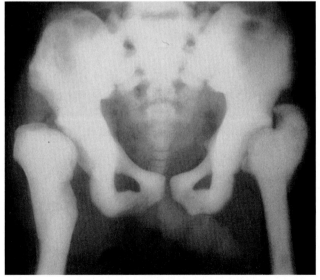

Figure 21-5 Osteopetrosis (marble bone disease). A frontal view of the pelvis demonstrates diffuse sclerosis of the bones in this 22-year-old patient with osteopetrosis, a rare defect in osteoclastic activity that results in an increase in bone density. Although the bones are dense, they are mechanically inferior to normal bone and subject to pathologic fractures. In the infantile form of this disease, the defective osseous material can replace normal bone marrow leading to anemia, thrombocytopenia, and leukopenia (pancytopenia).

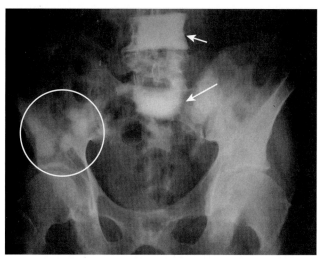

Figure 21-6 Focal sclerotic metastases from carcinoma of the prostate. There are sclerotic lesions seen in the L4 and S1 vertebral bodies (*solid white arrows*). It is no longer possible to distinguish the junction between the cortex and the medullary cavity in either of those vertebral bodies. Also present are multiple sclerotic lesions in the right ilium (*white circle*) and scattered throughout the pelvis. Sclerotic lesions in bone are a common finding in carcinoma of the prostate.

Box 21-2 Focal Increase in Bone Density

Carcinoma of the prostate (which can also cause a diffuse increase in bone density)

Avascular necrosis of bone

Paget disease

RECOGNIZING A FOCAL INCREASE IN BONE DENSITY

Focal sclerotic lesions can affect the cortex and medullary cavity. Those that affect the **cortex** will usually produce **periosteal new-bone formation (periosteal reaction)**, which leads to an appearance of **thickening of the cortex**. Those that affect the **medullary cavity** will result in **punctate, amorphous sclerotic lesions** surrounded by the normal medullary cavity (Fig. 21-6).

- Examples of diseases that cause a **focal increase in bone density** are shown in Box 21-2.

Carcinoma of the Prostate

- A substance secreted by tumor cells from **metastatic carcinoma of the prostate may stimulate osteoblastic activity** and produce focal areas of localized increased density, i.e., **sclerotic bone lesions.** The lesions may also be diffuse. These lesions are **most often seen in the vertebrae, ribs, pelvis, humeri, and femora** (Fig. 21-7).
- The **radionuclide bone scan is currently the study of choice for detecting skeletal metastases**, regardless of the suspected primary (Box 21-3).

Avascular Necrosis of Bone

- Avascular necrosis (AVN) of bone (also called *ischemic necrosis, aseptic necrosis, osteonecrosis*) results from cellular death and leads to collapse of the affected bone. It

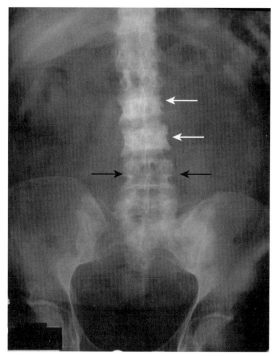

Figure 21-7 Focal increase in bone density from carcinoma of the breast. A frontal view of the lumbar spine and pelvis demonstrates abnormally dense vertebral bodies most marked at L2 and L3 (*solid white arrows*). Notice how the pedicles are obscured by the abnormally increased density of the vertebral body compared to the normal pedicles at L4 (*solid black arrows*). Dense, white vertebrae are called *ivory vertebrae*. Osteoblastic metastases from carcinoma of the breast and prostate are two causes of an ivory vertebra.

Box 21-3 Finding Metastases to Bone—Bone Scan

Bone scans use intravenous administration of a minute amount of Technetium 99m MDP, a radioactively tagged tracer that affixes to bone.

Technetium 99m is the radionuclide used to tag methylene diphosphonate (MDP), the portion that directs the tracer to bone.

Activity in bone depends, in part, on its blood supply and rate of bone turnover: processes with extremely high or extremely low bone turnover may produce false-negative scans.

Osteoblastic lesions almost always show increased activity (greater uptake of radiotracer). Even osteolytic metastases usually show increased uptake because of the repair that occurs in most, but not all, osteolytic processes.

The bone scan is much less sensitive in detecting multiple myeloma because of its purely lytic nature, so conventional radiographic surveys of the skeleton are the initial study of choice when searching for myeloma lesions

Bone scans are highly sensitive, but not very specific. A positive scan almost always requires another imaging procedure (conventional radiographs, CT, or MRI) to rule out nonmalignant causes of a positive bone scan (e.g., fractures or infection).

---

usually involves those bones that have a relatively poor collateral blood supply (e.g., scaphoid in the wrist or the head of the femur) and tends to affect the hematopoietic elements of marrow earliest so that **MRI is the most sensitive modality for detecting AVN.**

- There are a myriad of causes of avascular necrosis. Some of the more common are shown in Table 21-2.
- On conventional radiographs, the **region of avascular necrosis appears denser than the surrounding bone.** On

TABLE 21-2 SOME CAUSES OF AVASCULAR NECROSIS OF BONE

Location	Example of Disease
Intravascular	Sickle-cell disease Polycythemia vera
Vascular	Vasculitis (lupus and radiation-induced)
Extravascular	Trauma (fractures)
Idiopathic	Exogenous steroids and Cushing disease Legg-Calvé-Perthes disease

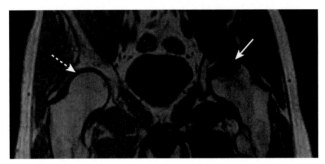

Figure 21-8 Avascular necrosis, MRI. A T1-weighted coronal view of both hips demonstrates normal high signal from the fatty marrow in the right femur (*dotted white arrow*) but decreased signal in the left femoral head extending to the subchondral bone of the left hip joint (*solid white arrow*). The joint space is preserved.

MRI, there is usually a **decrease from the normal high signal** produced by fatty marrow (Fig. 21-8).

- The **devascularized bone becomes denser** and therefore appears more sclerotic than the remainder of the bone. This especially occurs in the **femoral head** (Fig. 21-9) and **humeral head** (Fig. 21-10).
- On conventional radiographs, old *medullary bone infarcts* are recognized as dense, amorphous deposits of bone within the medullary cavities of long bones, frequently marginated by a thin, sclerotic membrane (Fig. 21-11).

Paget Disease

- Paget disease is a **chronic disease of bone**, most often occurring in older men, now believed to be due to chronic paramyxoviral infection. It is **characterized by varying degrees of increased bone resorption and increased bone formation** with the latter predominating in those cases seen in more progressive forms of the disease.
- The end result is almost always a **denser bone** that, despite its density, is **mechanically inferior** to normal bone and thus **susceptible to pathologic fractures** or bone-softening deformities such as *bowing*. The **pelvis is most frequently involved,** followed by the **lumbar spine, thoracic spine, proximal femur, and calvarium.**

Paget disease is usually diagnosed using conventional radiography. **The imaging hallmarks of Paget disease:**

- **Thickening of the cortex.** To recognize thickening of the cortex, compare the thickness of the cortex of the suspicious area with another part of the same bone or, if visible, the same bone on the opposite side of the body.

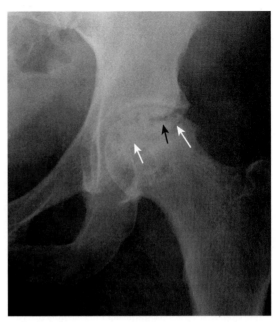

Figure 21-9 Avascular necrosis of the left femoral head in a patient on long-term steroids for lupus erythematosus. A close-up view of the left femoral head shows a zone of increased sclerosis in the superior aspect of the femoral head (*solid white arrows*), a characteristic finding of avascular necrosis of the head. The linear, subcortical lucency (*solid black arrow*) represents subchondral fractures seen with this disease, called the ***crescent sign***. Notice that the disease is isolated to the femoral head and involves neither the joint space nor the acetabulum, i.e., this it is not an arthritis.

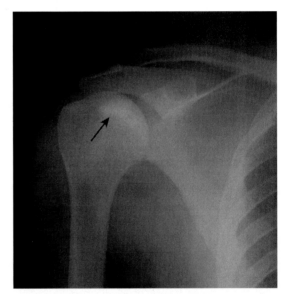

Figure 21-10 Avascular necrosis of humeral head. There is increased density seen at the very top of the humeral head (*solid black arrow*) in this patient with sickle cell disease who developed avascular necrosis of the humeral head. Because the white cap on the bone looks like snow on a mountaintop, this sign of avascular necrosis has been called **snow-capping.**

- **Accentuation of the trabecular pattern.** There is coarsening and thickening of the trabeculae (Fig. 21-12).
- **Increase in the size of the bone involved.** The "classical" history for Paget disease, rendered less useful as fashions have changed, was a gradual increase in a man's hat size as the calvarium increased in size from this disease.

RECOGNIZING A GENERALIZED DECREASE IN BONE DENSITY

- The bones will have an **overall increase in lucency.** There may be a **diffuse loss of the normal network of bony trabeculae in the medullary cavity** because of the decrease in, and thinning of, many of the smaller trabecular structures.

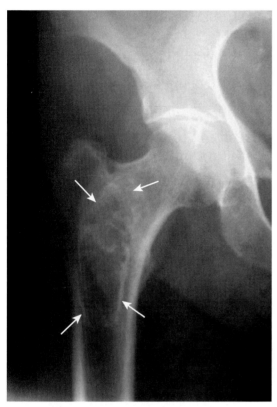

Figure 21-11 Old medullary bone infarct. Amorphous calcification is seen in the medullary cavity of the proximal femur (*solid white arrows*). In general, the differential diagnosis for such an intramedullary calcification includes bone infarct or enchondroma. The characteristic thin sclerotic membrane surrounding this lesion identifies it as a bone infarct.

- **Accentuation of the normal corticomedullary junction** may be present in which the **cortex,** although thinner than normal, **stands out more strikingly** because of the decreased density of the medullary cavity (Fig. 21-13).
- **Compression of vertebral bodies** may be present.
- **Pathologic fractures** may occur in the hip, pelvis, or vertebral bodies.
- Examples of diseases that cause a **diffuse decrease in bone density** are shown in Box 21-4.

Osteoporosis

- *Osteoporosis* is defined as a systemic skeletal disorder **characterized by low bone mineral density** (BMD) and generally divided into *postmenopausal* and *age-related bone loss.*
  - Postmenopausal osteoporosis is characterized by **increased bone resorption** due to osteoclastic activity.
  - Age-related bone loss begins around age 45-55 and is characterized by a **loss of total bone mass.**
- Additional factors that **increase the risk of osteoporosis** include exogenous steroid administration, Cushing disease, estrogen deficiency, inadequate physical activity, and alcoholism.
- Osteoporosis **predisposes to pathologic fractures** in the femoral neck, can lead to compression fractures of the vertebral bodies, and fractures of the distal radius (Colles' fractures).
- **Conventional radiographs** are relatively **insensitive for detecting osteoporosis.** Almost **50% of bone mass must be lost** before it is **recognizable** on conventional radiographs. Findings on conventional radiographs include **overall lucency of bone, thinning of the cortex, and decrease in the visible number of trabeculae in the medullary cavity.**
- Currently, **DEXA (dual-energy x-ray absorptiometry) scans are the most accurate** and widely recommended method for bone mineral density measurements.
  - DEXA scans are obtained by using a filtered x-ray source that produces two distinct energies which are differentially absorbed by bone and soft tissue respectively, allowing for the more accurate calculation of bone

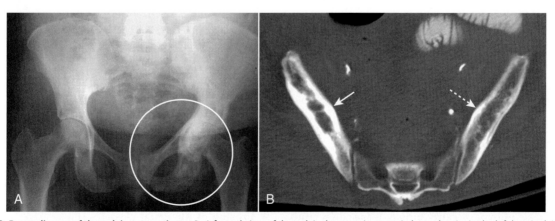

Figure 21-12 Paget disease of the pelvis, two patients. A, A frontal view of the pelvis shows an increase in bony density in the left hemipelvis, accentuation and coarsening of the trabeculae, and thickening of the cortex (*white circle*), the hallmarks of Paget disease of bone. Compare the left hemipelvis with the normal right side. **B,** Axial CT scan of the pelvis of another patient with Paget disease demonstrates thickening of the cortex and accentuation of the trabeculae in the right ilium (*solid white arrow*). Compare it with the normal left side (*dotted white arrow*).

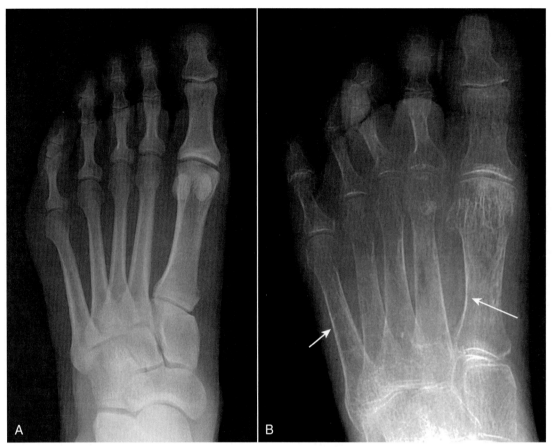

Figure 21-13 Normal and osteoporotic foot. Normal frontal view of the foot **(A)** to contrast with **(B),** which shows overall decreased density of the bone and thinning of the cortices (*solid white arrows*) secondary to disuse osteoporosis. Conventional radiographs are insensitive in diagnosing osteoporosis, and they are subject to technical variations that can mimic the disease even in a healthy individual. More sensitive methods, such as a DEXA scan, should be used to confirm the diagnosis.

Box 21-4 Diffuse Decrease in Bone Density

Osteoporosis
Hyperparathyroidism
Rickets (children)
Osteomalacia (adults)

---

density by subtracting out the error introduced by varying amounts of overlying soft tissue.
• The x-ray dose is very low and the spine or hip is generally used for density measurements.

Hyperparathyroidism

- *Hyperparathyroidism* is a condition caused by excessive secretion of *parathormone (PTH)* by the parathyroid glands. Parathormone exerts its effects on bones, the kidneys, and the GI tract. Its **effect on bones is to increase resorption** by stimulating osteoclastic activity. Calcium is removed from the bone and deposited in the bloodstream.
- There are **three forms** of hyperparathyroidism (Table 21-3).
- The **diagnosis of hyperparathyroidism is based on clinical and laboratory findings** but there are numerous findings of the disease on conventional radiographs and there are other imaging studies utilized to direct surgery on the

TABLE 21-3 FORMS OF HYPERPARATHYROIDISM

Type	Remarks
Primary	Usually caused by a single adenoma in most patients (80% to 90%) and almost always results in hypercalcemia.
Secondary	Results from hyperplasia of the glands secondary to imbalances in calcium and phosphorous levels, seen mostly with chronic renal disease.
Tertiary	Occurs in patients with long-standing secondary hyperparathyroidism in whom autonomous hypersecretion of parathyroid hormone develops, leading to hypercalcemia.

glands, if indicated. Imaging studies of the parathyroid glands themselves may include ultrasound, nuclear medicine parathyroid scans, and MRI scans.

 Some of the **findings of hyperparathyroidism on conventional radiographs:**

- Overall **decrease in bony density**
- *Subperiosteal bone resorption*, especially on the radial side of the middle phalanges of the index and middle fingers (Fig. 21-14)
- **Erosion of the distal clavicles** (Fig. 21-15)
- **Well-circumscribed lytic lesions** in the long bones called *brown tumors* and a *salt-and-pepper appearance* of the skull (Fig. 21-16)

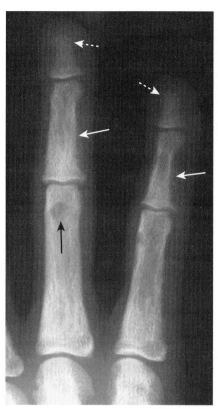

Figure 21-14 Subperiosteal resorption in hyperparathyroidism. The radiologic hallmark of hyperparathyroidism is **_subperiosteal bone resorption_**, seen especially well on the radial aspect of the middle phalanges of the index and middle fingers (*solid white arrows*). Here the cortex appears shaggy and irregular, compared to the cortex on the opposite side of the same bone which is well defined. This patient also displays two other findings of hyperparathyroidism: a small brown tumor (*solid black arrow*) and resorption of the terminal phalanges (**_acroosteolysis_**) (*dotted white arrows*).

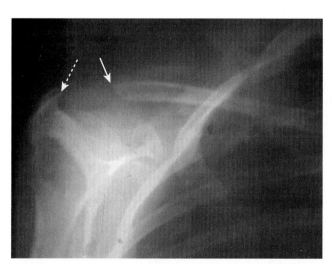

Figure 21-15 Erosion of distal clavicle in hyperparathyroidism. Another relatively common site of bone resorption in hyperparathyroidism is the distal end of the clavicle. Here the distal clavicle (*solid white arrow*), which should articulate with the acromion (*dotted white arrow*), has been resorbed, increasing the distance between it and the acromion. Other sites of bone resorption might include the terminal phalanges as in Fig. 21-14, the lamina dura of the teeth and the medial aspect of the tibia, humerus, and femur.

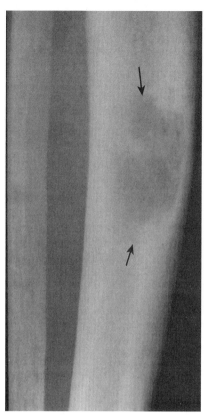

Figure 21-16 Brown tumor. There is a geographic, lytic lesion in the midshaft of the tibia (*solid black arrows*). Brown tumors (also called **_osteoclastomas_**) are benign lesions that represent the osteoclastic resorption of a localized area of (usually) cortical bone and its replacement with fibrous tissue and blood. Their high hemosiderin content gives them a characteristic brown color; they were not named after a "Dr. Brown." The lesions can look like osteolytic metastases or multiple myeloma, so that the clinical history of hyperparathyroidism is key. They can be seen with both primary and secondary hyperparathyroidism.

Rickets

- Rickets is caused by a wide variety of disorders, mostly related to abnormalities in vitamin D ingestion, absorption, or activation, the end result of which is a **failure to calcify the osteoid matrix of bone, especially at the sites of maximal growth in children.**
- Rickets usually **results either from a deficiency, or abnormal metabolism, of vitamin D** or from **abnormal metabolism or excretion of inorganic phosphate.**
- By definition, **rickets occurs only in children** whose growth plates have not closed (which occurs at approximately 17 years of age in females and 19 years of age in males).

➡️ **The imaging hallmarks of rickets:**

- **Fraying and cupping at the metaphyses of long bones** including the anterior ends of the ribs (*rachitic rosary*) (Fig. 21-17).
  - This is especially pronounced at the ends of bones where the maximum growth occurs such as the knees, wrists, and ankles.
- **Widening and irregularity of the epiphyseal plates.**
- **The bones are soft and pliable** so there can be **bowing of the femur and tibia.**

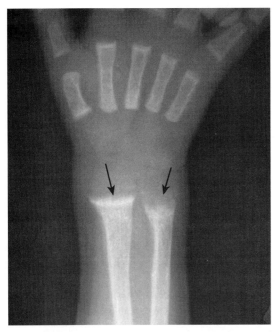

Figure 21-17 Rickets. Frontal view of the wrist shows cupping and fraying (*solid black arrows*) of the metaphyses of the distal radius and ulna, characteristic findings of rickets. Rickets will first affect the bones growing most quickly so it is most common around the knee, distal tibia, and distal radius. It may also be seen at the growing end of the ribs.

Osteomalacia

- *Osteomalacia* is characterized by the failure to calcify the osteoid matrix of bone in **adults**, most commonly as the result of chronic renal disease.

 Findings of osteomalacia on conventional radiographs:

- **Overall decrease in bone density**
- **Thinning of the cortex**
- **Coarsening of the trabecular pattern** due to resorption of secondary trabeculae
- The **imaging hallmark of osteomalacia is the *pseudofracture* (*Looser line*)**, which is a fracture that frequently **occurs at multiple sites** at the same time and is **associated with nonunion** due to inadequate calcification of the healing fracture.
- **Common locations for pseudofractures** are the medial femoral neck and shaft, pubic and ischial rami, metatarsals, and calcaneus. They typically appear as **short, lucent bands, at right angles to the cortex** with **sclerotic margins** in later stages. They are **frequently bilateral and symmetrical** (Fig. 21-18).

RECOGNIZING A FOCAL DECREASE IN BONE DENSITY

- These lesions are most often produced by **focal infiltration of bone by cells other than osteocytes.**
- Examples of diseases that cause a **focal decrease in bone density** are shown in Box 21-5.

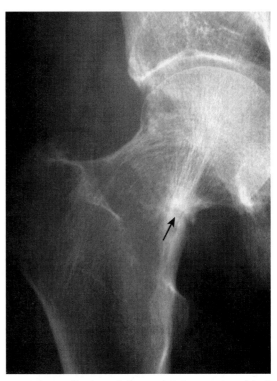

Figure 21-18 Looser line (pseudofracture). A close-up view of the femoral neck shows the typical features of a Looser line: short, lucent bands, at right angles to the cortex with sclerotic margins (*solid black arrow*). Looser lines are the hallmark of osteomalacia in adults. They are frequently bilateral and symmetrical.

Box 21-5 Focal Decrease in Bone Density

Metastatic disease to bone (osteolytic)

Multiple myeloma

Osteomyelitis

Box 21-6 Metastatic Disease to Bone

Metastases to bone are far more common than primary bone tumors.

Metastases to bone fall into two major categories: those that stimulate the production of new bone are called **osteoblastic**, and those that destroy bone are called **osteolytic**; some metastases include lesions in which osteoblastic and osteolytic changes are both present.

Metastatic bone lesions from any source are very uncommon distal to the elbow or the knee; when present in these locations, they are usually widespread and due to lung or breast cancer.

The radionuclide bone scan is currently the study of choice for detecting skeletal metastases.

Osteolytic Metastatic Disease

- **Osteolytic metastatic disease** can produce focal destruction of bone (Box 21-6).
- The **medullary cavity is almost always involved** and from there the disease may erode into and destroy the cortex as well. When the medullary cavity alone is involved, there must be almost a 50% reduction in bone mass in order for the lesion to be recognizable on conventional radiographs when viewed *en face*.
- MRI, on the other hand, is excellent at demonstrating the status of the medullary cavity and so is much more sensitive

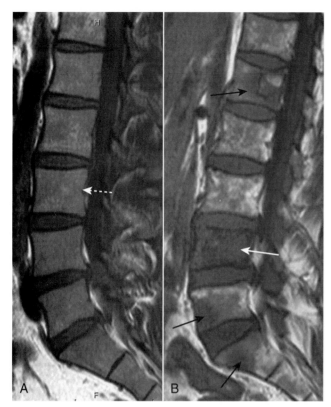

Figure 21-19 Metastases to lumbar spine, MRI. A, There is normal signal in the lumbar vertebral bodies on this T1-weighted sagittal view of the lumbar spine (*dotted white arrow*). **B,** In this patient with a primary breast carcinoma, there are multiple metastatic deposits replacing the normal marrow in the lumbar spine and sacrum (*solid black arrows*). The body of L4 is completely replaced by tumor (*solid white arrow*).

to the presence of metastatic disease than conventional radiography (Fig. 21-19).

■ In **some cases, only the cortex is involved.** Cortical metastases may be easier to visualize on conventional radiographs because relatively less cortical destruction is needed for them to become apparent, especially if the lesions happen to be viewed in tangent.

 On conventional radiographs, the **classical findings of osteolytic metastases** include:

■ **Irregularly shaped, lucent bone lesions,** which can be single or multiple.
■ These lytic lesions are frequently characterized as belonging to one (or sometimes more) of three patterns: *permeative, mottled,* or *geographic* in order of increasing size of the smallest and most discrete lesion visible (Fig. 21-20).
■ Osteolytic metastases **typically incite little or no reactive bone formation** around them. They can be **expansile** and *soap-bubbly* (i.e., contain bony septations) especially in renal and thyroid carcinoma (Fig. 21-21).
■ In the spine, they may preferentially **destroy the pedicles,** because of the blood supply to the pedicles (the *pedicle sign*), which can help to differentiate metastases from multiple myeloma (see below), which tends to spare the pedicle early in the disease (Fig. 21-22).

■ The most common causes of osteoblastic and osteolytic bone metastases are listed in Table 21-4.

Multiple Myeloma

■ **Multiple myeloma,** the most common primary malignancy of bone in adults, can occur in a **solitary form,** often seen as a soap-bubbly, expansile lesion in the spine or pelvis (called a *solitary plasmacytoma*), or a **disseminated form** with multiple, *punched-out* lytic lesions throughout the axial and proximal appendicular skeleton.

 Findings of multiple myeloma on conventional radiographs:

■ The most common early manifestation is **diffuse and usually severe osteoporosis.**
■ **Plasmacytomas** appear as **expansile, septated lesions, frequently with associated soft tissue masses** (Fig. 21-23).
■ Later, in its disseminated form, **multiple, small, sharply circumscribed** (described as *punched out*) **lytic lesions of approximately the same size** are present, usually without any accompanying sclerotic reaction around them (Fig. 21-24).
■ Classically, **conventional radiographs are more sensitive in detecting the lesions of multiple myeloma than radio-nuclide bone scans,** which tend to underestimate the number and extent of lesions due to the absence of reactive bone formation.

Osteomyelitis

■ *Osteomyelitis* refers to the **focal destruction of bone** most often by a blood-borne **infectious agent,** the most common of which is *Staphylococcus aureus.*
■ **In children,** the osteolytic lesion **tends to occur at the metaphysis** because of its rich blood supply.

 Findings of acute osteomyelitis on conventional radiographs:

■ **Focal cortical bone destruction.**
■ **Periosteal new bone formation** (Fig. 21-25).
■ Inflammatory changes accompanying the infection may produce **soft tissue swelling** and **focal osteoporosis** from hyperemia.
■ In **adults,** the **infection tends to involve the joint space** more often than in children producing not only osteomyelitis but also *septic arthritis* (see Chapter 24, *Arthritis*).
■ **Conventional radiographs can take up to 10 days to display the first findings of osteomyelitis** so that other imaging modalities, such as MRI and nuclear medicine studies, are frequently used for earlier diagnosis.
■ A variety of radionuclide bone scans can demonstrate osteomyelitis. The most specific is currently a **tagged, white-cell scan** in which a sample of the patient's white blood cells is tagged with a radioactive isotope (frequently indium), before the patient is imaged with a camera specific for nuclear studies to detect a site of abnormally increased radioactive tracer uptake.

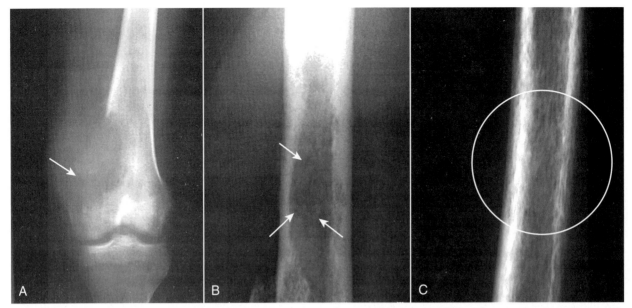

Figure 21-20 Three patterns of lytic bone lesions. A, A solitary bone lesion with a gradual zone of transition between it and the normal bone and complete destruction of the cortex (*solid white arrow*) is called a ***geographic lesion*. B,** Several ill-defined lytic lesions (*solid white arrows*) with indistinct margins imply a more aggressive malignancy. This is called a ***moth-eaten pattern*. C,** A close-up of the femur shows innumerable, small, irregular holes in the bone (*white circle*) called a ***permeative pattern*.** Permeative lesions are called ***round cell lesions*** for the shape of the cells that produce them. Such lesions include Ewing sarcoma, neuroblastoma, myeloma, and leukemia.

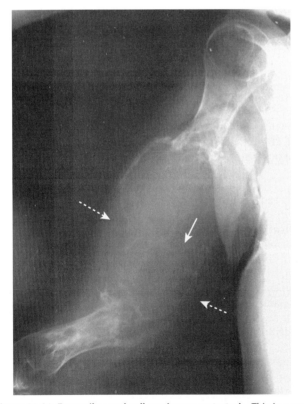

Figure 21-21 Expansile renal cell carcinoma metastasis. This is a very aggressive and expansile osteolytic metastasis in the humerus from a primary renal cell carcinoma. Notice that the cortex has been destroyed in several areas (*dotted white arrows*) and the lesion has a characteristic **soap-bubbly** appearance produced by fine septae (*solid white arrow*). Metastatic thyroid carcinoma and a solitary plasmacytoma could also produce these findings.

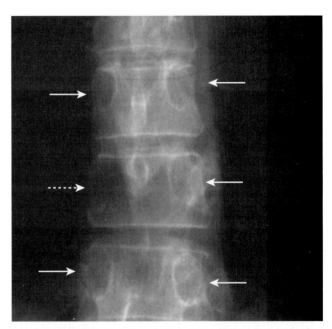

Figure 21-22 Pedicle sign. There is destruction of the right pedicle of T10 (*dotted white arrow*). Each vertebral body should normally have two, oval-shaped pedicles, one on each side, visible on the frontal radiograph of the spine (*solid white arrows*). In the spine, osteolytic metastases may preferentially destroy the pedicles, because of their blood supply, producing the pedicle sign, although most metastatic lesions to the spine will also involve the vertebral body as well. In multiple myeloma, the pedicle tends to be spared early in the disease.

TABLE 21-4 CAUSES OF OSTEOBLASTIC AND OSTEOLYTIC BONE METASTASES

Osteoblastic	Osteolytic
Prostate carcinoma (most common in older males)	Lung cancer (most common osteolytic lesion in males)
Breast carcinoma is usually osteolytic but can be osteoblastic, especially if treated	Breast cancer (most common osteolytic lesion in females)
Lymphoma	Renal cell carcinoma
Carcinoid tumors	Thyroid carcinoma

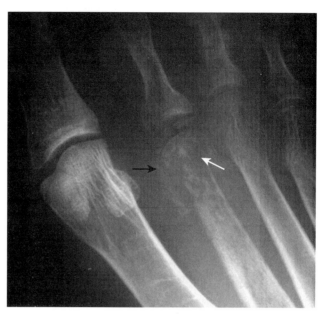

Figure 21-25 Acute osteomyelitis of 2ⁿᵈ metatarsal. Close-up view of the 2ⁿᵈ toe in this 59-year-old female with diabetes shows the hallmarks of bone destruction (*solid white arrow*) and periosteal new bone formation (*solid black arrow*) in osteomyelitis.

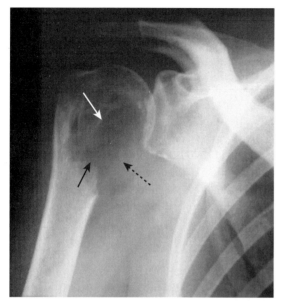

Figure 21-23 Solitary plasmacytoma, shoulder. There is a lytic lesion in the proximal humerus (*solid black arrow*), which destroys the cortex (*dotted black arrow*) and contains multiple septations (*solid white arrow*). This is the so-called **soap-bubbly** appearance and can be seen with expansile metastases and solitary plasmacytomas, a precursor to the more disseminated form of multiple myeloma.

> **Box 21-7 Insufficiency Fractures**
>
> Insufficiency fractures are a type of pathologic fracture in which mechanically weakened bone fractures from a normal or physiologic stress.
>
> They are most common in postmenopausal women secondary to osteoporosis.
>
> Common sites include the pelvis, thoracic spine, sacrum, tibia, and calcaneus.
>
> Unlike other fractures that manifest themselves by a lucency in the bone, most insufficiency fractures display a sclerotic band (representing healing) on conventional radiographs.
>
> CT, MRI, or nuclear medicine bone scans are more sensitive than conventional radiographs in detecting insufficiency fractures (see Fig. 21-26).

PATHOLOGIC FRACTURES

- Pathologic fractures are those that **occur in bone with a preexisting abnormality.** Pathologic fractures tend to occur with **minimum or no trauma.**
- *Insufficiency fractures* are a type of pathologic fracture (Box 21-7; Fig. 21-26).
- Diseases that produce either an increase or a **decrease** in bone density tend to **weaken the normal architecture** of bone and predispose to pathologic fractures.
- Diseases that predispose to pathologic fractures may be **local** (e.g., metastases) or **diffuse** (e.g., rickets). In general, pathologic fractures occur more often in the **ribs, spine, and proximal appendicular skeleton** (humeri and femurs).
- **Recognizing pathologic fractures** (Fig. 21-27)
  - First, there has to be a fracture present.
  - The bone surrounding the fracture will demonstrate abnormal density or architecture.
  - **Delayed healing** is **common** in pathologic fractures.

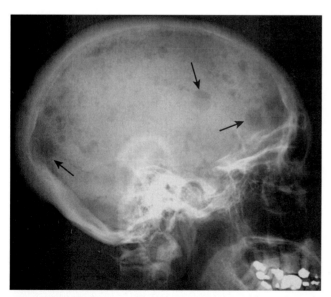

Figure 21-24 Multiple myeloma. Innumerable lytic lesions (*solid black arrows*) are seen in the skull. They are small, uniform in size, and have sharply marginated edges, the so-called **punched out** lytic defect seen in multiple myeloma.

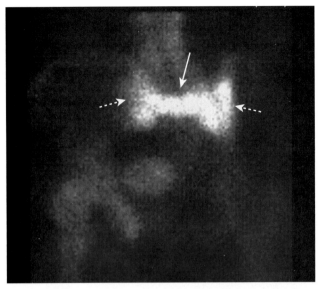

Figure 21-26 Sacral insufficiency fractures seen with bone scintigraphy. There is increased radiotracer uptake in vertical fractures through the sacral ala (*dotted white arrows*) and a horizontal fracture through the body of the sacrum (*solid white arrow*). This has been called the **Honda sign** because it resembles the carmaker's insignia. Insufficiency fractures occur in abnormal bones that undergo normal stress. The sacrum is a common site for such fractures in osteoporosis.

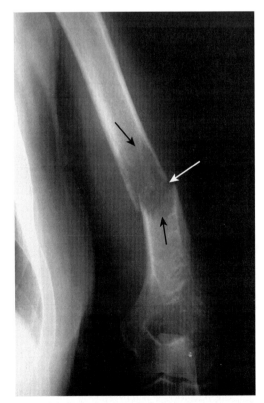

Figure 21-27 Pathologic fracture. Pathologic fractures are those that occur with minimal stress in bones with preexisting abnormalities. In this patient with metastatic renal cell carcinoma to the humerus, there is a geographic, lytic lesion seen in the distal humerus (*solid black arrows*) through which a transverse fracture has occurred (*solid white arrow*).

- Attempts to predict impending fractures in diseased bone have, by and large, proven to be unreliable.
- The treatment of a pathologic fracture depends in part on successful treatment of the underlying condition that produced it, e.g., vitamin D replacement in rickets.

WEBLINK

Registered users may obtain more information on Recognizing Abnormalities of Bone Density on StudentConsult.com.

TAKE-HOME POINTS

Recognizing Abnormalities of Bone Density

Bones consist of a *cortex* of compact bone surrounding a *medullary cavity* containing cancellous bone arranged as trabeculae, separated by blood vessels, hematopoietic cells, and fat.

On conventional radiographs, the cortex is best seen in tangent. On CT, the entire cortex is visualized. MRI is particularly sensitive to assessment of the marrow. Both CT and MRI are superior to conventional radiographs in evaluating soft tissues.

Bone is undergoing continuous change from a combination of biochemical and mechanical forces.

Increased **osteoclastic** activity can produce focal or generalized decrease in bone density. Increased **osteoblastic** activity can produce focal or diffuse increased bone density. Osteoblastic metastases, especially from carcinoma of the prostate and breast, can produce focal or generalized increase in bony density.

Other diseases that can increase bone density include osteopetrosis, avascular necrosis of bone, and Paget disease.

Hallmarks of *Paget disease* include thickening of the cortex, accentuation of the trabecular pattern, and enlargement and increased density of the affected bone.

Osteolytic metastases, especially from lung, renal, thyroid, and breast cancer, can produce focal areas of decreased bone density as can solitary plasmacytomas, considered to be a precursor to multiple myeloma, the most common primary tumor of bone.

Examples of diseases that can cause a generalized decrease in bone density include osteoporosis, hyperparathyroidism, rickets (in children), and osteomalacia (in adults).

Osteoporosis is characterized by low bone mineral density and is most often either postmenopausal or age-related. Osteoporosis predisposes to pathologic fractures.

Pathologic fractures are those that occur with minimal or no trauma in bones that had a preexisting abnormality.

Examples of diseases that can cause a focal decrease in bone density include metastases, multiple myeloma, and osteomyelitis.

The radionuclide bone scan is the modality of choice in screening for skeletal metastases. MRI is used primarily to solve specific questions related to a lesion's composition and extent.

There must be almost a 50% reduction in the mass of bone in order for a difference in density to be perceived on conventional radiographs; MRI is much more sensitive to the presence of medullary metastatic disease.

Chapter 22

Recognizing Fractures and Dislocations

RECOGNIZING AN ACUTE FRACTURE

- Everyone, it seems, is fascinated by a broken bone or two. Fractures are a favorite among those learning radiology, perhaps because of how common they are. Fractures due to moderate trauma are much more common than those due to severe trauma or pathologic fractures.
- A fracture is described as a **disruption in the continuity of all or part of the cortex of a bone.**
  - If the **cortex** is **broken through and through**, the fracture is called *complete*.
  - If **only a part of the cortex** is fractured, it is called *incomplete*. Incomplete fractures tend to occur in bones that are "softer" than normal such as those in children, or in adults with bone-softening diseases such as *osteomalacia* or *Paget disease* (see Chapter 21, *Recognizing Abnormalities of Bone Density*).
  - Examples of incomplete fractures in children are **the greenstick fracture,** which involves only one part of, but not the entire, cortex, and the ***torus fracture* (buckle fracture),** which represents compression of the cortex (Fig. 22-1).

 Radiologic features of acute fractures (Box 22-1)

- **Fracture lines,** when viewed in the correct plane, **tend to be "blacker" (more lucent)** than other lines normally found in bones, such as *nutrient canals* (Fig. 22-2A).
- There may be an **abrupt discontinuity of the cortex,** sometimes associated with **acute angulation of the normally smooth contour of bone** (Fig. 22-2B).
- Fracture lines tend to be **straighter in their course yet more acute in their angulation** than any naturally occurring lines (such as *epiphyseal plates*) (Fig. 22-3).
- The **edges of a fracture tend to be jagged and rough.**

 Pitfalls: sesamoids, accessory ossicles, and unhealed fractures (Table 22-1)

- *Sesamoids* are bones that form in a tendon as it passes over a joint. The **patella** is the largest and most famous sesamoid bone.
- *Accessory ossicles* are accessory epiphyseal or apophyseal ossification centers that do not fuse with the parent bone.
- **Old, unhealed fracture fragments** can sometimes mimic acute fractures (Fig. 22-4A).
- Unlike fractures, these small bones are **corticated** (i.e., there is a white line that completely surrounds the bony fragment) and their edges are usually **smooth.**

- In the case of sesamoids and accessory ossicles, they are **usually bilaterally symmetrical** so that a view of the opposite extremity will usually demonstrate the same bone in the same location. They also **occur at anatomically predictable sites.**
- There are almost always sesamoids present in the thumb, the posterolateral aspect of the knee (*fabella*), and the great toe (Fig. 22-4B).
- Accessory ossicles are most common in the foot (Fig. 22-4C).

RECOGNIZING DISLOCATIONS AND SUBLUXATIONS

- In a **dislocation,** the bones that originally formed the two components of a joint are no longer in apposition to each other. Dislocations occur only at joints (Fig. 22-5A).
- In a **subluxation,** the bones that originally formed the two components of a joint are in **partial contact** with each other. Subluxations also occur only at joints (Fig. 22-5B).
- Some characteristics of dislocations of the shoulder and hip are shown in Table 22-2.

DESCRIBING FRACTURES

- There is a common lexicon used in describing fractures to facilitate a reproducible description and to assure reliable and accurate communication.
- **Fractures are usually described using four major parameters** (Table 22-3):
  - The **number of fragments**
  - The **direction of the fracture line**
  - The **relationship of the fragments** to each other
  - By **communication of the fracture with the outside atmosphere**

How Fractures are Described: by the Number of Fracture Fragments

- If the fracture produces **two fragments**, it is called a **simple fracture.**
- If the fracture produces **more than two** fragments, it is called a **comminuted fracture.** Some comminuted fractures have special names.
  - A **segmental fracture** is a comminuted fracture in which a portion of the shaft exists as an isolated fragment (Fig. 22-6A).
  - A **butterfly fragment** is a comminuted fracture in which the central fragment has a triangular shape (Fig. 22-6B).

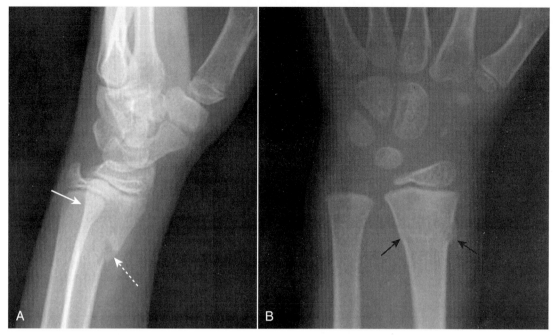

Figure 22-1 Greenstick and torus fractures. Incomplete fractures are those that involve only a portion of the cortex. They tend to occur in bones that are "softer" than normal, such as those in children or in adults with bone-softening diseases, such as osteomalacia or Paget disease. There is a greenstick fracture of the distal radius **(A)**, which involves only one part of (*dotted white arrow*), but not the entire, cortex (*solid white arrow*). **B**, In this torus fracture (buckle fracture) of the distal radius, buckling of the cortex is seen (*solid black arrows*).

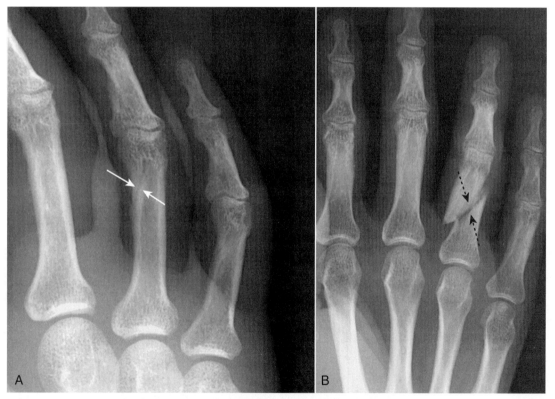

Figure 22-2 Nutrient canal versus fracture. Fracture lines, when viewed in the correct orientation, tend to be "blacker" (more lucent) than other lines normally found in bones, such as nutrient canals. This is a nutrient canal **(A)** (*solid white arrows*) while a true fracture is seen in another patient in **(B)** (*dotted black arrows*). Notice how the nutrient canal has a sclerotic (whiter) margin, which is not the case with fracture lines. The edges of a fracture tend to be jagged and rough.

Box 22-1 **Characteristics of an Acute Fracture**
Abrupt disruption of all or part of the cortex
Acute changes in the smooth contour of a normal bone
Fracture lines are black and linear
Where fracture lines change their course, they tend to be sharply angulated
Fracture fragments are jagged and not corticated

How Fractures are Described: by the Direction of the Fracture Line (Table 22-4)

- In a **transverse fracture**, the fracture line is perpendicular to the long axis of the bone. Transverse fractures are caused by a force directed **perpendicular to shaft** (Fig. 22-7A).
- In a **diagonal or oblique fracture**, the fracture line is diagonal in orientation relative to the long axis of the bone.

Diagonal or oblique fractures are caused by a force usually applied along the **same direction as the long axis** of the affected bone (Fig. 22-7B).

- With a **spiral fracture**, a twisting force or torque produces a fracture like those that might be caused by planting the foot in a hole while running. Spiral fractures are usually unstable and often associated with soft tissue injuries such as tears in ligaments or tendons (Fig. 22-7C).

How Fractures are Described: by the Relationship of One Fracture Fragment to Another

By convention, abnormalities of the position of bone fragments secondary to fractures describe **the relationship of the distal fracture fragment relative to the proximal fragment.** These descriptions are based on the position the distal fragment would have normally assumed had the bone not been fractured.

- There are four major parameters most commonly used to describe the relationship of fracture fragments. Most fractures display more than one of these abnormalities of position. The four parameters are:
  - **Displacement**
  - **Angulation**

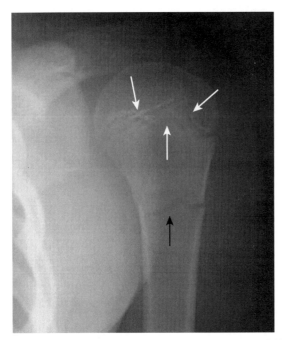

Figure 22-3 Fracture versus epiphyseal plate. Fracture lines (*solid black arrow*) tend to be straighter in their course and more acute in their angulation than any naturally occurring lines, such as the epiphyseal plate in the proximal humerus (*solid white arrows*). Because the top of the metaphysis has irregular hills and valleys, the epiphyseal plate has an undulating course that will allow you to see it in tangent both on the anterior and posterior margins of the humeral head. This gives the mistaken appearance that there is more than one epiphyseal plate.

TABLE 22-1 DIFFERENTIATING FRACTURES, OSSICLES, AND SESAMOIDS

Finding	Acute Fracture	Sesamoids and Accessory Ossicles*
Abrupt disruption of cortex	Yes	No
Bilaterally symmetrical	Almost never	Almost always
"Fracture line"	Unsharp, jagged	Smooth
Bony fragment has a cortex completely around it	No	Yes

*Old, unhealed fractures will not be bilaterally symmetrical.

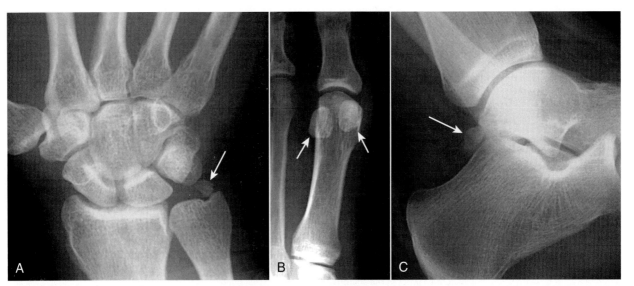

Figure 22-4 Pitfalls in fracture diagnosis. A, Old, unhealed fracture fragments (*solid white arrow*). **B,** Sesamoids are bones that form in a tendon as it passes over a joint (*solid white arrows*). **C,** Accessory ossicles are accessory epiphyseal or apophyseal ossification centers that do not fuse with the parent bone, (like this os trigonum, *open white arrow*). Unlike fractures, these small bones are corticated (i.e., there is a white line that completely surrounds the bony fragment) and their edges are usually smooth. Sesamoids and accessory ossicles are usually bilaterally symmetrical.

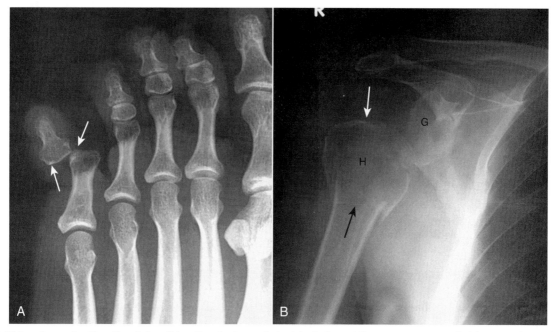

Figure 22-5 Dislocation and subluxation. A, In a dislocation, the bones that originally formed the two components of a joint are no longer in apposition to each other (*solid white arrows*). The terminal phalanx is dislocated lateral compared to the middle phalanx. **B,** In a subluxation, the bones that originally formed the two components of a joint are in partial contact with each other. The humeral head (*H*) is subluxed inferiorly (*solid white arrow*) in the glenoid (*G*) because of large hematoma in the joint secondary to a fracture of the humeral neck (*solid black arrow*). The hematoma itself is not visible by conventional radiography.

TABLE 22-2 DISLOCATIONS OF THE SHOULDER AND HIP

Shoulder	Hip
Anterior, subcoracoid most common	Posterior and superior more common
Caused by a combination of abduction, external rotation, and extension	Frequently caused by knee striking dashboard transmitting force to hip
Associated with fractures of humeral head (Hill-Sachs lesion) and glenoid (Bankart lesion)	Associated with fractures of posterior rim of the acetabulum

- Shortening
- Rotation
- **Displacement** describes the **amount by which the distal fragment is offset,** front to back and side to side, from the proximal fragment. Displacement is most often described either in terms of *percent* (*the distal fragment is displaced by 50% of the width of the shaft*) or by *fractions* (*the distal fragment is displaced half the width of the shaft of the proximal fragment*) (Fig. 22-8A).
- **Angulation** describes the **angle between the distal and proximal fragments** as a function of the degree to which the distal fragment is deviated from the position it would have assumed were it in its normal position. Angulation is described in degrees and by position (*the distal fragment is angulated 15° anteriorly relative to the proximal fragment*) (Fig. 22-8B).
- **Shortening** describes **how much, if any, overlap there is of the ends of the fracture fragments,** which translates into how much shorter the fractured bone is than it would be had it not been fractured (Fig. 22-8C).
  - The term opposite from shortening is *distraction,* which refers to the **distance the bone fragments are separated from each other** (Fig. 22-8D).

TABLE 22-3 HOW FRACTURES ARE DESCRIBED

Parameter	Terms Used
Number of fracture fragments	Simple or comminuted
Direction of fracture line	Transverse, oblique (diagonal), spiral
Relationship of one fragment to another	Displacement, angulation, shortening, and rotation
Open to the atmosphere (outside)	Closed or open (compound)

- Shortening (overlap) or distraction (lengthening) is usually described by a number of centimeters (*there are 2 cm of shortening of the fracture fragments*).
- **Rotation** is an unusual abnormality in fracture positioning almost always involving the **long bones,** such as the femur or humerus. Rotation describes the orientation of the joint at one end of the fractured bone relative to the orientation of the joint at the other end of the same bone.
  - Normally, for example, when the hip joint is pointing forward, the knee joint is also pointing forward.
  - If there is **rotation** about a fracture of the femoral shaft, the hip joint could be pointing forward while the knee joint is oriented in another direction (Fig. 22-9).
  - To appreciate rotation, both the joint above and the joint below a fracture must be included, preferably on the same radiograph.

How Fractures are Described: by the Relationship of the Fracture to the Atmosphere

- A **closed fracture** is the **more common** type of fracture in which there is **no communication** between the fracture fragments and the outside atmosphere.

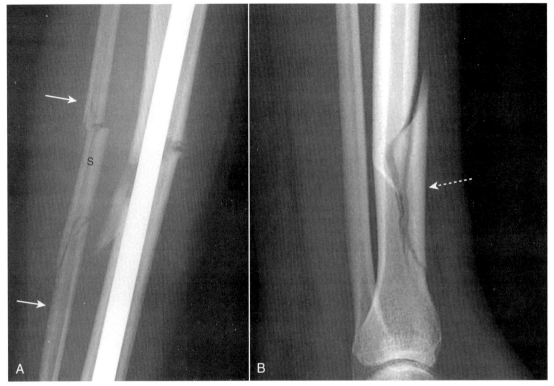

Figure 22-6 Segmental fracture and butterfly fractures. These are two comminuted fractures. **A,** This is a segmental fracture in which a portion of the shaft exists as an isolated fragment. Notice how the fibula has a center segment (*S*) and two additional fragments, one on either side (*solid white arrows*). **B,** A butterfly fragment is a comminuted fracture in which the central fragment has a triangular shape (*dotted white arrow*).

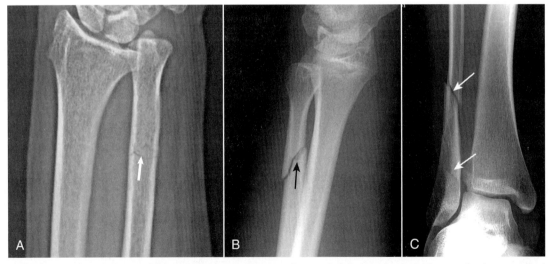

Figure 22-7 Transverse, diagonal, and spiral fracture lines. A, In a transverse fracture (*solid white arrow*), the fracture line is perpendicular to the long axis of the bone. **B,** Diagonal or oblique fractures (*solid black arrow*) are diagonal in orientation relative to the normal axis of the bone. **C,** Spiral fractures (*solid white arrows*) are usually caused by twisting or torque injuries.

TABLE 22-4 DIRECTION OF FRACTURE LINE AND MECHANISM OF INJURY

Direction of Fracture Line	Mechanism
Transverse	Force applied perpendicular to long axis of bone; fracture occurs at point of impact
Diagonal (also known as oblique)	Force applied along the long axis of bone; fracture occurs somewhere along shaft
Spiral	Twisting or torque injury

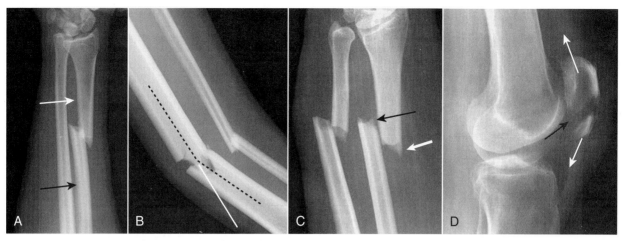

Figure 22-8 Fracture parameters. The orientation of fracture fragments is described by using these four parameters. **A,** ***Displacement*** describes the amount by which the distal fragment (*solid white arrow*) is offset, front to back and side to side, from the proximal fragment (*solid black arrow*). **B,** ***Angulation*** describes the angle between the distal and proximal fragments (*dotted black line*) as a function of the degree to which the distal fragment is deviated from its normal position (*solid white line*). **C,** ***Shortening*** describes how much, if any, overlap occurs at the ends of the fracture fragments (*solid white and black arrows*). **D,** The term that is opposite from shortening is ***distraction,*** which refers to the distance the bone fragments are separated from each other (*two white arrows* show pull of tendons on fracture fragments of patella, *black arrow* points to distraction of fracture).

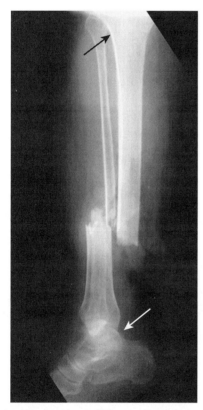

Figure 22-9 Rotation. An unusual abnormality in fracture positioning, almost always involving the long bones, which describes the orientation of the joint at one end of the fractured bone relative to the orientation of the joint at the other end of the fractured bone. To appreciate rotation, both the joint above and the joint below a fracture must be included, preferably on the same radiograph. In this patient, the proximal tibia (*solid black arrow*) is oriented in the frontal projection while the distal tibia and ankle (*solid white arrow*) are rotated and oriented laterally.

- In an **open or compound fracture**, there is **communication between the fracture and the outside** atmosphere, i.e., a fracture fragment penetrates the skin (Fig. 22-10). Compound fractures have implications regarding the way in which they are treated in order to avoid the complication

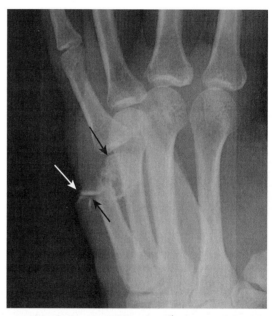

Figure 22-10 Open (compound) fracture, 5th metacarpal. Most fractures are closed, meaning there is no communication between the fracture fragments and the outside atmosphere. Open or compound fractures (*solid black arrows*) have communication between the fracture and the outside (*solid white arrow*). Whether a fracture is open or not is best evaluated clinically. Treatment of a compound fracture must consider the higher incidence of infection that can occur in these injuries.

of osteomyelitis. Whether a fracture is open or not is best diagnosed clinically.

AVULSION FRACTURES

- Avulsion is a **common mechanism of fracture production** in which the fracture fragment (***avulsed fragment***) is pulled from its parent bone by contraction of a tendon or ligament.
- Although avulsion fractures can and do occur at any age, they are **particularly common in younger individuals**

TABLE 22-5 AVULSION FRACTURES AROUND THE PELVIS

Avulsed Fragment	Muscle that Inserts on that Fragment
Anterior, superior iliac spine	Sartorius muscle
Anterior, inferior iliac spine	Rectus femoris muscle
Ischial tuberosity	Hamstring muscles
Lesser trochanter of femur	Iliopsoas muscle

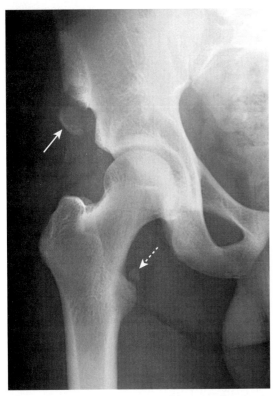

Figure 22-11 Avulsion fractures, ASIS and lesser trochanter. Avulsion fractures are common fractures in which the avulsed fragment is pulled from its parent bone by contraction of a tendon or ligament. Although avulsion fractures can occur at any age, they are particularly common in younger individuals who engage in athletic endeavors. There is an avulsion of the anterior superior iliac spine (ASIS) (*solid white arrow*), which is the site of the insertion of the sartorius muscle. There is also an avulsion of a portion of the lesser trochanter, on which the iliopsoas muscle inserts (*dotted white arrow*). The patient had participated in track and field events a week prior to this radiograph.

SALTER-HARRIS FRACTURES: EPIPHYSEAL PLATE FRACTURES IN CHILDREN

- In growing bone, the hypertrophic zone in the **growth plate** (*epiphyseal plate* or *physis*) is most vulnerable to shearing

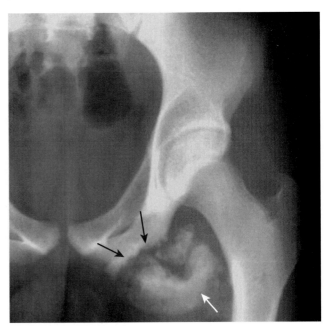

Figure 22-12 Healing avulsion fracture of ischial tuberosity. Avulsion fractures of the pelvis occur in anatomically predictable locations (tendons insert on bones in known locations) and they are typically small fragments. Sometimes they heal with such exuberant callus formation that they can be mistaken for a bone tumor. This is a healing fracture (*solid black arrows*) of the ischial tuberosity originally caused by contraction of the hamstring muscles. There is a great deal of external callus present (*solid white arrow*).

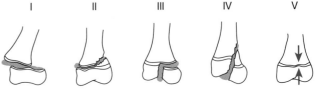

Figure 22-13 The Salter-Harris classification of epiphyseal plate fractures helps in recognizing the likelihood of complications based on the type of fracture. All of these fractures involve the epiphyseal plate (growth plate). Type I are fractures of the epiphyseal plate alone. Type II fractures, the most common of the epiphyseal plate fractures, involve the epiphyseal plate and metaphysis. These first two types have a favorable prognosis. Type III are fractures of the epiphyseal plate and the epiphysis and have a less favorable prognosis. Type IV is a fracture of the epiphyseal plate, epiphysis, and metaphysis. It has an even less favorable prognosis. Type V is a crush injury of the epiphyseal plate. It has the worst prognosis. (Adapted from Robertson J, Shilkofski N, editors: *The Johns Hopkins Hospital: The Harriet Lane Handbook*, ed 17, Philadelphia, 2005, Mosby.)

engaging in athletic endeavors—in fact, they derive many of their names from the type of athletic activity that produces them, e.g., *dancer's fracture*, *skier's fracture*, and *sprinter's fracture*.

- They **occur in anatomically predictable locations** because tendons insert on bones in a known location (Table 22-5) and the avulsed fragment is **typically small** (Fig. 22-11).
- They sometimes **heal with such exuberant callus formation** that they can be mistaken for a bone tumor (Fig. 22-12).

injuries. Epiphyseal plate fractures are common and **account for as many as 30% of childhood fractures.** By definition, since these are all fractures through an open epiphyseal plate, they **can only occur in children.**

- The **Salter-Harris classification of epiphyseal plate injuries** is a commonly used method of describing such injuries that helps identify the type of treatment required and predicts the likelihood of complications based on the type of fracture (Fig. 22-13; Table 22-6).

 Types I and II heal well.

- Type III fractures can develop arthritic changes or asymmetric growth plate fusion.

TABLE 22-6 SALTER-HARRIS CLASSIFICATION OF EPIPHYSEAL PLATE FRACTURES

Type	What's Fractured	Remarks
I	Epiphyseal plate	Seen in phalanges, distal radius, SCFE; good prognosis
II	Epiphyseal plate and metaphysis	Most common of all Salter-Harris fractures; frequently distal radius; displays corner sign; good prognosis
III	Epiphyseal plate and epiphysis	Intraarticular fracture; frequently distal tibia; prognosis is less favorable
IV	Epiphyseal plate, epiphysis, and metaphysis	Seen in distal humerus and distal tibia; poor prognosis
V	Crush injury of epiphyseal plate	Worst prognosis; difficult to diagnose until healing begins

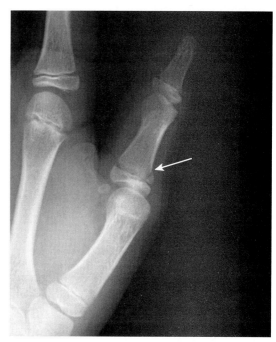

Figure 22-15 **Salter-Harris II fracture.** In type II fractures, there is a fracture of the epiphyseal plate and a fracture of the metaphysis. This is the most common type of Salter-Harris fracture. The small metaphyseal fracture fragment (*solid white arrow*) produces the so-called **corner sign**.

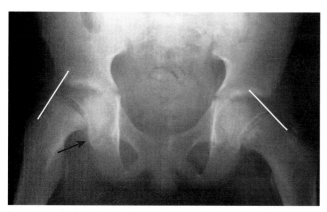

Figure 22-14 **Slipped capital femoral epiphysis.** Slipped capital femoral epiphysis (SCFE) is a manifestation of a Salter-Harris type I injury. It occurs more often in taller and heavier teenage boys and produces inferior, medial, and posterior slippage of the proximal femoral epiphysis (*solid black arrow*) relative to the neck of the femur. A line drawn parallel to the neck of the femur (*solid white lines*) should intersect a portion of the head. It does so on the normal left side, but does not on the right side because the epiphysis has slipped.

- Types IV and V are more likely to develop early fusion of the growth plate with angular deformities and shortening of that bone.
- **Type I: Fractures of the epiphyseal plate alone**
  - Salter-Harris type I fractures are often **difficult to detect without the opposite side for comparison.** Fortunately, these fractures have a **favorable prognosis.**
  - *Slipped capital femoral epiphysis (SCFE)* is a manifestation of a Salter-Harris type I injury.
    - Slipped capital femoral epiphysis **occurs most often in taller and heavier teenage boys** and involves the inferior, medial, and posterior slippage of the proximal (capital) femoral epiphysis relative to the neck of the femur (Fig. 22-14).
    - It is **bilateral in about 25% of cases** and can result in **avascular necrosis** of the slipped femoral head because of interruption of the blood supply **in up to 15% of cases.**
- **Type II: Fracture of the epiphyseal plate and fracture of the metaphysis**

- This is the **most common type of Salter-Harris fracture (75%),** seen especially in the distal radius. The small metaphyseal fracture fragment of a Salter-Harris type II fracture produces the so-called *corner sign* (Fig. 22-15).
- **Type III: Fracture of the epiphyseal plate and the epiphysis**
  - There is a **longitudinal fracture through the epiphysis itself,** which means the fracture invariably enters the joint space and fractures the articular cartilage.
  - This type of injury can have long-term implications for the development of **secondary osteoarthritis** (see Chapter 23, *Arthritis*) and can result in **asymmetric and premature fusion of the growth plate** with subsequent deformity of the bone (Fig. 22-16).
- **Type IV: Fracture of the epiphyseal plate, metaphysis, and epiphysis**
  - Type IV fractures have a **poorer prognosis** than other Salter-Harris fractures—i.e., premature and possibly asymmetric closure of the epiphyseal plate, especially in bones of the lower extremity that may lead to differences in leg length, angular deformities, and secondary osteoarthritis (Fig. 22-17).
- **Type V: Crush fracture of epiphyseal plate**
  - Type V Salter-Harris fractures are a **rare,** crush-type injury of the epiphyseal plate that **are associated with vascular injury** and almost always **result in growth impairment** through early focal fusion of the growth plate.
  - They are **most common in the distal femur,** proximal tibia, and distal tibia. They are **difficult to diagnose on conventional radiographs** until later in their course when complications ensue (Fig. 22-18).

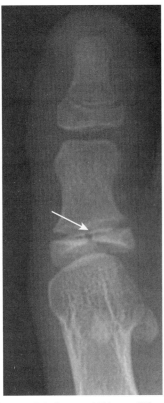

Figure 22-16 Salter-Harris III fracture. With type III fractures, a fracture of the epiphyseal plate as well as a longitudinal fracture through the epiphysis itself is seen (*solid white arrow*), which means the fracture invariably enters the joint space and fractures the articular cartilage. This can have long-term implications for the development of secondary osteoarthritis and can result in asymmetric and premature fusion of the growth plate with subsequent deformity of the bone.

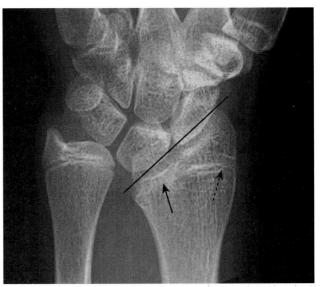

Figure 22-18 Salter-Harris V fracture. Type V fractures are crush fractures of the epiphyseal plate. They are frequently not diagnosed until after they produce their growth impairment through early focal fusion of the growth plate leading to angular deformity. In this child, the medial portion of the distal radial epiphyseal plate has fused (*solid black arrow*) while the lateral portion remains open (*dotted black arrow*). This premature fusion of the medial growth plate has resulted in an angular deformity of the distal radius (*black line*).

TABLE 22-7 SKELETAL TRAUMA SUSPICIOUS FOR CHILD ABUSE

Site(s)	Remarks
Distal femur, distal humerus, wrist, ankle	Metaphyseal corner fractures
Multiple	Fractures in different stages of healing
Femur, humerus, tibia	Spiral fractures <1 year of age
Posterior ribs, avulsed spinous processes	Unusual "naturally occurring" fractures <5 years of age
Multiple skull fractures	Multiple fractures of occipital bone should suggest child abuse
Fractures with abundant callous formation	Implies repeated trauma and no immobilization
Metacarpal and metatarsal fractures	Unusual "naturally occurring" fractures <5 years of age
Sternal and scapular fractures	
Vertebral body fractures and subluxations	

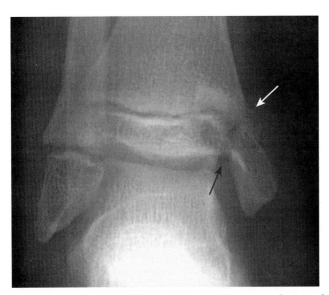

Figure 22-17 Salter-Harris IV fracture. In type IV fractures, a fracture of the epiphyseal plate, metaphysis (*solid white arrow*), and the epiphysis (*solid black arrow*) is present. These have a poorer prognosis than other Salter-Harris fractures because of increased likelihood of premature and possibly asymmetric closure of the epiphyseal plate. Salter-Harris IV fractures are most often seen in the distal humerus and distal tibia.

CHILD ABUSE

- Salter-Harris fractures are examples of accidental injuries in children. Certain kinds of fractures at other sites or of other types can be highly suggestive for nonaccidental injuries produced by abuse. **Radiologic evaluations are key in diagnosing child abuse.**

 There are several fracture sites and characteristics that should raise the suspicion for child abuse (Table 22-7).

- **Metaphyseal corner fractures.** Small, avulsion-type fractures of the metaphyses due to rapid rotation of ligamentous insertions, corner fractures are considered

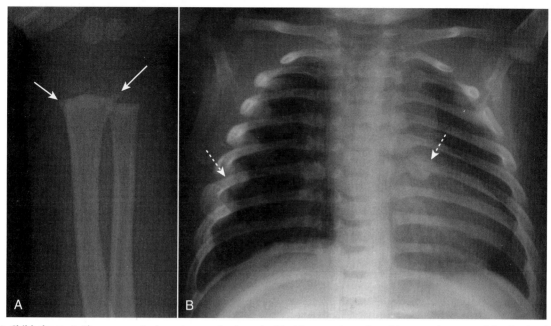

Figure 22-19 Child abuse. A, There are metaphyseal corner fractures (*solid white arrows*), small avulsion-type fractures of the distal radius, a finding characteristic of child abuse. **B,** There are several healing rib fractures (*dotted white arrows*), including one involving the left 6th posterior rib. Fractures of the posterior ribs are unusual, even in accidental trauma, and should raise suspicion for child abuse.

diagnostic of physical abuse. They can parallel the metaphysis and have a **bucket-handle appearance** (Fig. 22-19A).

- **Rib fractures**, especially multiple fractures and fractures of the posterior ribs (which rarely fracture even due to accidental trauma) (Fig. 22-19B).
- **Head injuries** are the most common cause of death in child abuse under age 2 years. Findings include **subdural and subarachnoid hemorrhage** and **cerebral contusions. Skull fractures** tend to be comminuted, bilateral, and may cross suture lines.

STRESS FRACTURES

- Stress fractures **occur as a result of numerous microfractures** in which bone is subjected to repeated stretching and compressive forces.

⮞ Although **conventional radiographs are usually the study first obtained,** they may **initially appear normal in as many as 85%** of cases, so it is common for a patient to complain of pain yet have a normal-appearing radiograph at first.

- The **fracture may not be diagnosable** until after periosteal new bone formation occurs or, in the case of a healing stress fracture of cancellous bone, **the appearance of a thin, dense zone of sclerosis across the medullary cavity** (Fig. 22-20).
- Radionuclide **bone scans will usually be positive much earlier** than conventional radiographs: **within 6 to 72 hours after the injury.**
- Some **common locations for stress fractures** are the **shafts of long bones** such as the proximal femur or proximal tibia, as well as the calcaneous and the 2nd and 3rd metatarsals (*march fractures*).

COMMON FRACTURE EPONYMS

- There are almost as many fracture eponyms as there are types of fractures. We will concentrate on five of the most commonly used eponyms.
- **Colles' fracture** is a **fracture of the distal radius with dorsal angulation** of the distal radial fracture fragment caused by a fall on the outstretched hand (sometimes abbreviated as *FOOSH*). There is frequently an associated fracture of the ulnar styloid (Fig. 22-21).
- **Smith's fracture** is a fracture of the distal radius with palmar angulation of the distal radial fracture fragment (a reverse Colles fracture). It is caused by a fall on the back of the flexed hand (Fig. 22-22).
- **Jones fracture** is a transverse fracture of the 5th metatarsal about 1 to 2 cm from its base caused by plantar flexion of the foot and inversion of the ankle. A Jones fracture may take longer to heal than the more common avulsion fracture of the base of the 5th metatarsal (Fig. 22-23).
- **Boxer's fracture** is a fracture of the head of the 5th metacarpal (little finger) with palmar angulation of the distal fracture fragment. It is most often the result of punching a person or wall (Fig. 22-24).
- **March fracture** is a type of *stress fracture* caused by repeated microfractures to the foot from trauma (such as marching), most often affecting the **shafts of the 2nd and 3rd metatarsals** (see Fig. 22-20).

SOME EASILY MISSED FRACTURES OR DISLOCATIONS

- Look at these areas carefully when evaluating for a possible fracture; then look a second and third time.
- **Scaphoid fractures (common)**
  - Scaphoid fractures are clinically suspected if there is tenderness in the *anatomic snuff box* after a fall on an

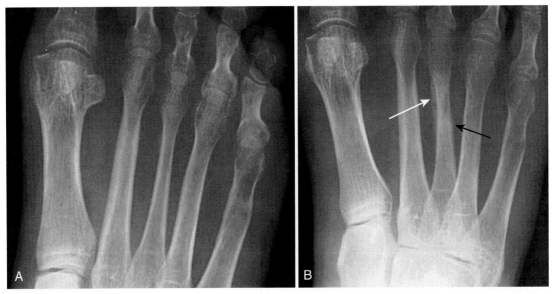

Figure 22-20 Stress fracture, two frontal views taken three weeks apart. A, Although conventional radiographs are the study of first choice, they may initially appear normal in as many as 85% of cases, so it is common for a patient to complain of pain yet have a normal-appearing radiograph, as occurs here one day after pain began. Radionuclide bone scan will usually be positive much earlier than conventional radiographs: within 6 to 72 hours after the injury. **B,** The fracture may not be diagnosable until after periosteal new bone formation forms (*solid white arrow*) or, in the case of a healing stress fracture of cancellous bone, the appearance of a thin, dense zone of sclerosis across the medullary cavity (*solid black arrow*). This radiograph was taken 3 weeks after the first.

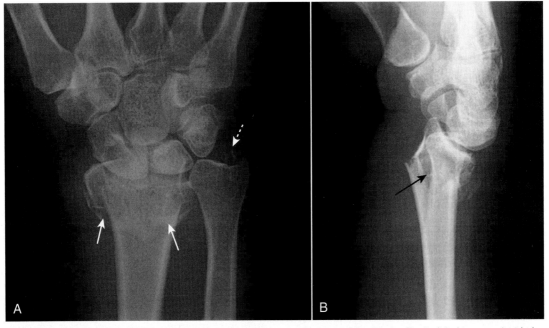

Figure 22-21 Colles' fracture, frontal (A) and lateral (B) views. Colles' fractures are fractures of the distal radius (*solid white arrows*) with dorsal angulation of the distal radial fracture fragments (*solid black arrow*) caused by a fall on the outstretched hand (sometimes abbreviated as **_FOOSH_**). There is frequently an associated fracture of the ulnar styloid (*dotted white arrow*).

outstretched hand. Look for **hairline-thin radiolucencies** on special angled views of the scaphoid (Fig. 22-25). Fractures across the waist of the scaphoid can lead to **avascular necrosis of proximal pole** of that bone.

- Because of peculiarities of vascularization, a fracture through the midportion (**waist**) of the scaphoid (**navicular**) bone in the wrist **interrupts blood supply to the proximal pole** while the other bones of the wrist continue to undergo the process of bone turnover. The result

is an **apparent relative increase in the density of the devascularized part compared to the remainder of the bone** (Fig. 22-26).

- **Buckle fractures of radius and ulna in children (common)**
  - Look for **acute and sudden angulation of the cortex,** especially near the wrist (see Fig. 22-1). These are impacted fractures and usually heal quickly with no deformity.

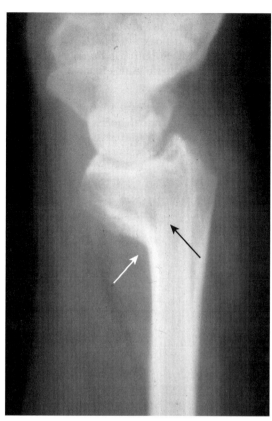

Figure 22-22 Smith's fracture. A Smith fracture is a fracture of the distal radius (*solid white arrow*) with palmar angulation of the distal radial fracture fragment (*solid black arrow*), the reverse of a Colles fracture. It is caused by a fall on the back of the flexed hand.

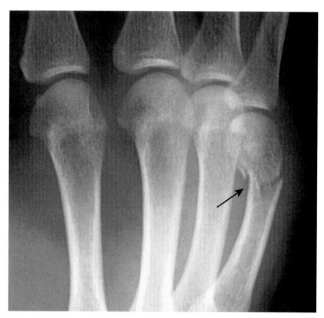

Figure 22-24 Boxer's fracture. A boxer's fracture is a fracture of the head of the 5th metacarpal with palmar angulation of the distal fracture fragment (*solid black arrow*). It is most often the result of punching a person (or a wall).

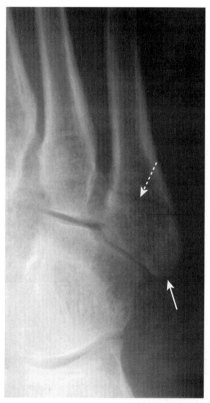

Figure 22-23 Jones fracture, base of 5th metatarsal. A Jones fracture is a transverse fracture of the base 5th metatarsal (*dotted white arrow*). It occurs about 1 to 2 cm from the tuberosity of the 5th metatarsal (*solid white arrow*) and frequently takes longer to heal than an avulsion fracture of the tuberosity. It is caused by plantar flexion of the foot and inversion of the ankle.

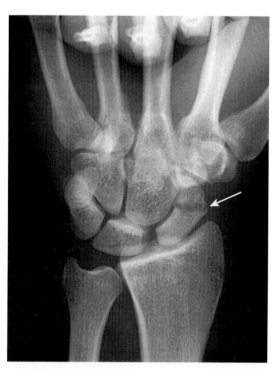

Figure 22-25 Scaphoid fracture. Scaphoid fractures are common. They are suspected clinically if there is tenderness in the anatomic snuff box after a fall on an outstretched hand. Look for linear fracture lines on special angled views of the scaphoid (*solid white arrow*). Fractures across the waist of the scaphoid can lead to avascular necrosis of proximal pole of that bone.

- Radial head fracture (common)
  - A fracture of the radial head is the **most common fracture of the elbow in an adult.** Look for a crescentic lucency of fat along the posterior aspect of the distal humerus produced by normally invisible **intracapsular, extrasynovial fat** that is lifted away from the bone by swelling of the joint capsule due to a **traumatic hemarthrosis**—the *positive posterior fat-pad sign* (Fig. 22-27).

- Supracondylar fracture of the distal humerus in children (common)
  - This is the **most common fracture of the elbow in a child.** Most of these fractures produce **posterior displacement** of the distal humerus.
  - On a true lateral film, the **anterior humeral line** (a line drawn tangential to the anterior humeral cortex) should bisect the middle third of the ossification center of capitellum. In a **supracondylar fracture, this line passes anterior to its normal location** (Fig. 22-28).

- Posterior dislocation of the shoulder (uncommon)
  - The humeral head is fixed in internal rotation and looks like a "lightbulb" in all views of the shoulder. Look at a view like the axillary or "Y" view to see if head still lies within the glenoid fossa. On the "Y" view (an oblique view of the shoulder), the head will lie lateral to the glenoid in a posterior dislocation (Fig. 22-29).

- Hip fractures in the elderly (common)
  - Hip fractures are frequently related to osteoporosis. Conventional radiographs of the femoral neck should be performed with the patient's leg in internal rotation so as to display the neck in profile. Look for **angulation of the cortex** or zones of **increased density indicating impaction** (Fig. 22-30).
  - Sometimes, hip fractures may be very subtle and require an MRI or radionuclide bone scan for diagnosis.

- **Look for indirect signs indicating the possibility of an underlying fracture** (Table 22-8, Fig. 22-31).

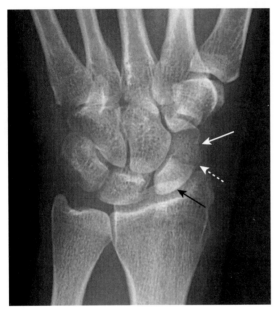

Figure 22-26 Avascular necrosis of the proximal pole of the scaphoid. A close-up frontal view of the wrist demonstrates that the proximal pole of the scaphoid (*solid black arrow*) is denser than the distal pole (*solid white arrow*). There is a fracture through the waist of the scaphoid (*dotted white arrow*). Because of the peculiar blood supply of the scaphoid (from distal to proximal), fractures through the waist may interrupt the proximal blood supply while the other bones of the wrist, having normal blood supply, become demineralized. This makes the proximal pole of the scaphoid appear denser relative to the other bones of the wrist.

FRACTURE HEALING

- Fracture healing is determined by many factors including the **age of the patient,** the **fracture site,** the **position of the fracture fragments,** the degree of **immobilization,** and the **blood supply** to the fracture site (Table 22-9).
- Immediately following a fracture, there is hemorrhage into the fracture site.

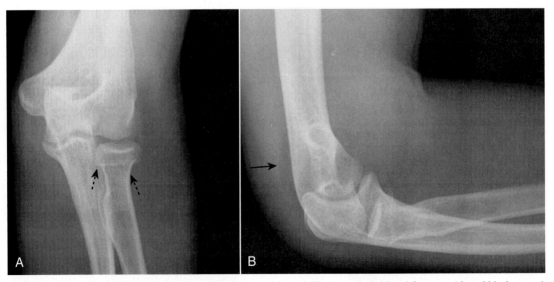

Figure 22-27 Fracture of radial head with joint effusion, frontal (A) and lateral (B) views. Radial head fractures (*dotted black arrows*) are the most common fractures of the elbow in an adult. Look for fat appearing as a crescentic lucency along the dorsal aspect of the distal humerus (*solid black arrow*) caused by intracapsular, extrasynovial fat that is lifted away from the bone by swelling of the joint capsule due to a traumatic hemarthrosis—the ***positive posterior fat-pad sign.*** Virtually all studies of bones will include at least two views at 90° angles to each other called ***orthogonal views.*** Many protocols call for two additional oblique views which enable you to visualize more of the cortex in profile.

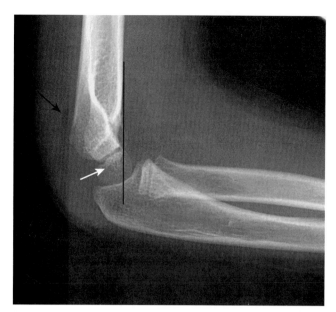

Figure 22-28 Supracondylar fracture. A supracondylar fracture of the distal humerus is a common fracture in children, and its findings may be subtle. Most of these fractures produce posterior displacement of the capitellum of the distal humerus. On a true lateral film, the anterior humeral line (a line drawn tangential to the anterior humeral cortex and *shown here in black*) should bisect the middle portion of the capitellum (*solid white arrow*). When there is a supracondylar fracture, this line will pass more anteriorly, as it does here. There is a positive posterior fat pad sign present (*solid black arrow*).

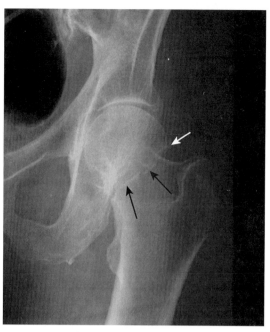

Figure 22-30 Impacted subcapital hip fracture. Hip fractures are relatively common fractures in the elderly and are frequently related to osteoporosis. Look for angulation of the cortex (*solid white arrow*) and zones of increased density (*solid black arrows*) indicating impaction. Conventional radiographs of the femoral neck should be obtained with the patient's leg in internal rotation (as shown here) so as to display the neck in profile. Hip fractures can be very subtle and sometimes require additional imaging such as MRI or bone scan for their diagnosis.

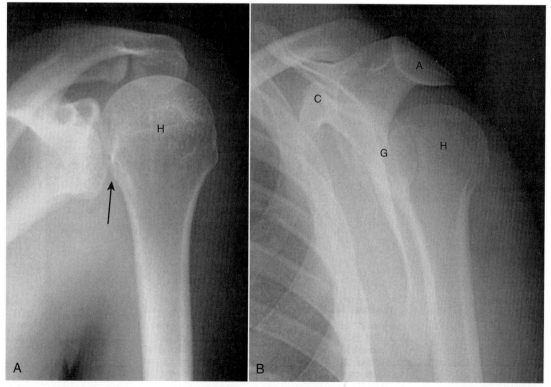

Figure 22-29 Posterior dislocation of the shoulder. Posterior dislocations of the shoulder are much less common than anterior dislocations but more difficult to diagnose. **A**, On the frontal view, look for the humeral head (*H*) to be persistently fixed in internal rotation and resemble a "lightbulb" no matter how the patient turns the forearm. There is also an increased distance between the head and the glenoid (*solid black arrow*). **B**, On the "Y" view, the head (*H*) will lie under the acromion (*A*), a posterior structure of the scapula. The coracoid process (*C*) is anterior. Normally, the head is centered between the coracoid and the acromion in the glenoid fossa (*G*).

- Over the next several weeks, osteoclasts act to remove the diseased bone. The **fracture line may actually minimally widen** at this time.
- Then, over the course of several more weeks, **new bone** (*callus*) begins to bridge the fracture gap (Fig. 22-32).
  - **Internal endosteal healing** is manifest by **indistinctness of the fracture line** leading to obliteration of the fracture line.
  - **External, periosteal healing** is manifest by external callus formation eventually leading to **bridging of the fracture site.**

TABLE 22-8 INDIRECT SIGNS OF POSSIBLE FRACTURE

Sign	Remarks
Soft tissue swelling	Frequently accompanies a fracture but does not necessarily mean that a fracture is present
Disappearance of normal fat stripes	The **pronator quadratus fat stripe** on the volar aspect of the wrist, for example, may be displaced with a fracture of the distal radius (see Fig. 22-31).
Joint effusion	The **positive posterior fat pad sign** seen on the dorsal aspect of the distal humerus from a traumatic joint effusion is an example (see Fig. 22-27B).
Periosteal reaction	Sometimes the healing of a fracture will be the first manifestation that a fracture was present, especially with stress fractures of the foot.

- **Remodeling** of bone **begins at about 8 to 12 weeks** post-fracture as mechanical forces, in part, begin to adjust the bone to its original shape.
  - In **children, this occurs much more rapidly** and usually leads to a bone that eventually appears normal. In **adults, this process may take years** and the healed fracture may never assume a completely normal shape.
- **Complications of the healing process**
  - **Delayed union.** The fracture **does not heal in the expected time** for a fracture at that particular site (e.g., 6 to 8 weeks for a fracture of the shaft of the radius). **Most cases of delayed union will eventually progress to complete healing** with further immobilization.
  - **Malunion.** Healing of the fracture fragments occurs in a **mechanically or cosmetically unacceptable position.**

TABLE 22-9 FACTORS THAT AFFECT FRACTURE HEALING

Accelerate Fracture Healing	Delay Fracture Healing
Youth	Old age
Early immobilization	Delayed immobilization
Adequate duration of immobilization	Too short a duration of immobilization
Good blood supply	Poor blood supply
Physical activity after adequate immobilization	Steroids
Adequate mineralization	Osteoporosis, osteomalacia

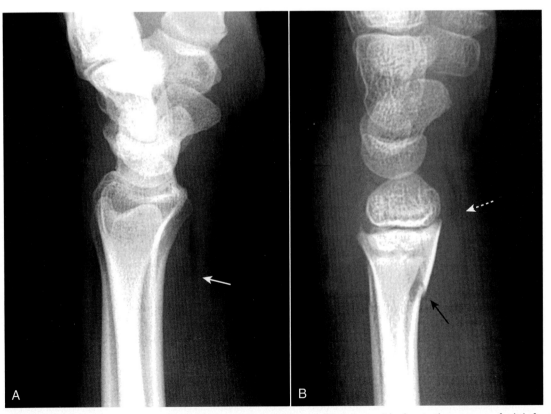

Figure 22-31 Normal and abnormal pronator quadratus fat plane. Soft tissue abnormalities can provide clues to the presence of subtle fractures or help confirm the significance of a questionable finding. Here is an example of a normal fascial plane **(A)** produced by the pronator quadratus (*solid white arrow* points to lucency) on the volar aspect of the wrist compared to the bulging fascial plane (*dotted white arrow*), which has occurred because of soft tissue swelling accompanying a fracture of the distal radius (*solid black arrow*) in **(B)**.

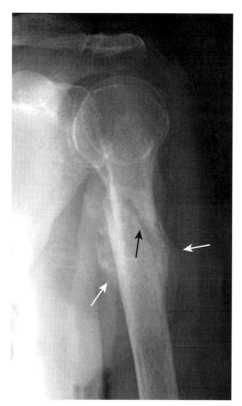

Figure 22-32 Healing humeral fracture. Immediately following a fracture, there is hemorrhage into the fracture site. Over the next several weeks, new bone (callus) begins to bridge the fracture gap. Internal endosteal healing is manifest by indistinctness of the fracture line (*solid black arrow*) eventually leading to obliteration of the fracture line. External, periosteal healing is manifest by external callus formation (*solid white arrows*) leading to bridging of the fracture site.

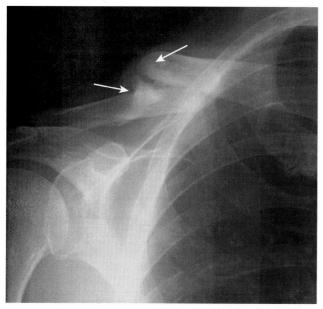

Figure 22-33 Nonunion of clavicular fracture. Nonunion is a radiologic diagnosis that implies fracture healing is not likely to occur because the processes leading to the repair of bone have ceased. It is characterized by smooth and sclerotic fracture margins with distraction of the fracture fragments (*solid white arrows*). A *pseudarthrosis*, complete with a synovial lining, may form at the fracture site.

- **Nonunion.** This implies that **fracture healing will never occur.** It is characterized by **smooth and sclerotic fracture margins** with **distraction of the fracture fragments** (Fig. 22-33). A *pseudarthrosis*, complete with a synovial lining, may form at the fracture site.
  - **Motion at the fracture site** may be demonstrated under fluoroscopic manipulation or on stress views.

WEBLINK

Registered users may obtain more information on Recognizing Fractures and Dislocations on StudentConsult.com.

TAKE-HOME POINTS

Recognizing Fractures and Dislocations

A *fracture* is described as a disruption in the continuity of all or part of the cortex of a bone.

Complete fractures involve the entire cortex, are more common, and typically occur in adults; *incomplete fractures* involve only a part of the cortex and typically occur in bones that are softer, such as those of children; *torus* and *greenstick fractures* are incomplete fractures.

Fracture lines tend to be blacker, more sharply angled, and more jagged than other lucencies in bones such as nutrient canals or epiphyseal plates.

Sesamoids, accessory ossicles, and unhealed fractures may mimic acute fractures but all will have smooth and corticated margins.

Dislocation is present when two bones that originally formed a joint are no longer in contact with each other; *subluxation* is present when two bones that originally formed a joint are in partial contact with each other.

Fractures are described in many ways including the number of fracture fragments, direction of the fracture line, relationship of the fragments to each other, and whether or not they communicate with the outside atmosphere.

Simple fractures have two fragments; *comminuted fractures* have more than two fragments; segmental and butterfly fractures describe two types of comminuted fracture.

The direction of fracture lines is described as *transverse*, *diagonal*, or *spiral*.

The relationships of the fragments of a fracture are described by four parameters: *displacement*, *angulation*, *shortening*, and *rotation*.

Closed fractures are those in which there is no communication between the fracture and the outside atmosphere; they are much more common than *open or compound fractures* in which there is communication with the outside atmosphere.

Avulsion fractures are produced by the forceful contraction of a tendon or ligament; they can occur at any age but are particularly common in younger, athletic individuals.

The *Salter-Harris classification* categorizes fractures through the epiphyseal plate that are graded by severity and prognosis, the more severe having an increased risk of resulting in angular deformities or shortening of the affected bone.

Child abuse should be suspected when there are multiple fractures in various stages of healing, metaphyseal corner fractures, rib fractures, and skull fractures, especially if multiple.

Stress fractures, such as march fractures in the metatarsals, occur as a result of numerous microfractures and frequently are not visible on conventional radiographs taken when the pain first begins; after some time, bony callus formation or a dense zone of sclerosis becomes visible.

Some common named fractures are *Colles' fracture* (of the radius), *Smith's fracture* (of the radius), *Jones fracture* (of the base of the 5th metatarsal), *boxer's fracture* (of the head of the 5th metacarpal), and *march fracture* (in the foot).

Some fractures are more difficult to detect than others; the easily missed fractures (and how common they are) include scaphoid fractures (common), buckle fractures of the radius and ulna (common), radial head fractures (common), supracondylar fractures (common), posterior dislocations of the shoulder (uncommon), and hip fractures (common).

Soft tissue swelling, the disappearance of normal fat stripes and fascial planes, joint effusions, and periosteal reaction are indirect signs that should alert you to the possibility of an underlying fracture.

Fractures heal with a combination of **endosteal callus**, recognized by a progressive indistinctness of the fracture line, and **external callus** that bridges the fracture site; many factors affect fracture healing, including the age of the patient, the degree of mobility of the fracture, and its blood supply.

Delayed union refers to a fracture that is taking longer to heal than is usually required for that site; *malunion* means the fracture is healing but in a mechanically or cosmetically unacceptable way; *nonunion* is a radiologic diagnosis that implies there is little if any likelihood the fracture will heal.

Chapter 23

Recognizing Joint Disease: An Approach to Arthritis

- Imaging studies play a key role in the diagnosis and management of arthritis and are the method by which many arthritides are first diagnosed. Other arthritides are initially diagnosed on clinical and laboratory grounds and imaging is used to document the severity, extent, and course of the disease (Table 23-1).
- Conventional radiographs demonstrate osseous abnormalities but provide only indirect and usually delayed evidence of abnormalities involving the soft tissues, such as the synovial lining of the joint, the articular cartilage, muscles, ligaments, and tendons surrounding the joint. MRI is used to demonstrate those soft tissue abnormalities.

ANATOMY OF A JOINT

- Figure 23-1 contains a diagram of a typical synovial joint and compares the structures visualized on conventional radiographs and MRI.
- The *articular cortex* is the thin, white line as seen on conventional radiographs that lies within the joint capsule and is usually capped by *hyaline cartilage*, called the *articular cartilage.* The bone immediately beneath the articular cortex is called *subchondral bone.*
- Lining the *joint capsule* is the *synovial membrane* containing *synovial fluid.* The synovial membrane is frequently the earliest structure involved by an arthritis.
- Conventional radiographs will demonstrate abnormalities of the **articular cortex** and the **subchondral bone** and will provide late, indirect evidence of the integrity of the articular cartilage.
- On conventional radiographs, the synovial membrane, synovial fluid, and the articular cartilage are usually not directly visible. All, however, are visible using MRI.
- While MRI is more sensitive in directly visualizing the soft tissues in and around a joint, **conventional radiographs remain the study of first choice** in evaluating for the presence of an arthritis.

CLASSIFICATION OF ARTHRITIS

- First, let's define **what an arthritis** is and then we'll outline a classification of arthritides. An **arthritis is a disease that affects a joint** and usually the bones on either side of the joint, almost always accompanied by **joint space narrowing** (Fig. 23-2).
- We will divide arthritides into three main categories: (Table 23-2)

- **Hypertrophic arthritis** is characterized, in general, by **bone formation** at the site of the involved joint(s). The bone formation may occur within the confines of the parent bone (*subchondral sclerosis*) or protrude from the parent bone (*osteophyte*) (Fig. 23-3A).
- **Erosive arthritis** indicates underlying inflammation and is characterized by tiny, marginal, irregularly shaped lytic lesions in or around the joint surfaces called *erosions* (Fig. 23-3B).
- **Infectious arthritis** is characterized by joint swelling, osteopenia, and **destruction of long, contiguous segments of the articular cortex** (Fig. 23-3C).
- Within each of these three main categories, we'll look at a few of the more common types of arthritis that also have characteristic imaging findings.

HYPERTROPHIC ARTHRITIS

- **Hypertrophic arthritis is characterized by bone formation,** either **within** the confines of preexisting bone (*subchondral sclerosis*) or by bony protrusions **extending from** the normal bone (*osteophytes*).
- **Hypertrophic arthritides** include:
  - Osteoarthritis (degenerative arthritis, degenerative joint disease), which is further divided into:
    - Primary osteoarthritis
    - Secondary osteoarthritis
  - Erosive osteoarthritis
  - Charcot arthropathy (neuropathic joint)
  - Calcium pyrophosphate deposition disease (CPPD)

Primary Osteoarthritis (Also Known as Primary Degenerative Arthritis, Degenerative Joint Disease)

- This is the **most common form of arthritis,** estimated to affect over 20 million Americans. It results from **intrinsic degeneration of the articular cartilage,** mostly from the mechanical stress of **excessive wear and tear** in weight-bearing joints.
- It mostly involves the **hips, knees, and hands** and increases in prevalence with increasing age.

 The imaging findings in osteoarthritis:

- **Marginal osteophyte formation. A hallmark of hypertrophic arthritis,** osseous transformation of cartilaginous excrescences and metaplasia of synovial lining cells lead to the production of these **bony protrusions at or near the joint** (Fig. 23-4).

- **Subchondral sclerosis.** This is a reaction of the bone to the mechanical stress to which it is subjected when its protective cartilage has been destroyed.
- **Subchondral cysts.** As a result of chronic impaction, necrosis of bone and imposition of synovial fluid into the subchondral bone, cysts of varying sizes form in the subchondral bone.
- **Narrowing of the joint space.** This is seen in all forms of arthritis.

TABLE 23-1 ARTHRITIS: WHO MAKES THE DIAGNOSIS?

Usually Diagnosed Clinically	Frequently Diagnosed Radiologically
Septic (pyogenic) arthritis	Osteoarthritis
Psoriatic arthritis	Early rheumatoid arthritis
Gout	Calcium pyrophosphate deposition disease
	Ankylosing spondylitis
Hemophilia	Septic (TB)
	Charcot (neuropathic) joint—late

- What joints are involved?
  - In osteoarthritis, destruction of the cartilaginous buffer between the apposing bones of a joint leads to narrowing of the joint space most often on the **weight-bearing** side of the joint: **hip (superior and lateral) and knee (medial)** (Fig. 23-5).
  - In most patients with osteoarthritis of the interphalangeal joints of the hands, the first carpometacarpal joint (base of thumb) is also affected (Fig. 23-6). It is also common for osteoarthritis to affect the distal interphalangeal joints, especially in older females.

Secondary Osteoarthritis (Secondary Degenerative Arthritis)

- Secondary osteoarthritis is a form of degenerative arthritis of synovial joints that occurs because of an underlying, predisposing condition, **most frequently trauma**, that damages or leads to damage of the articular cartilage.
- The radiographic findings of secondary osteoarthritis are the same as those for the primary form with several special clues to help suggest secondary osteoarthritis:
  - It **occurs at an atypical age** for primary osteoarthritis (e.g., a 20-year-old with osteoarthritis) (Box 23-1).

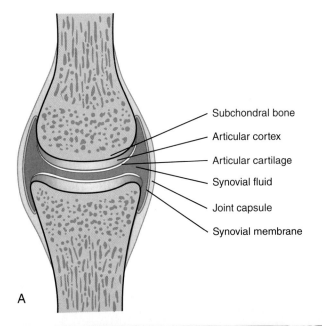

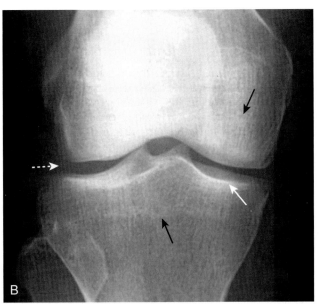

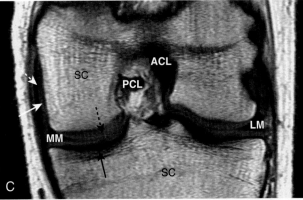

Figure 23-1 Diagram, radiograph, and MRI image of a true joint. A, A representation of a synovial joint shows the *articular cortex,* which corresponds to the thin, white line within the *joint capsule* that is usually capped by *articular cartilage.* The bone immediately beneath the articular cortex is called *subchondral bone.* Within the joint capsule is the *synovial membrane* and *synovial fluid.* **B,** On conventional radiographs, the articular cortex (*solid white arrow*) and subchondral bone (*solid black arrows*) are visible but the cartilage and synovial fluid are not (*dotted white arrow*). **C,** A T1-weighted coronal MRI of the knee shows the medial (*MM*) and lateral (*LM*) menisci, anterior (*ACL*) and posterior (*PCL*) cruciate ligaments, articular cartilage (*dotted black arrow*), joint capsule (*dotted white arrow*), synovial fluid (*solid white arrow*), and marrow in the subchondral bone (*SC*). The cortex of the bone (*solid black arrow*) produces little signal and is dark.

Labels on diagram (A): Subchondral bone, Articular cortex, Articular cartilage, Synovial fluid, Joint capsule, Synovial membrane

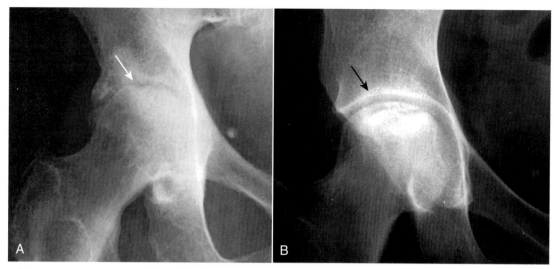

Figure 23-2 Arthritis or not? An arthritis is a disease that affects a joint and usually the bones on either side of the joint, almost always accompanied by joint space narrowing. **A,** This disease meets those specifications. There is narrowing of the hip joint, and both the femoral head and the acetabulum are abnormal (*solid white arrow*). This is osteoarthritis of the hip. **B,** There is an abnormality of the femoral head (sclerosis) but the joint space is normal as is the acetabulum (*solid black arrow*). This is avascular necrosis of the femoral head.

TABLE 23-2 CLASSIFICATION OF ARTHRITIS

Category	Hallmarks	Types	Remarks
Hypertrophic arthritis	Bone formation Osteophytes	Primary osteoarthritis	Most common; mechanical stress; hands, hips, and knees most common
		Secondary osteoarthritis	Degenerative joint disease (DJD) secondary to prior trauma, or avascular necrosis
		Charcot arthropathy	Fragmentation; joint destruction; sclerosis; most often secondary to diabetes
		CPPD	Chondrocalcinosis; DJD in unusual sites
Erosive arthritis	Erosions	Rheumatoid	Carpals, metacarpal-phalangeal joints, proximal interphalangeal joints of hands; osteoporosis; soft-tissue swelling
		Gout	Juxtaarticular erosions with overhanging edges; long-latency; metatarsal-phalangeal joint of big toe; no osteoporosis
		Psoriatic	Juxtaarticular erosions of distal interphalangeal joints of hands; pencil-in-cup deformity; enthesophytes
		Hemophilia	Remodeling from hemarthroses and hyperemia; same changes in knee in female—think of juvenile rheumatoid arthritis
		Ankylosing spondylitis	HLA-B27+; bilateral sacroiliac (SI) joints; syndesmophytes
		Seronegative spondyloarthropathies	Rheumatoid factor negative; HLA- B27+; SI joints; syndesmophytes reactive arthritis, psoriasis
Infectious arthritis	Osteopenia and soft tissue swelling; early and marked destruction of most or all of the articular cortex	Pyogenic	Early destruction of articular cortex; osteoporosis
		TB	Gradual and late destruction of articular cortex; marked osteoporosis

- It has an **atypical appearance for primary osteoarthritis** (e.g., primary osteoarthritis is usually bilateral and often symmetrical; severe osteoarthritic changes of one hip while the opposite appears perfectly normal should alert you to the possibility of secondary osteoarthritis).
- It may **appear in an unusual location** for primary arthritis, (e.g., the elbow joint) (Fig. 23-7).

⮕ **Eventually any arthritis that affects the articular cartilage, no matter what the etiology, can lead to changes of secondary osteoarthritis.**

Erosive Osteoarthritis

- Erosive osteoarthritis is a **type of primary osteoarthritis** characterized by more **severe inflammation** and by the

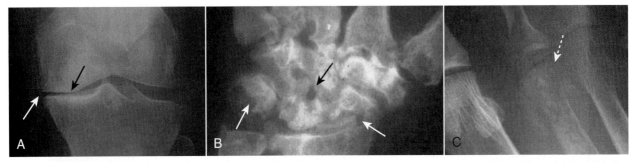

Figure 23-3 The imaging hallmarks of the three major categories of arthritis. A, Hypertrophic arthritis features subchondral sclerosis (*solid black arrow*) and marginal osteophyte production (*solid white arrow*). **B,** Erosive (inflammatory) arthritis features characteristic marginal lytic erosions (*solid white and black arrows*). **C,** Infectious arthritis features destruction of the articular cortex (*dotted white arrow*).

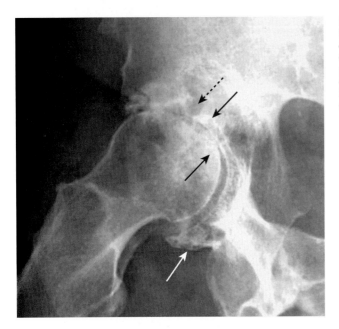

Figure 23-4 Osteoarthritis. The hallmarks of osteoarthritis are demonstrated in this patient's right hip. There is marginal osteophyte formation (*solid white arrow*), a process by which osseous transformation of cartilaginous excrescences and metaplasia of synovial lining cells leads to the production of bony protrusions at or near the joint. There is also subchondral sclerosis (*solid black arrows*), representing reaction of the bone to the mechanical stress to which it is subjected when its protective cartilage has been destroyed. Subchondral cyst formation is also present(*dotted black arrow*).

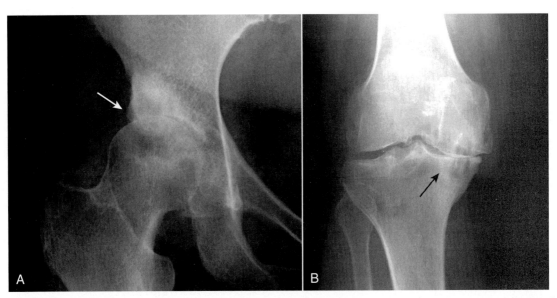

Figure 23-5 Osteoarthritis of hip (A) and knee (B). In osteoarthritis, destruction of the cartilaginous buffer between the apposing bones of a joint leads to narrowing of the joint space most often on the weight-bearing side of the joint. In the hip **(A),** the superior and lateral surface is most affected (*solid white arrow*) while in the knee **(B),** the medial compartment is more affected (*solid black arrow*).

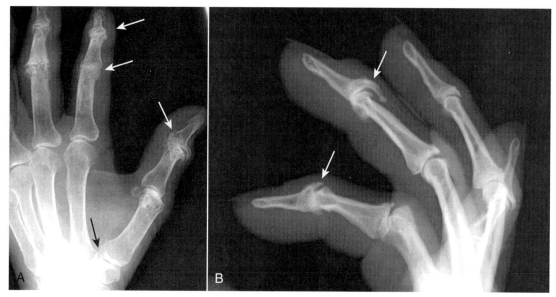

Figure 23-6 Osteoarthritis of the hands (A and B). In the hands, osteoarthritis affects primarily the distal and then proximal interphalangeal joints. There are osteophytes at the distal and proximal phalangeal joints (*solid white arrows*) and the joint spaces are narrowed. There is also subchondral sclerosis present at the carpal-metacarpal joint of the thumb (*solid black arrow*). Osteoarthritis of the hands occurs most often in older women.

Box 23-1 **Some Causes of Secondary Osteoarthritis**
Trauma
Infection
Avascular necrosis
Calcium pyrophosphate deposition disease
Rheumatoid arthritis

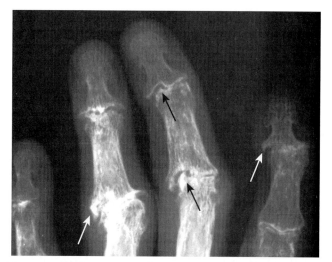

Figure 23-8 Erosive osteoarthritis. A type of primary osteoarthritis characterized by more severe inflammation and by the development of erosive changes, erosive osteoarthritis may feature bilaterally symmetrical changes like the osteophytes of DJD but with marked inflammation (swelling and tenderness). The erosions are typically centrally located within the joint (*solid black arrows*) and, combined with the small osteophytes associated with the disease (*solid white arrows*), produce what has been called the ***gull-wing deformity***.

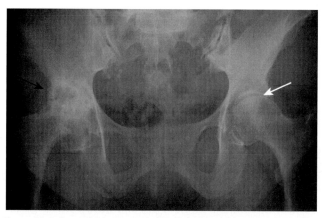

Figure 23-7 Secondary osteoarthritis, right hip. Notice the marked discrepancy between the two hips with severe and advanced osteoarthritis of the right hip (*solid black arrow*) and a normal left hip (*solid white arrow*). The radiographic findings of secondary osteoarthritis are the same as those for the primary form except it occurs at an atypical age for primary osteoarthritis, it has an atypical appearance for primary osteoarthritis, and it may appear in an unusual location for primary osteoarthritis. This patient had a slipped capital femoral epiphysis on the right, and it was never attended to medically.

development of **erosive changes.** It occurs most often in **perimenopausal females**.

- Erosive osteoarthritis may feature bilaterally symmetrical changes such as the osteophytes of primary osteoarthritis but with **marked inflammation (swelling and tenderness) and erosions** at the affected joints.
  - The **erosions are typically centrally located within the joint** and, combined with the small osteophytes

associated with the disease, may produce the so-called ***gull-wing deformity*** (Fig. 23-8).
- Erosive osteoarthritis most commonly occurs at the **proximal and distal interphalangeal joints of the fingers, 1ˢᵗ carpal-metacarpal and the interphalangeal joint of the thumb.**
- **Bony ankylosis may occur,** an uncommon finding in primary osteoarthritis.

Charcot Arthropathy (Neuropathic Joint)

- Charcot arthropathy develops from a **disturbance in sensation** that leads to **multiple microfractures** as well as an

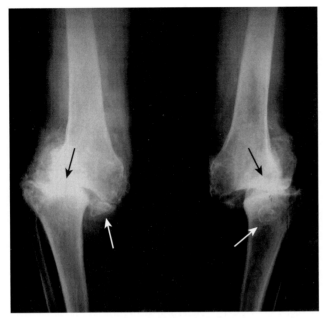

Figure 23-9 Charcot arthropathy of knees. As a hypertrophic arthritis, a Charcot joint will demonstrate extensive subchondral sclerosis. The hallmark findings of a Charcot joint, however, are fragmentation of the bones surrounding the joint, which produces numerous small, bony densities within the joint capsule (*solid white arrows*) as well as joint space destruction (*solid black arrows*). The most common cause of a Charcot joint of the knee is diabetes.

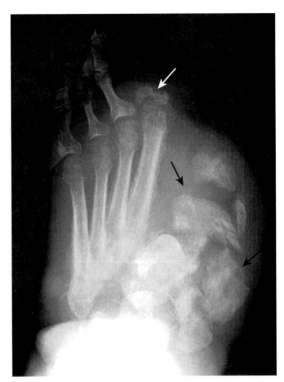

Figure 23-10 Charcot arthropathy of foot. This patient had previously undergone an amputation of the phalanges of the second toe (*solid white arrow*) for diabetic gangrene but the destruction and marked fragmentation of the great toe are manifestations of Charcot neuropathy (*solid black arrows*). Charcot neuropathy can produce some of the most dramatic examples of total joint destruction of any arthritis.

autonomic imbalance that leads to hyperemia, **bone resorption, and fragmentation of bone.**

- Even though the joint lacks sensory feedback, almost three out of four patients with a Charcot joint **complain of some degree of pain,** although it is usually far less than would be expected for the degree of joint destruction present.
- **Soft tissue swelling is a prominent feature.**
- The **most common cause of a Charcot joint today is diabetes,** and most Charcot joints are found in the **lower extremities, particularly in the feet and ankles.**
- Causes of Charcot joints by location:
  - **Shoulders**—syrinx, spinal tumor, and syphilis
  - **Hips**—tertiary syphilis, diabetes
  - **Ankles and feet**—diabetes (common) and syphilis (uncommon)

 Radiographic findings in Charcot arthropathy:

- As a hypertrophic arthritis, a Charcot joint will demonstrate **extensive subchondral sclerosis.**
- The **hallmark findings of a Charcot joint:**
  - **Fragmentation** of the bones surrounding the joint, which produces numerous small, bony densities within the joint capsule. Sometimes, **many—if not all—of the fragments may be resorbed** and no longer be visible (Fig. 23-9).
  - Eventual **destruction of the joint.** Charcot neuropathy is responsible for some of the **most dramatic examples of total joint destruction of any arthritis** (Fig. 23-10).
- A Charcot joint shares findings with osteomyelitis, and the two may mimic each other in that they both produce **bone destruction** and **periosteal reaction (from**

fracture healing). A radioactive Indium-tagged white-cell bone scan can help to differentiate infection from Charcot joint.

Calcium Pyrophosphate Deposition Disease (Pyrophosphate Arthropathy)

- Calcium pyrophosphate deposition disease is an arthropathy resulting from the deposition of **calcium pyrophosphate dihydrate (CPPD)** crystals in and around joints, **mostly in hyaline cartilage and fibrocartilage.** This is especially common in the **triangular fibrocartilage of the wrist** and the **menisci of the knee.**
- The terminology associated with describing this disease can be confusing.
  - *Chondrocalcinosis* refers only to **calcification** of the articular cartilage or fibrocartilage and is seen in about 50% of adults over the age of 85, most of whom are **asymptomatic.** Chondrocalcinosis can occur in other diseases besides CPPD, such as hyperparathyroidism or hemochromatosis (Fig. 23-11).
  - *Pseudogout* is a **clinical syndrome** consisting of **acute, monarticular arthropathy** characterized by **redness, pain, and swelling** of the affected joint (most commonly the knee) from which **calcium pyrophosphate dihydrate** crystals can be aspirated.
  - *Pyrophosphate arthropathy* is a radiologic diagnosis and the most common form of CPPD.

Pyrophosphate arthropathy may be indistinguishable from primary osteoarthritis but differs from it in several important respects:

- CPPD affects joints **not usually affected by primary osteoarthritis** such as the **patellofemoral joint space of the knee**, the **radiocarpal joint**, the **metacarpalphalangeal joints of the hands**, and the **joints of the wrist**.

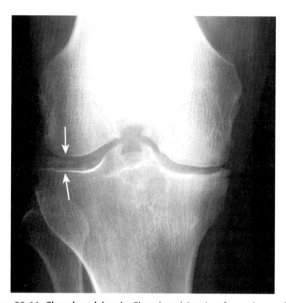

Figure 23-11 Chondrocalcinosis. Chondrocalcinosis refers only to calcification of the articular cartilage (*solid white arrows*) or fibrocartilage and is seen in about 50% of adults over the age of 85, most of whom are asymptomatic. If this patient had acute pain, redness, swelling, and limitation of motion, the combination would be called **pseudogout**.

- **Chondrocalcinosis is usually present** in pyrophosphate arthropathy, but is not required for the diagnosis.
- **Subchondral cysts** are more common, larger, more numerous, and more widespread than in primary osteoarthritis.
- **Hook-shaped bony excrescences** along the 2nd and 3rd metacarpal heads are a common finding in this form of CPPD (Fig. 23-12A).
- **In the wrist**, characteristic findings include **calcification of the triangular fibrocartilage**, narrowing of the radiocarpal joint, separation of the scaphoid and the lunate by more than 3 mm (*scapholunate dissociation*), and collapse of the distal carpal row towards the radius (*scapholunate advanced collapse*) (Fig. 23-12B).

EROSIVE ARTHRITIS

- **Erosive arthritis** comprises a large number of arthritides, all of which are associated with some degree of *inflammation* and *synovial proliferation* (*pannus formation*), which participates in the production of **lytic lesions in or near the joint** called *erosions*, especially in the small joints of the hands and feet.
- **Pannus** acts like a mass of growing and enlarging synovial tissue, which leads to **marginal erosions** of the **articular cartilage and underlying bone**.
- Box 23-2 lists some of the many causes of erosive arthritis. We shall talk about only four of the more common.

Rheumatoid Arthritis

- Rheumatoid arthritis (RA) is **more common in females**, frequently involving the **proximal joints of the hands and wrists**. It is **usually bilateral and symmetrical**.

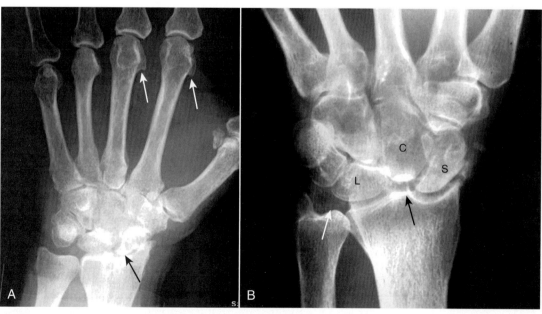

Figure 23-12 Calcium pyrophosphate deposition disease (CPPD). CPPD arthropathy produces changes similar to osteoarthritis but differs from it in that CPPD affects joints not usually affected by primary osteoarthritis. **A,** Hook-shaped bony excrescences along the 2nd and 3rd metacarpal heads are a common finding in CPPD (*solid white arrows*). The radiocarpal joint is narrowed (*solid black arrow*). **B,** In the wrist, characteristic findings include calcification of the triangular fibrocartilage (*solid white arrow*), separation of the scaphoid (*S*) and the lunate (*L*) (*scapholunate dissociation*) and collapse of the capitate (*C*) toward the radius (*solid black arrow*) called *scapholunate advanced collapse (SLAC)*.

■ Conventional radiographs remain the study of first choice in imaging RA.

 The **earliest** radiographic changes are **soft tissue swelling** of the affected joints and **osteoporosis**, which tends to be most severe on both sides of the joint space (*periarticular osteoporosis* or *periarticular deminer*alization).

■ **In the hand**, the **erosions tend to involve the proximal joints:** the carpal-metacarpal, metacarpal-phalangeal, and proximal interphalangeal joints (Fig. 23-13).
  • **Late findings in the hands** include deformities such as **ulnar deviation of the fingers at the MCP joints, subluxation of the MCP joints,** and ligamentous laxity leading to deformities of the fingers (*swan-neck* and *boutonnière deformities*).
■ **In the wrist**, erosions of the **carpals, ulnar styloid,** and **narrowing of the radio-carpal joint** space are frequently seen.
■ Elsewhere in the body, the larger joints usually show no erosions, but there may be **marked uniform narrowing of the joint space with little or no subchondral sclerosis** (Fig. 23-14).

Box 23-2 **Some Causes of Erosive Arthritis**
Rheumatoid arthritis
Gout
Psoriatic arthritis
Ankylosing spondylitis (spine)
Rheumatoid variants
Reactive arthritis (formerly known as Reiter syndrome)
Sarcoid
Hemophilia

■ In the spine, RA tends to involve the **cervical spine** by producing **ligamentous laxity**, which can lead to forward subluxation of C1 on C2 (*atlantoaxial subluxation*). Atlantoaxial subluxation can produce cord compression if severe (Fig. 23-15).
  • **RA may also cause narrowing, sclerosis, and eventual fusion of the facet joints in the cervical spine.**

Gout

■ Gout represents the **inflammatory changes incited by the deposition of calcium urate crystals in the joint.** There is **characteristically an extremely long latent period (5 to 7 years)** between the onset of symptoms and the visualization of bone changes, so **gout is usually a clinical and not a radiologic diagnosis** (see Table 23-1).
■ Gout tends to be **monoarticular** at its onset and **asymmetric later** in its course.
■ It is **more common in males** and **most commonly affects the metatarsal-phalangeal joint of the great toe** at the time of symptom onset.

 Imaging findings of gout:

■ As an erosive arthritis, the **hallmark of gout is the sharply marginated, juxtaarticular erosion which tends to have a sclerotic border.** The overhanging edges of gouty erosions have been called *rat bites.*
■ **Joint space narrowing may be a late finding** in the disease, and there is **characteristically little or no periarticular osteoporosis** (Fig. 23-16).
■ **Tophi,** collections of urate crystals in the soft tissues, are a late finding in gout and **rarely calcify.**
■ **Olecranon bursitis is common** (Fig. 23-17).

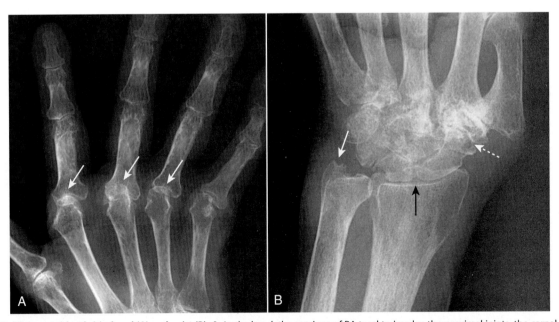

Figure 23-13 Rheumatoid arthritis, hand (A) and wrist (B). A, In the hand, the erosions of RA tend to involve the proximal joints: the carpal-metacarpal joints, metacarpal-phalangeal (*solid white arrows*), and proximal interphalangeal joints. Late findings in the hands include deformities such as ulnar deviation of the fingers at the MCP joints, subluxation of the MCP joints, and ligamentous laxity leading to deformities of the fingers, which are also present in this hand. **B,** In the wrist, erosions of the carpals (*dotted white arrow*), ulnar styloid (*solid white arrow*), and narrowing of the radiocarpal joint space (*solid black arrow*) are commonly seen.

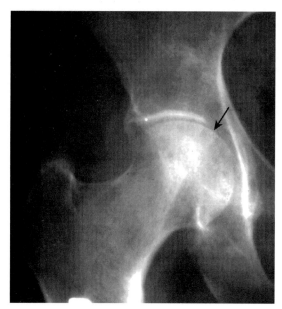

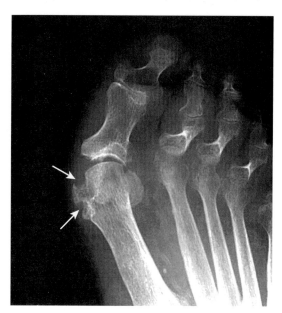

Figure 23-14 Rheumatoid arthritis of the hip. The larger joints (hips and knees) usually show no erosions, but there may be marked uniform narrowing of the joint space with little or no subchondral sclerosis (*solid black arrow*). If this were primary osteoarthritis, you would expect far more subchondral sclerosis and osteophyte production for this degree of joint space narrowing.

Figure 23-16 Gout. Gout most commonly affects the metatarsalphalangeal joint of the great toe, as in this patient. As an erosive arthritis, the hallmark of gout is the sharply marginated, juxtaarticular erosion which may have a sclerotic border (*solid white arrows*). The overhanging edges of gouty erosions have been called ***rat bites***. The metatarsalphalangeal joint space is not particularly narrowed, and there is no periarticular osteoporosis.

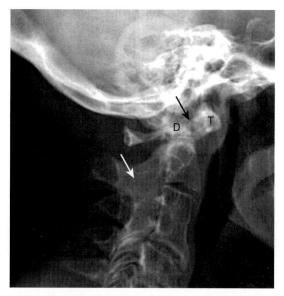

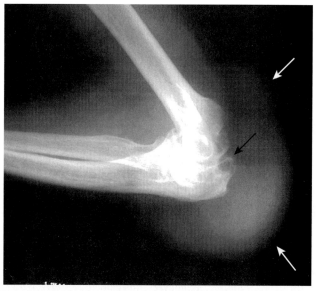

Figure 23-15 Rheumatoid arthritis of the cervical spine. RA tends to involve the cervical spine by producing ligamentous laxity, which can lead to forward subluxation of C1 on C2 (***atlantoaxial subluxation***). The distance between the anterior border of the dens (*D*) and the posterior border of the anterior tubercle of C1 (*T*) is called the ***predentate space*** and is normally no more than 3 mm. This patient's predentate space measured 8 mm (*solid black arrow*). RA may also cause fusion of the facet joints (*solid white arrow*).

Figure 23-17 Olecranon bursitis in gout. Olecranon bursitis is a common manifestation of gout (large soft tissue mass around elbow shown by *solid white arrows*) and its presence alone should alert you to the possibility of underlying gout. This patient also displays erosions adjacent to the elbow joint (*solid black arrow*).

Psoriatic Arthritis

■ **Most patients** with psoriatic arthritis **also have skin and nail changes of psoriasis** for many years, although, for some, the joint manifestations may be the initial presentation of the disease. About 25% of patients with longstanding psoriasis develop psoriatic arthritis. It is **usually polyarticular.**

■ Psoriatic arthritis **typically involves the small joints of the hands, especially the distal interphalangeal (DIP) joints**.

 The **hallmarks of psoriatic arthritis:**

■ **Juxtaarticular erosions, especially of the DIP joints** of the hands.

■ **Bony proliferation at the sites of tendon insertions (enthesophytes).**

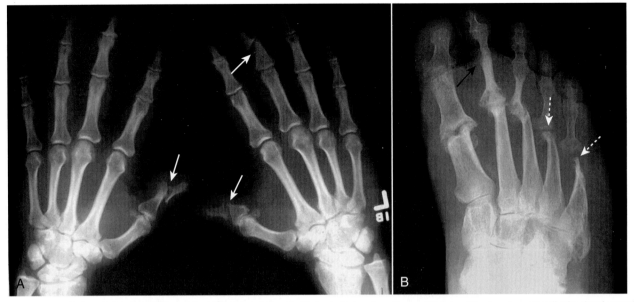

Figure 23-18 Psoriatic arthritis, hand (A) and foot (B). A, Psoriatic arthritis typically involves the small joints of the hands, especially the distal interphalangeal (DIP) joints (*solid white arrows*) leading to telescoping of one phalanx into another (***pencil-in-cup deformity***). **B,** In the foot of another patient with psoriasis, there is ankylosis of the 2nd toe (*solid black arrow*) and more pencil-in-cup deformities (*dotted white arrows*).

- **Periosteal reaction along the shafts of the bone** (not common).
- **Resorption of the terminal phalanges** or the DIP joints with telescoping of one phalanx into another (***pencil-in-cup deformity***) (Fig. 23-18).
- **Absence of osteoporosis.**
- In the **sacroiliac joints,** psoriasis can produce **bilateral, but asymmetric, sacroiliitis.** The SI joints do not usually completely fuse as they do in ankylosing spondylitis.

Ankylosing Spondylitis

- Ankylosing spondylitis is a chronic and progressive arthritis characterized by **inflammation and eventual fusion of the sacroiliac joints** along with the spinal facet joints and involvement of the paravertebral soft tissues.
- More **common in young males,** the disease characteristically ascends the spine starting in the SI joints and moving to the lumbar, thoracic, and finally cervical spine.
- Almost all patients with ankylosing spondylitis test positive for the **human leukocyte antigen B27 (HLA-B27)** as opposed to only about 5 to 10% of the general population.
- **Conventional radiographs** of the affected areas are the **usual study performed for diagnosis and follow-up** of patients with ankylosing spondylitis.
- Ankylosing spondylitis is an *enthesopathy,* a process that **produces inflammation, with subsequent calcification and ossification at and around the *entheses,*** which are the insertion **sites of tendons, ligaments, and joint capsules.**

 Sacroiliitis is the hallmark of ankylosing spondylitis.

- It is usually **bilaterally symmetrical** and **eventually leads to bony fusion** or *ankylosis* of these joints until they

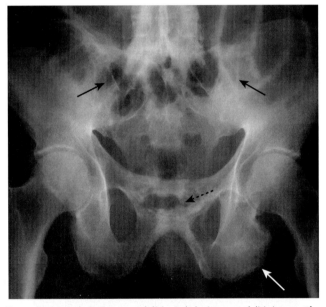

Figure 23-19 Ankylosing spondylitis. Ankylosing spondylitis is an ***enthesopathy,*** a process that produces inflammation with subsequent calcification and ossification at and around the ***entheses,*** which are the insertion sites of tendons, ligaments, and joint capsules (*solid white arrow* points to bony overgrowth at the ischial tuberosity). Bilaterally symmetrical ***sacroiliitis*** is the hallmark of ankylosing spondylitis. This eventually leads to bony fusion or ***ankylosis*** of the SI joints until they disappear as joints altogether (*solid black arrows*). The symphysis pubis is also ankylosed (*dotted black arrow*).

appear either as a thin white line (instead of a joint space) or they disappear altogether (Fig. 23-19).
- In the spine, **ossification of the outer fibers of the annulus fibrosis** produces **thin, bony bridges** from the corners of one vertebra to another called **syndesmophytes.** Progressive syndesmophytes production connecting adjacent vertebral bodies produces a *bamboo-spine* appearance (Fig. 23-20).

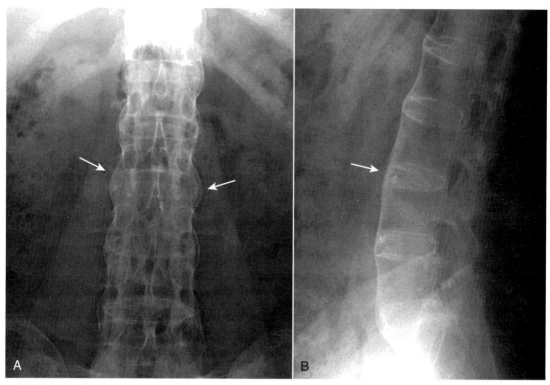

Figure 23-20 Ankylosing spondylitis, frontal (A) and lateral (B) spine. In the spine, there is ossification of the outer fibers of the annulus fibrosus producing thin, bony bridges joining the corners of adjacent vertebrae called **syndesmophytes** (*solid white arrows*). Progressive ossification connecting adjacent vertebral bodies produces the **bamboo-spine** appearance seen in this case, which is characteristic of ankylosing spondylitis.

INFECTIOUS ARTHRITIS

- **Infectious arthritis** usually **occurs as a result of hematogenous seeding of the synovial membrane from an infected source elsewhere in the body,** such as a wound infection or from direct, contiguous extension from osteomyelitis adjacent to the joint.
- It is usually subdivided into **pyogenic (septic) arthritis,** due mostly to *Staphylococcal* and *Gonococcal* organisms and **nonpyogenic arthritis,** due mostly to infection with *Mycobacterium tuberculosis.*
- **Risk factors** include intravenous drug use, steroid injections or oral administration, joint prostheses, and recent joint trauma, including joint surgery.
  - **In children and adults, the knee is frequently affected; in children,** the hip is another **common** site of infection. Hands may be infected from human bites and the feet from diabetes.
- Although **conventional radiographs** are obtained as the initial study, they are **relatively insensitive** to the early findings of the disease except for soft tissue swelling and osteopenia.
  - If septic arthritis is strongly suspected, aspiration of the joint will usually confirm the diagnosis.

The **hallmark of infectious arthritis,** especially the pyogenic form, is **destruction of the articular cartilage and long, contiguous segments of the adjacent articular cortex** from proteolytic enzymes released by the inflamed synovium.

- This **destruction,** unlike other arthritides, **is usually quite rapid.**

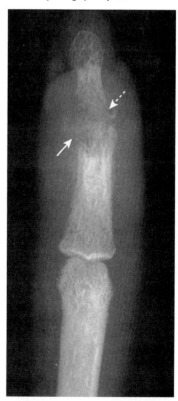

Figure 23-21 Septic arthritis and osteomyelitis, middle finger. The hallmark of infectious arthritis, especially the pyogenic form, is destruction of the articular cartilage and long contiguous segments of the adjacent articular cortex from proteolytic enzymes released by the inflamed synovium. This patient has septic arthritis (the distal interphalangeal joint is destroyed) which has extended to the subjacent bone as osteomyelitis and destroyed either side of the joint space as well (*solid and dotted white arrows*). The time course of septic arthritis, unlike other arthritides, is usually quite rapid. This infection was the result of a human bite.

- Infectious arthritis tends to be **monoarticular** and is associated with **soft tissue swelling** and **osteopenia** from the hyperemia of inflammation (Fig. 23-21).
- Because of its sensitivity, MRI is now used extensively after conventional radiography in diagnosing septic joints. **Enhancement of the synovium** and the **presence of a joint effusion** have the best correlation with the clinical diagnosis of a septic joint.
- **Nonpyogenic infectious arthritis** is most often caused by *Mycobacterium tuberculosis*, which **spreads via the bloodstream from the lungs.**
- Unlike pyogenic arthritis, **tuberculous arthritis** has an **indolent and protracted course** resulting in **gradual loss of the joint space** and **late destruction of the articular cortex.**
- Nonpyogenic infectious arthritis is **usually monarticular. Severe osteoporosis is a common finding. In children, the spine is most often affected; in adults, the knee.**
- Healing with fibrous and bony ankylosis occurs in both pyogenic and nonpyogenic infectious arthritis.

WEBLINK

Registered users may obtain more information on Recognizing Joint Disease: An Approach to Arthritis on StudentConsult.com.

TAKE-HOME POINTS

Recognizing Joint Disease: An Approach to Arthritis

An arthritis is a disease of a joint that invariably leads to joint space narrowing and changes to the bones on both sides of the joint.

Arthritides can be roughly divided into *hypertrophic, infectious,* and *erosive* (inflammatory) categories.

Hypertrophic arthritis features subchondral sclerosis, marginal osteophyte production, and subchondral cyst formation.

Primary osteoarthritis, the most common form of arthritis, is a type of hypertrophic arthritis. It typically occurs on weight-bearing surfaces of the hip and knee and the distal interphalangeal joints of the fingers.

Other hypertrophic arthritides include CPPD, Charcot joints, and osteoarthritis secondary to prior trauma, AVN, or superimposed on another underlying arthritis.

Pyrophosphate arthropathy (CPPD) occurs with the deposition of calcium pyrophosphate crystals (chondrocalcinosis). It can produce large and multiple subchondral cysts, narrowing of the patellofemoral joint space, metacarpal hooks, and proximal migration of the distal carpal row.

Charcot or neuropathic joints feature fragmentation, sclerosis, and soft tissue swelling. Diabetes is the most frequent cause of a Charcot joint.

Erosive (or inflammatory) arthritis is associated with inflammation and synovial proliferation (pannus formation) which produces lytic lesions in or near the joint called erosions.

Rheumatoid arthritis, gout, and psoriasis are three examples of erosive arthritis; the site of involvement is helpful in differentiating among the causes of erosive arthritides.

Rheumatoid arthritis affects the carpals and proximal joints of the hand, can widen the predentate space in the cervical spine, and produces fusion of the posterior elements in the cervical spine.

Gout most often affects the metatarsal-phalangeal joint of the great toe with juxtaarticular erosions and little or no osteoporosis. Tophi are late manifestations of the disease and usually do not calcify.

Psoriatic arthritis usually occurs in patients with known skin changes and affects the distal joints primarily in the hands producing characteristic erosions that resemble a pencil in cup.

Ankylosing spondylitis is a chronic and progressive arthritis characterized by symmetric fusion of the SI joints and ascending involvement of the spine eventually producing a bamboo-spine appearance.

Infectious arthritis features soft tissue swelling and osteopenia and, in the case of pyogenic arthritis, relatively early and marked destruction of most or all of the articular cortex. It is due mostly to staphylococcal and gonococcal organisms.

Chapter 24

Recognizing Some Common Causes of Neck and Back Pain

CONVENTIONAL RADIOGRAPHY, MRI, AND CT

- **Conventional radiographs** remain an important method of evaluating certain spinal lesions because they are **inexpensive** and **rapidly available,** even on a portable basis if needed, and they **demonstrate bony anatomy well.** They are utilized as a **screening method** for most spinal trauma.
- Nevertheless, they provide little if any information about the important soft tissues of the spine and they use ionizing radiation to produce an image.

> **MRI,** with its superior soft tissue differentiation, **is the study of choice for most diseases of the spine** because of its **ability to visualize, and detect abnormalities in, soft tissues** such as bone marrow, the spinal cord, and the intervertebral disks, its **ability to display images in any plane,** and the **lack of exposure to radiation.**

- But MRI has its limitations. The study **remains relatively expensive** and its **availability is not as widespread** as CT or conventional radiographs, **patients with pacemakers** and certain internal ferromagnetic materials (aneurysm clips) **are not able to be scanned,** the procedure **takes more time** to complete, and some patients cannot tolerate the **claustrophobia** they experience in some of the high-field strength MRI scanners (see Chapter 20).
- **CT,** with its ability to reformat images in different planes and provide additional information about the soft tissues, now supplements and, in some cases, **has replaced conventional radiography in the evaluation of spinal trauma.** CT is utilized to determine the **extent of the injury** in any patient in whom a traumatic spinal injury has already been demonstrated by conventional radiographs.
- CT is also utilized to **detect bony lesions** not visible on **conventional radiographs** and to **evaluate soft tissue abnormalities** in patients who are unable to undergo an MRI examination.

THE NORMAL SPINE

- There are normally 7 cervical vertebrae, 12 thoracic vertebrae—all of which normally bear ribs—5 lumbar vertebrae, and 5 fused sacral vertebrae.

Vertebral Body

- Each vertebra (well, almost every vertebra) has a *body* composed of inner cancellous bone and marrow and *posterior elements* made of compact, dense bone consisting of the pedicles, laminae, facets, transverse processes, and a spinous process (Fig. 24-1A).
- From the level of **C3** through the level of **L5** the vertebral bodies are more or less **rectangular in shape** and of about equal height posteriorly as anteriorly.
- The **endplates of contiguous vertebral bodies are roughly parallel to each other.**
- The articular facets of the *superior and inferior articular processes* are lined with cartilage, and these facet joints are **true synovial joints.**
- In the frontal projection, **each vertebral body displays two ovoid pedicles** visible on each side of the vertebral body. The **pedicles of L5** are frequently **difficult to visualize, even in normal individuals** due to the lordosis of the lumbar spine (Fig. 24-1B).

> In the cervical spine, three parallel arcuate lines should smoothly join (1) all of the *spinolaminar white lines* (the junction between the lamina and the spinous process), (2) the **posterior aspects of the vertebral bodies,** and (3) all of the **anterior aspects of the vertebral bodies.** Alterations in the smooth curvature of these three lines may indicate forward or backward displacement of all or part of the vertebral body (Fig. 24-2).

- On conventional radiographs of the **lumbar spine** performed in the oblique projection, the anatomic structures normally superimpose to produce a shadow that resembles the front end of a Scottish terrier, the famous *Scottie dog* sign (Fig. 24-3).

Intervertebral Disks

- The intervertebral disks have a central gelatinous *nucleus pulposus* surrounded by an outer *annulus fibrosus* that is, in turn, made up of inner fibrocartilaginous fibers and outer cartilaginous fibers (*Sharpey fibers*). The nucleus pulposus is located near the posterior aspect of the disk.

> The relative height of the disk space varies in each part of the spine.

- In the **cervical spine,** the **disk spaces** are about **equal** to each other in height.
- In the **thoracic spine,** they are usually slightly **decreased** in size from the **cervical spine,** but **equal** in height **to each other.**
- In the **lumbar spine,** the disk spaces **progressively increase in height** with each successive interspace, except

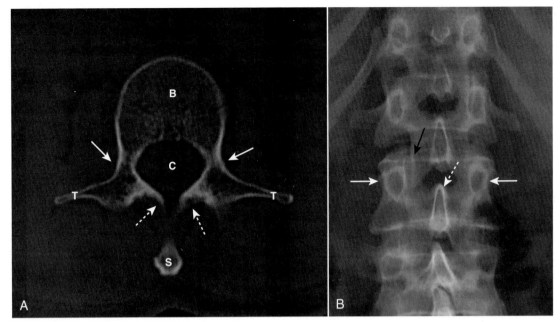

Figure 24-1 Normal spine, axial CT (A), and frontal conventional radiograph (B). A, In this CT scan of a "typical" vertebral body, we see the body (*B*), pedicles (*solid white arrows*), laminae (*dotted white arrows*), transverse processes (*T*), spinal canal (*C*), and spinous process (*S*). **B,** Each vertebral body has two pedicles that project as small ovals on either side of the vertebral body (*solid white arrows*). The spinous process (*dotted white arrow*) may be visualized slightly below the body to which it is attached. The facet joint is seen here *en face* (*solid black arrow*).

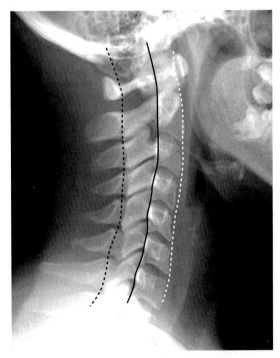

Figure 24-2 The three cervical lines. The lateral view of the cervical spine enables a quick assessment for spinal fracture/subluxation before further studies are performed that might involve motion of the patient's neck. Three parallel arcuate lines should smoothly join all of the spinolaminar white lines, which are the junctions between the laminae and the spinous processes (*dotted black line*), a second line should join all of the posterior aspects of the vertebral bodies (*solid black line*), and a third should join all of the anterior aspects of the vertebral bodies (*dotted white line*).

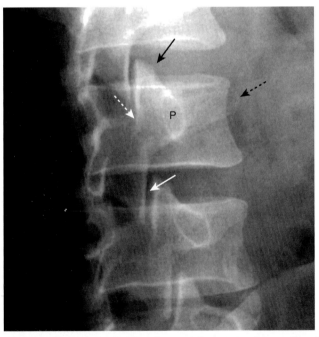

Figure 24-3 Normal Scottie dog. This is a left posterior oblique view of the lumbar spine (the patient is turned about halfway toward her own left). The "Scottie dog" is made up of the following: the "ear" (*solid black arrow*) is the superior articular facet, the "leg" (*solid white arrow*) is the inferior articular facet, the "nose" (*dotted black arrow*) is the transverse process, the "eye" (*P*) is the pedicle and the "neck" (*dotted white arrow*) is the pars interarticularis. All of these structures are paired—an identical set should be visible on the patient's right side.

for L5-S1, which can be equal to or slightly less than the height of L4-L5 on conventional radiographs.

Spinal Cord and Spinal Nerves

- The spinal cord extends from the medulla oblongata to the level of L1-L2, ending as the *conus medullaris*. The *cauda equina* extends inferiorly from that point as a collection of nerve roots with each root exiting below its respectively numbered vertebral body.
- Each of the paired **neural foramina** of the spine contains a **spinal nerve, blood vessels,** and **fat.**
- **Spinal nerves** are named and numbered **according to the site they exit** from the spinal canal. **From C1-C7** nerves exit **above** their respective vertebrae. The **C8** nerve exits **between the 7th cervical and 1st thoracic** vertebrae. The **remaining nerves exit below** their respectively numbered vertebrae.

Spinal Ligaments

- There are several ligaments that traverse the spine (Table 24-1).

Normal MRI Appearance of the Spine

On **T1-weighted** sagittal MRI images of the spine, the **vertebral bodies,** containing bone marrow, will normally be of **high signal intensity (bright),** the **disks** will be **lower in signal intensity,** and **CSF** in the thecal sac will have a **low signal intensity** (dark) (Fig. 24-4A).

- On conventional **T2-weighted images,** the **vertebral body** will be slightly **lower in signal** intensity than the disks, while the **CSF will appear bright** (the reverse of T1) (Fig. 24-4B).
- Cortical bone is dark (has a low signal) on all sequences.

BACK PAIN

- It has been estimated that **almost 80% of all Americans will have some episode of back pain** during their lifetime. The causes of back pain are numerous and the anatomic and physiologic interrelationships that produce it in many cases are still not known.
- Some causes of back pain:
  - **Muscle and ligament strain**
  - **Herniation of an intervertebral disk**
  - **Degeneration of an intervertebral disk**
  - **Arthritis involving the synovial joints of the spine**
  - **Compression fractures, usually from osteoporosis**

TABLE 24-1 LIGAMENTS OF THE SPINE

Ligament	Connects
Anterior longitudinal ligament	Anterior surfaces of vertebral bodies
Posterior longitudinal ligament	Posterior surfaces of vertebral bodies
Ligamentum flavum	Laminae of adjacent vertebral bodies and lies in posterior portion of spinal canal
Interspinous ligament	Between spinous processes
Supraspinous ligament	Tips of spinous processes

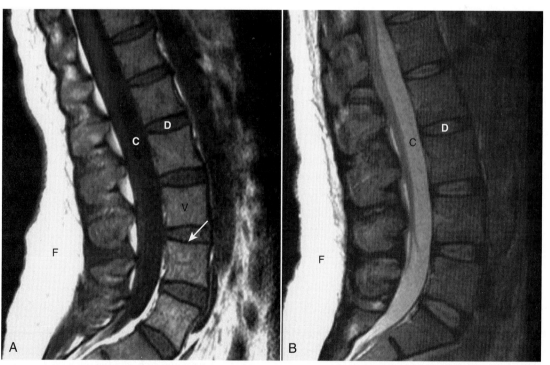

Figure 24-4 Normal MRI lumbar spine, T1-weighted and T2-weighted images. A, Sagittal T1-weighted image demonstrates the normal dark appearance of the disks (*D*) relative to the vertebral body (*V*). The CSF in the spinal canal is dark (*C*), and the subcutaneous fat of the back is bright (*F*). Cortical bone has a low signal (*solid white arrow*). **B,** Sagittal T2-weighted image demonstrates the normal appearance of the disks (*D*), which are slightly higher intensity (brighter) than the vertebral bodies. The CSF (*C*) in the spinal canal is now bright, and the subcutaneous fat (*F*) of the back remains bright.

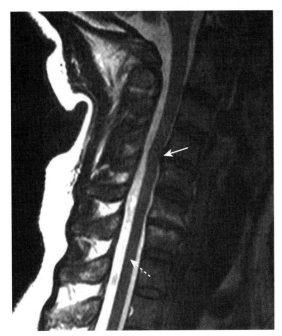

Figure 24-5 Herniated disk, C4-C5 on MRI. The spinal cord is dark (*dotted white arrow*) relative to the high intensity (whiter) signal surrounding it which is the cerebrospinal fluid in the spinal canal. A herniated disk (*solid white arrow*) extends posteriorly from the C4-C5 disk space and compresses the cord.

- **Trauma to the spine**
- **Malignancy involving the spine**
- **Infection of the spine**
- ■ We will discuss all except muscle and ligament strains.

HERNIATED DISKS

- ■ Only about 2% of patients with acute low back pain have a herniated disk. In the **lumbar region**, disk herniation may lead to **back pain** and **sciatica**, while herniation of a **cervical disk** may produce **radiculopathy** and **myelopathy. MRI is the study of choice for evaluating herniated disks.**
- ■ In the **cervical spine, disk herniations occur most frequently at C4-C5, C5-C6, and C6-C7** (Fig. 24-5).
- ■ Compared with the cervical and lumbar spine, **thoracic disks are very stable**, in part because they are protected by the rib cage that surrounds them.

➡ The majority of **disk herniations occur at** the lower three lumbar disk levels, **L3-L4, L4-L5 (most common), and L5-S1. More than 60% of disk herniations occur posterolaterally,** the location of the herniation determining the clinical presentation depending on which nerve roots are compressed.

- ■ **Degeneration** of the outer annular fibers of the disk or **trauma** can lead to an interruption in those fibers and allow the disk material to bulge, which may or may not be associated with back pain.
- ■ When the annular fibers rupture, the **nucleus pulposus may herniate** (usually posterolaterally) **through a weakened area of the posterior longitudinal ligament.**

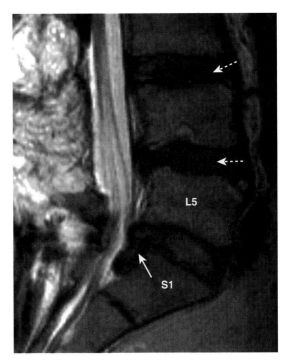

Figure 24-6 Disk herniation, L5-S1. Sagittal T2-weighted image of the lower lumbar spine demonstrates disk material (*solid white arrow*) beyond the confines of the *L5-S1* intervertebral disk space representing a disk herniation extending inferiorly. Notice that degeneration and desiccation of the other disks has led them to become darker than normal on this T2-weighted image (*dotted white arrows*).

- ■ The herniated material may **protrude** but remain in contact with the parent disk from which it originated or it may be completely **extruded** into the spinal canal.
- ■ Symptoms are caused by acute compression of the nerve root.
- ■ Disk herniations can be visualized on both **CT and MRI.** CT demonstrates disk material compressing nerve roots or the thecal sac. On MRI, the herniated disk material is usually a **focal, asymmetric protrusion of hypointense disk material** that extends beyond the confines of the annulus fibrosus (Fig. 24-6).
- ■ **Postlaminectomy syndrome** (also called *failed back surgery syndrome*) is persistent pain in the back or legs following spine surgery. In some studies, it has been estimated to occur in 40% of postoperative patients. Gadolinium-enhanced MRI studies of the spine are useful in differentiating persistent or recurrent disk herniation from scar formation as a cause of the pain.

DEGENERATIVE DISK DISEASE

- ■ With increasing age, the normally gelatinous nucleus pulposus becomes dehydrated and degenerates. This gradually leads to **progressive loss of the height of the intervertebral disk space.** At times, desiccation of the disk leads to **release of nitrogen** from tissues surrounding the disk resulting in the appearance of **air density in the disk space** called a *vacuum-disk phenomenon.* A vacuum-disk represents a **late sign of a degenerated disk** (Fig. 24-7).
- ■ **Degenerative disk disease (DDD) on MRI:** The decrease in water content of the nucleus pulposus results in a lower

signal intensity of the disk on T2-weighted images (see Fig. 24-6).

- **Degenerative disk disease on conventional radiographs:**
  - There is **disk space narrowing**. There are also changes in the vertebral bodies themselves.

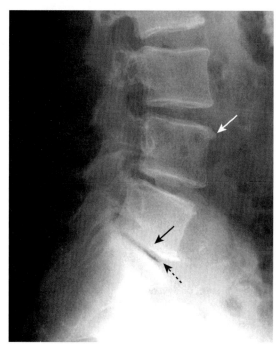

Figure 24-7 Degenerative disk disease. With increasing age, there is progressive loss of the height of the intervertebral disk space. The endplates of contiguous vertebral bodies become sclerotic (*solid black arrow*), small osteophytes are produced at the margins of the vertebral bodies (*solid white arrow*), and there is desiccation of the disk with a vacuum-disk phenomenon (gas in the disk space) recognized by the air density in place of the disk seen at L5-S1 (*dotted black arrow*).

- The endplates of contiguous vertebral bodies become **eburnated** or sclerotic. **Small osteophytes are produced** at the margins of the vertebral bodies at each disk space (see Fig. 24-7).
- At the same time, there is typically **degeneration of the outer annulus fibrosus**. This leads to the production of **larger marginal osteophytes** at the endplates than those seen with degeneration of the nuclear material.
- It should be noted that osteophytes are an extremely common finding, increasing in prevalence with increasing age, and that most patients with osteophytes of the spine are **asymptomatic.**

OSTEOARTHRITIS OF THE FACET JOINTS

- The *facet joints* (also known as the *apophyseal joints*) are **true joints** in that they have cartilage, a synovial lining, and synovial fluid. As such, they are **subject to developing osteoarthritis**, similar to true joints in the appendicular skeleton.
- Some consider the small jointlike structures at the lateral edges of C3 to T1, called the **uncovertebral joints** or the **joints of Luschka**, to be true joints, but others do not.
  - In either case, they are frequent sites of osteophyte formation. Osteophytes at the uncovertebral joints are frequently associated with both degenerative disk disease and osteophytes of the facet joints.

In the **cervical spine, osteophytes that develop at the uncovertebral joints** can produce **protrusions of bone into the** normally oval-shaped **neural foramina**, which are visualized on conventional radiographs taken in the oblique projection (Fig. 24-8A).

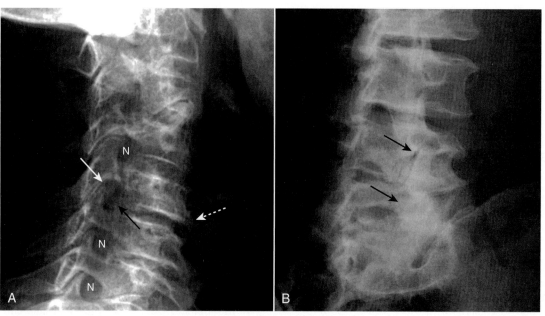

Figure 24-8 Uncovertebral osteophytes and facet arthritis. A, In the cervical spine, osteophytes may develop at the uncovertebral joints (*solid black arrow*) producing bony protrusions into the normally oval-shaped neural foramina (*N*), in this radiograph taken in the oblique projection. Osteophytes at the uncovertebral joints are frequently associated with both degenerative disk disease (*dotted white arrow*) and osteophytes of the facet joints (*solid white arrow*). **B,** There is sclerosis and osteophyte formation involving the lower facet joints of the lumbar spine (*solid black arrows*) representing facet arthritis.

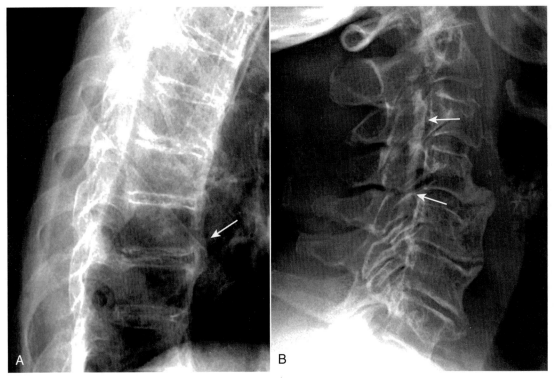

Figure 24-9 **Diffuse idiopathic skeletal hyperostosis (DISH) and ossification of the posterior longitudinal ligament (OPLL). A,** DISH is manifest by thick, bridging or flowing calcification/ossification of the anterior longitudinal ligament (*solid white arrow*). This ossification is visualized along the anterior or anterolateral aspects of at least four contiguous vertebral bodies. **B,** OPLL, here shown by a long linear ossific density inside the spinal canal (*solid white arrows*), can be associated with DISH and may contribute to the production of spinal stenosis.

- There is usually a **complex interrelationship between degenerative disk disease and facet arthritis** such that the two frequently occur together. The **osteophytes** formed by osteoarthritis of the facet joints **may also encroach on the neural foramina and produce radicular pain.**
- In the **lumbar spine,** facet osteoarthritis may cause **narrowing** and **sclerosis of the facet joints,** best seen on oblique views of the spine. Facet arthritis is easier to visualize on CT scans of the spine than on conventional radiographs, and actual nerve compression is easier to visualize on MRI of the spine (Fig. 24-8B).

DIFFUSE IDIOPATHIC SKELETAL HYPEROSTOSIS

- Diffuse idiopathic skeletal hyperostosis (DISH) is a common disorder characterized by bone or calcium formation at the sites of ligamentous insertions (*enthesopathy*).
- It usually affects **men** over the age of **50,** can occur **anywhere in the spine,** but **most often** affects the **lower thoracic and lower cervical spine.**
- Frequently patients with DISH complain of back stiffness but may have **no pain** or **only mild back pain.**
- **Conventional radiographs of the spine are sufficient** to make the diagnosis of DISH.

➡ DISH is manifest **by thick, bridging, or flowing calcification/ossification** of the **anterior** or sometimes **posterior longitudinal ligaments.**

- This ossification is visualized along the anterior or anterolateral aspects **of at least four contiguous vertebral bodies.** Unlike degenerative disk disease, **the disk spaces** and usually the **facet joints are preserved.** The flowing ossification seen in DISH is **separated slightly from the vertebral body** (Fig. 24-9A).
  - Unlike ankylosing spondylitis, which may radiographically resemble DISH in the spine, the **sacroiliac joints are normal.**
- **Ossification of the posterior longitudinal ligament (OPLL)** is often present with DISH and better visualized on CT and MRI than on conventional radiographs. It may cause compression of the spinal cord, especially in the cervical spine, due to narrowing of the spinal canal (see Fig. 24-9B).

COMPRESSION FRACTURES OF THE SPINE

- Vertebral compression fractures are **common,** affecting **women more than men,** and typically secondary to **osteoporosis.** They may be **asymptomatic** or they may produce **pain** in the midthoracic or upper lumbar area that typically disappears in 4 to 6 weeks. Sometimes they are first noticed because of increasing **kyphosis** or **loss of overall body height.**
- **Conventional spine radiographs are usually the study of first choice.** MRI can be utilized for differentiating osteoporotic compression fractures from malignancy. Both MRI and nuclear bone scans can help in establishing the age of a compression abnormality that might be impossible on conventional radiographs alone.

Recognizing Some Common Causes of Neck and Back Pain | **267**

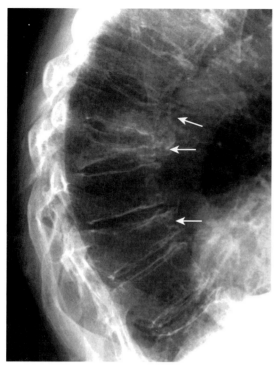

Figure 24-10 Compression fractures secondary to osteoporosis. Vertebral compression fractures are common, affecting women more than men, and typically secondary to osteoporosis. Osteoporotic compression fractures usually involve the anterior and superior aspects of the vertebral body sparing the posterior aspect (*solid white arrows*). This produces a wedge-shaped deformity that leads to accentuation of the kyphosis in the thoracic spine. Progressive loss of overall body height is a common finding with compression fractures in the elderly.

 Osteoporotic compression fractures usually **involve the anterior and superior aspects** of the vertebral body **sparing the posterior body**. There will usually be a difference in the height between the **anterior and posterior** aspects of the same vertebral body in **excess of 3 mm**. Alternatively, the compressed body is typically >20% shorter than the body above or below it.

- This compression pattern produces a **wedge-shaped deformity** that leads to accentuation of the normal kyphosis in the thoracic spine (the so-called *dowager's hump*) (Fig. 24-10).
- There is **usually no neurologic deficit** associated with an osteoporotic compression fracture because the fracture involves the anterior part of the vertebral body, away from the spinal cord.

SPONDYLOLISTHESIS AND SPONDYLOLYSIS

- *Spondylolisthesis* is defined as **slippage** (typically forward) **of one vertebral body** (with the spine above it) **on another.** Forward slipping spondylolisthesis is also called *anterolisthesis.* Posterior slippage is called *retrolisthesis.* Spondylolisthesis is graded according to the degree one body has slipped on the adjacent body.

 In general, spondylolisthesis can occur if there are **bilateral breaks in the pars interarticularis**

(*spondylolytic spondylolisthesis*) or if there is osteoarthritis of the facet joints (*degenerative spondylolisthesis*) (Fig. 24-11).

- **Conventional radiographs of the lumbar spine are usually the initial imaging study.** CT may be more helpful in detecting spondylolysis whereas MRI may demonstrate soft tissue abnormalities but be less effective in detecting spondylolysis.
- **Spondylolysis** is believed to be due to a combination of a **congenitally dysplastic pars** that is then subjected to the strains of an upright posture which eventually leads to a **stress fracture of the pars.** A **family history** of spondylolysis is relatively **common.**
- **Facet osteoarthritis** may be associated with spondylolisthesis (*degenerative spondylolisthesis*) through a complex interaction between the **ligaments, disks,** and **facet joints** wherein disease in any one (or more) of these components increases the stress on the others which can lead to spondylolisthesis.
- In **degenerative spondylolisthesis,** there is **no break in the pars interarticularis**. The degree of spondylolisthesis is usually less from this etiology than in those with spondylolisthesis from spondylolysis. Degenerative spondylolisthesis is more common in women and usually affects the **L4-L5 disk space.**
  - **Posterior slippage** of one vertebral body on the body below (**retrolisthesis**) may also occur from **facet osteoarthritis.**
- Other causes of spondylolisthesis include trauma, malignancy, and congenital vertebral anomalies.
- **Recognizing spondylolisthesis/spondylolysis**
  - The **lateral (sagittal) view is best** at demonstrating **spondylolisthesis,** which will be visible as slippage of one vertebral body on the body below, usually anteriorly.
  - If the slippage approximates 25% of the anteroposterior (AP) diameter of the vertebral body below, it is called a *grade I spondylolisthesis.* If the slippage approximates 50% of the AP diameter of the vertebral body below, it is called a grade II spondylolisthesis, and so on for grade III and grade IV (see Fig. 24-11).
  - **Spondylolysis** is easiest to visualize on an **oblique conventional radiograph of the lumbar spine** or CT in which a **lucency** representing the break in the "neck" of the Scottie dog (the "collar" on the Scottie dog) may be seen **in the pars interarticularis** (Fig. 24-12).

SPINAL STENOSIS

- Spinal stenosis refers to **narrowing of the spinal canal** or the neural foramina secondary to **soft tissue or bony abnormalities,** either on an **acquired or a congenital** basis. **Acquired etiologies** such as those from **degenerative changes** are **more common** than congenital causes.
- **Soft tissue abnormalities** that can lead to **spinal stenosis** include hypertrophy of the ligamentum flavum, bulging disk(s) and ossification of the posterior longitudinal ligament (OPLL).
- **Bony abnormalities** that can lead to **spinal stenosis** include a congenitally narrow spinal canal, osteophytes,

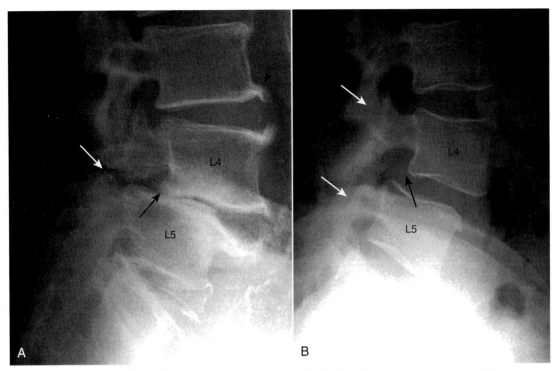

Figure 24-11 Spondylolytic spondylolisthesis (A) and degenerative spondylolisthesis (B). A, There is forward slippage of *L4* on *L5* equal to about half the AP diameter of L5 (*solid black arrow*), so this is classified as a Grade II spondylolisthesis. Spondylolysis is present (*solid white arrow*) that has allowed the slip to take place. There are also incidental large osteophytes at the corners of the vertebral bodies (*dotted black arrow*). **B,** Facet osteoarthritis (*solid white arrows*) may be associated with spondylolisthesis through a complex interaction between the ligaments, disks, and facet joints. In degenerative spondylolisthesis, there is no break in the pars interarticularis and the degree of spondylolisthesis (*solid black arrow*) is usually less in this group than in those with spondylolisthesis from bilateral spondylolysis. The L4-L5 disk space is most commonly affected.

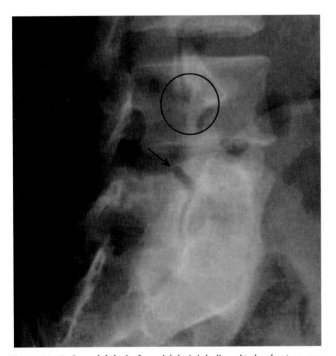

Figure 24-12 Spondylolysis. Spondylolysis is believed to be due to a combination of factors including a congenitally dysplastic pars that is subjected to certain strains that eventually lead to a stress fracture of the pars (*solid black arrow*). You might recognize the break as a "collar" on the "neck" of the Scottie dog (see Fig. 24-3). A normal pars is shown in the *black circle*. Spondylolysis allows the affected vertebral body to slip forward on the body below it (spondylolisthesis).

facet osteoarthritis, or spondylolisthesis. A spinal canal that was borderline normal in size may become stenotic when any of these processes superimposes to further narrow the canal.

Spinal stenosis is **most common in the cervical and lumbar areas** and can lead to radicular pain, myelopathy, or, in the lumbar region, neurogenic claudication. **Neurogenic claudication** is intermittent pain and paresthesias radiating down the leg worsened by standing or walking and relieved by flexing the spine by lying supine or squatting.

- **Conventional radiographs are usually obtained first** in evaluating for spinal stenosis, but **MRI is the study of choice** because the bony dimensions alone do not account for the soft tissues that can produce stenosis.
- **Conventional radiographic** findings may include an **AP diameter of the spinal canal of 10 mm or less, facet joint arthritis,** and **spondylolisthesis** (Fig. 24-13).
- **CT** provides an excellent method of demonstrating bony abnormalities, but **MRI is the best imaging modality for detecting lumbar spinal stenosis.**

MALIGNANCY INVOLVING THE SPINE

- Metastases to bone are 25 times more common than primary bone tumors. Metastases usually occur where **red marrow** is found, with 80% of metastatic bone lesions occurring

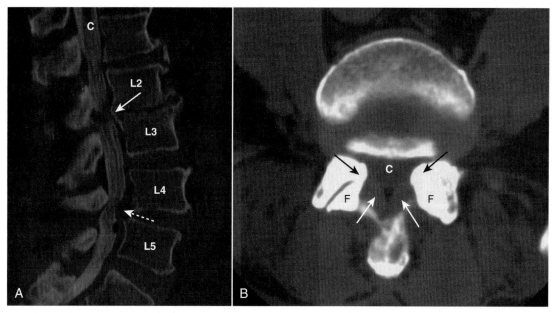

Figure 24-13 **Spinal stenosis, CT. A,** At the level of L2-L3, there are osteophytes that narrow the canal (*C*) (*solid white arrow*). There is a protruding disk (*dotted white arrow*) at L4-L5 that reduces the size of the spinal canal at this level. **B,** The canal (*C*) is narrowed by thickening of the ligamenta flava (*solid white arrows*) and by bony overgrowth (*solid black arrows*) from osteoarthritis of the facet joints (*F*). Spinal stenosis refers to narrowing of the spinal canal or the neural foramina secondary to soft tissue or bony abnormalities.

in the **axial skeleton** (i.e., spine, pelvis, skull, and ribs) because that is where, with normal aging, the red marrow exists.

Because of the **rich blood supply** in the posterior portion of vertebral bodies, hematogenous **metastatic deposits to that part of the spine are common**, especially from **lung** and **breast** carcinoma.

- In the spine, **metastases may lead to compression fractures. Metastases** tend to **destroy the vertebral body,** including and especially the posterior aspect and the pedicles, which is different from **osteoporotic compression fractures** in which the **posterior vertebral body and pedicles remain intact** (see Fig. 21-22).
- **Metastatic disease** can either be mostly bone-producing, i.e., *osteoblastic*, or mostly bone-destroying, i.e., *osteolytic*. Metastases that contain both osteolytic and osteoblastic processes occurring simultaneously are called *mixed metastatic lesions.*
- **Osteoblastic metastases** will appear **denser** (whiter) than the surrounding normal bone on conventional radiographs. If **focal**, they may appear as **punctate regions of increased density.** When **widespread**, they may **produce diffuse sclerosis of bone** (see Fig. 21-3).
- **Prostate cancer** is the prototype example of a primary malignancy that produces **osteoblastic metastases**; the prototype of such a primary malignancy **in a female is breast cancer.**
- **Osteolytic metastases** will appear **less dense** (blacker) than the surrounding normal bone on conventional radiographs. They **destroy all or part of a bone,** e.g., a portion of a bone may be absent, a rib may be destroyed, a pedicle may be missing.
- The **most common** causes of primary malignancies that produce **osteolytic metastatic lesions** are **lung** and **breast**

cancer. Thyroid and renal carcinomas may **produce osteolytic lesions** that are also **expansile** (see Fig. 21-21).

- The spine is also a frequent site of **multiple myeloma,** the most common primary malignancy of bone. Multiple myeloma is known for its tendency to produce almost **totally lytic lesions.** One of the hallmarks of multiple myeloma is osteoporosis, so that myeloma may be associated with **diffuse spinal osteoporosis** and **multiple compression fractures** (Fig. 24-14).

The current **screening study of choice** for the detection of spinal metastases is a **Technetium-99m (Tc 99m) bone scintiscan** (radionuclide bone scan). The technetium is most commonly bound to **methylene diphosphonate (MDP)** that transports the Tc 99m to bone. A radionuclide bone scan is relatively inexpensive, widely available, and screens the entire body. While bone scans are **highly sensitive** to the presence of metastatic deposits, they are **not very specific.** In many cases, a confirmatory study, usually a conventional radiograph, is needed to exclude other causes of abnormal radiotracer uptake such as fractures, infection, and arthritis (Fig. 24-15).

MRI IN METASTATIC SPINE DISEASE

- MRI can detect changes of spinal metastases even **earlier than a radionuclide scan,** and techniques are being described that may allow for a rapid, whole-body screening similar to radionuclide bone scanning.

With neoplastic infiltration of the bone marrow, there is a **decrease** in the normally high signal of the vertebrae on **T1-weighted images** and there is usually a **high signal on T2-weighted** images (Fig. 24-16).

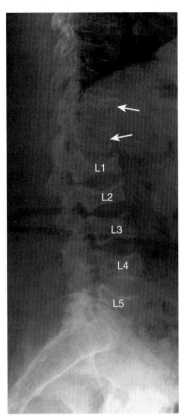

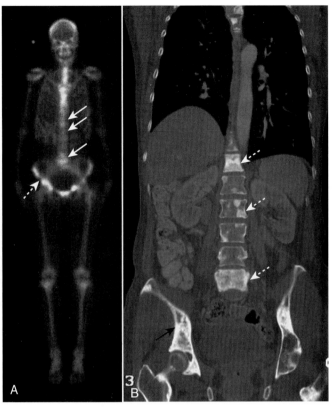

Figure 24-14 Multiple myeloma of the spine. One of the hallmarks of multiple myeloma is osteoporosis, so that myeloma may be associated with diffuse spinal osteoporosis (*solid white arrows*) and multiple compression fractures (L1-L5). Notice how the posterior aspects of the vertebral bodies remain essentially normal in height in osteoporotic fractures while the central and anterior aspects collapse.

Figure 24-15 Metastases, radionuclide bone scan, and CT. A, A Technetium-99m methylene diphosphonate (MDP) bone scan demonstrates abnormal tracer uptake in numerous areas including the spine (*solid white arrows*) and pelvis (*dashed white arrow*). Because of the nonspecific nature of positive bone scans, a confirmatory study, usually conventional radiography, is obtained as well. **B,** In this case the patient had undergone a CT scan and the coronal reformatted image shows numerous osteoblastic lesions in the spine (*dotted white arrows*) and the pelvis (*solid black arrow*) corresponding to the lesions seen on bone scan. This patient had known breast carcinoma.

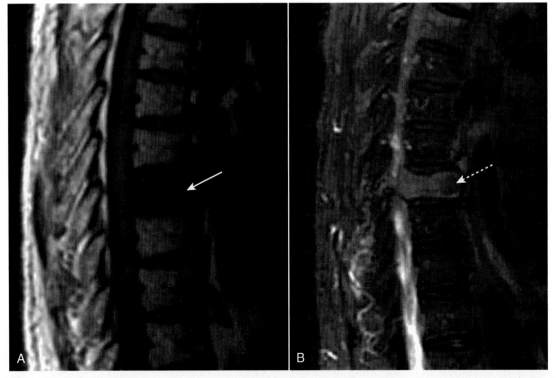

Figure 24-16 Metastases to the spine, MRI. A, T1-weighted sagittal MRI of the thoracic spine demonstrates marrow replacement in the T8 vertebral body (*solid white arrow*). The signal is decreased compared to the normal bodies above and below it. **B,** T2-weighted sagittal MRI shows abnormally high signal in the compressed vertebral body (*dotted white arrow*). The entire vertebral body is involved. The patient had primary breast carcinoma.

- Unlike osteoporotic compression fractures which tend to spare the posterior aspects of the bodies while the central and anterior portions collapse, **spinal metastases** will more often **affect the entire body** including the posterior portion.

INFECTIONS OF THE SPINE: DISKITIS AND OSTEOMYELITIS

- Spinal infection is **usually due to** *Staphylococcus*. It is also frequently caused by *Enterobacter*. In **adults**, infection most often occurs subsequent to **spinal instrumentation** such as surgery or spinal tap. In **children**, the disease is usually **hematogenously spread**.
- In children, the disk is involved directly most often. In adults, the vertebral body **endplates** are usually **involved first** (*osteomyelitis*) and infection will then spread to the adjacent **intervertebral disk** (*diskitis*).
- An exception to this pattern can be **tuberculosis**, which can affect multiple vertebral bodies without involvement of the disks because the infection spreads silently beneath the longitudinal ligaments of the spine.
- **Epidural abscess** or phlegmon may form due to **direct extension** into, or **hematogenous seeding** of, the epidural space. Epidural abscesses are potentially life threatening and have a significant morbidity.
- **Recognizing vertebral body osteomyelitis and diskitis on MRI** (Fig. 24-17).
  - Think of diskitis when a process involves two adjacent vertebral bodies and the intervening disk.
  - On MRI, the involved vertebral body **endplates will be T1-dark, often T2-bright**, and will **enhance on postgadolinium images** (these findings alone are not specific and can, in fact, also be seen in the setting of degenerative disk disease).
  - The **involved disk will be diffusely T2-bright and will enhance on postgadolinium images** (**specific for diskitis**).
  - **Epidural abscesses** will be T2-bright fluid collections that rim enhance after administration of gadolinium.

SPINAL TRAUMA

- Fractures of the spine are infrequent compared to fractures of other parts of the skeleton. When they occur, they have particular importance because of the implications for associated spinal cord injury. The most **commonly fractured vertebrae are L1, L2, and T12**, accounting for more than half of all thoracolumbar spine fractures. In the thoracic spine, compression fractures are the most common type of spinal fracture.
- **The three cervical lines** (see Fig. 24-2).
  - Many trauma protocols include a *cross-table* **lateral view of the cervical spine** (the patient's neck is immobilized, the patient remains on the stretcher or examining table, and the x-ray beam is directed **horizontally** so that the patient's **head is not moved**).
  - This view enables a **quick assessment for spinal fracture/subluxation** before further studies which might involve motion of the patient's neck are performed.

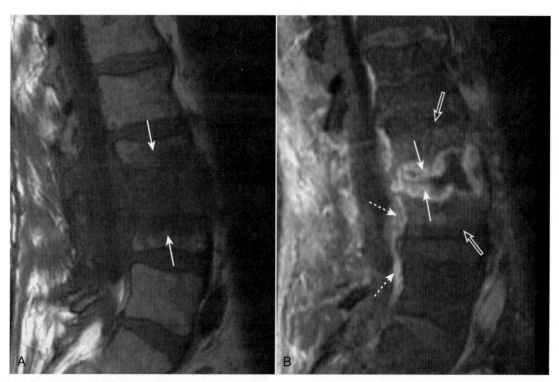

Figure 24-17 Osteomyelitis and diskitis, lumbar spine. A, Sagittal T1-weighted image demonstrates extensive abnormal T1-dark signal indicating destruction of the endplates of the L3 and L4 vertebral bodies and the intervening disk (*solid white arrows*). **B,** Sagittal T1-weighted postgadolinium image demonstrates abnormal disk enhancement (*solid white arrows*) and, more importantly for this diagnosis, enhancement of the adjacent L3 and L4 vertebral bodies (*open white arrows*). In addition, there is extension to the anterior epidural space (*dotted white arrows*).

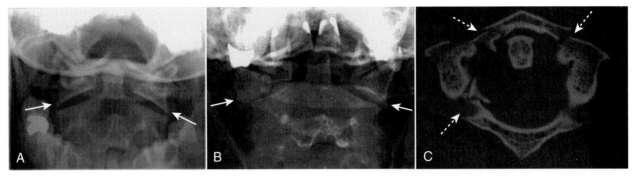

Figure 24-18 Normal open-mouth view, Jefferson's fracture open-mouth view, and CT. A Jefferson's fracture is a fracture of C1 usually involving both the anterior and posterior arches. **A,** The normal "open-mouth" view of C1 and C2 demonstrates that the lateral margins of C1 (*solid white arrows*) line up with the lateral margins of C2. **B,** The hallmark of a Jefferson's fracture is bilateral, lateral offset of the lateral masses of C1 (*solid white arrows*) relative to C2. **C,** The fracture is confirmed utilizing CT, which shows fractures of both the right and left anterior arch and the right posterior arch of C1 (*dotted white arrows*).

At the beginning of this chapter, we talked about the three cervical lines. **Three parallel arcuate lines** should smoothly join (1) all of the *spinolaminar white lines* (the junction between the lamina and the spinous process), (2) all of the **posterior aspects of the vertebral bodies,** and (3) all of the **anterior aspects of the verte**bral bodies.

- Deviation from the normal parallel curvature of these **lines should suggest a subluxed or fractured vertebral body.**
- Some of the more common spinal fractures:
  - **Compression fractures**, the most common fractures of the spine, were previously discussed.
  - **Jefferson's fracture**
  - **Hangman's fracture**
  - **Burst fracture**

Jefferson's Fracture

- A Jefferson's fracture is a **fracture of C1** usually involving both the anterior and posterior arches. In its classical presentation, there are **bilateral fractures of both the anterior and posterior arches of C1** producing four fractures in all.
- It is **caused by an axial loading injury** (such as diving into a swimming pool and hitting one's head on the bottom).

On conventional radiographs, the hallmark of a Jefferson fracture is **bilateral**, *lateral* offset of the lateral masses of C1 relative to C2 as seen on the *open-mouth view* (atlantoaxial view) of the cervical spine. The fracture is **confirmed utilizing CT** (Fig. 24-18).

- A Jefferson's fracture is a "self-decompressing" fracture in that the spinal canal at the level of the fracture is wide enough to accommodate any swelling of the cord. There is **usually no neurologic deficit** associated with this type of fracture.

Hangman's Fracture

- A hangman's fracture is a **fracture of the posterior elements of C2.**

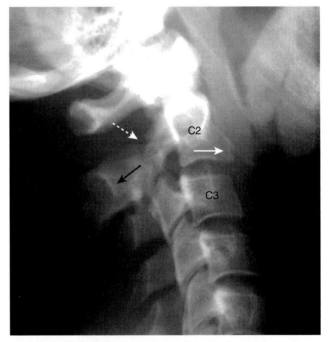

Figure 24-19 Hangman's fracture. A hangman's fracture results from a hyperextension-compression injury. It involves fractures through the posterior elements of C2 best evaluated on the lateral view. The fracture (*dotted white arrow* shows fracture line) effectively separates the posterior aspect of the C2 vertebral body from the anterior aspect of C2 allowing the anterior aspect to sublux forward on the body of C3. Notice that the spinolaminar line of C2 lies posterior to the other vertebral bodies (*solid black arrow*) and the anterior aspect of C2 lies forward of the anterior body of C3 (*solid white arrow*).

- Hangman's fractures **result from a hyperextension-compression injury** typically occurring in an unrestrained occupant in a motor vehicle accident who strikes his forehead on the windshield.
- They are **best evaluated on the lateral view** of the cervical spine on conventional radiography and the **sagittal view** on CT.

The fracture effectively **separates the posterior aspect of the C2 vertebral body** from the **anterior aspect of C2** allowing the **anterior aspect of C2 to sublux forward on the body of C3** (Fig. 24-19).

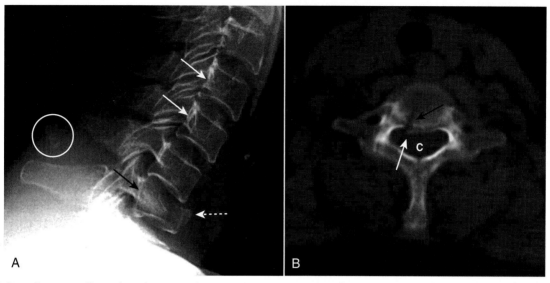

Figure 24-20 Burst fracture, radiograph, and CT. A, Findings include a comminuted, compression fracture of the vertebral body in which the anterior vertebral body is displaced forward (*dotted white arrow*) while the posterior aspect of the body is propelled dorsally toward the spinal canal (*solid black arrow*). Notice how the posterior aspects of vertebral bodies are normally concave inward (*solid white arrows*). Calcification of the ligamentum nuchae is of no clinical consequence (*white circle*). **B,** Axial CT scan of the spine shows a fracture of the body (*solid black arrow*) and the retropulsed fragment (*solid white arrow*) protruding into the spinal canal (*C*).

- Some hangman fractures are less displaced, so that CT may be needed for their detection.
- Because hangman fractures lead to overall **widening of the bony canal**, they are usually **not associated with neurologic deficits**. This is in contradistinction to the injury after which this fracture is named, the fracture incurred during a *judicial hanging* in which there was hyperextension leading to a fracture of C2 **and marked distraction** of C2 from C3 associated with distraction of the spinal cord itself.

Burst Fractures

- Burst fractures can occur at any level but are most common in the **cervical spine, thoracic spine, and upper lumbar spine**.
- They are high-energy **axial loading injuries**, typically secondary to motor vehicle accidents or falls, in which the disk above is driven into the vertebral body below and the vertebral body bursts. This in turn drives bony fragments **posteriorly into the spinal canal** (*retropulsed fragments*) while the anterior aspect of the vertebral body is displaced forward.
- Because these fractures involve incursion on the spinal canal, the **majority of burst fractures are associated with a neurologic deficit**.

Findings of burst fractures include a **comminuted, compression fracture of the vertebral body** in which the **posterior aspect of the body is bowed backward toward the spinal canal**. CT is the **best imaging modality** for identifying **bony fragments** in the spinal canal (Fig. 24-20).

Locked Facets

- Bilateral locking of the facets in the cervical spine can occur as a result of a **hyperflexion injury** in which the **inferior facets of one vertebral body slide over and in front of the superior facets of the body below**. In this position, the slipped facets cannot return to their normal position without medical intervention; thus, the term "locked."
- Locked facets occur with **forward slippage** of the affected vertebral body on the body below it **by at least 50% of its AP diameter**.

On **lateral (sagittal) imaging** of the cervical spine, the **inferior articular facets will lie in front of the superior facets** of the body below. This is the reverse of the normal anatomic relationship between adjacent facets (Fig. 24-21).

- Since the superior articular facets are no longer "covered" by the inferior facets above them, this appearance was described on CT as the *naked facet sign*.
- This injury virtually **always results in neurologic impairment**.

WEBLINK

Registered users may obtain more information on Recognizing Some Common Causes of Neck and Back Pain on StudentConsult.com.

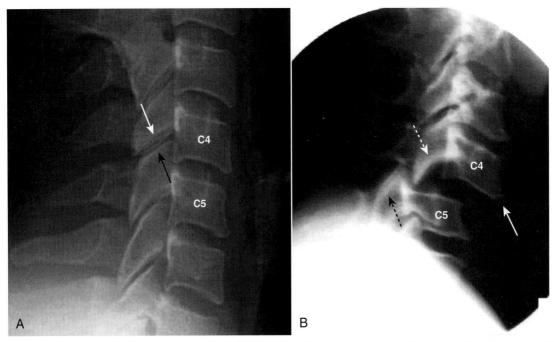

Figure 24-21 Normal and bilateral locked facets. A, Normally, the inferior articular facet of the body above (in this case C4, *solid white arrow*) lies posterior to the superior articular facet of the body below (in this case C5, *solid black arrow*). **B,** The inferior articular facet of C4 (*dotted white arrow*) lies anterior to the superior articular facet of C5 (*dotted black arrow*), the reverse of normal. Locking of the facets in the cervical spine can occur as a result of a hyperflexion injury that results in forward slippage of the affected vertebral body on the body below it by at least 50% of its AP diameter (*solid white arrow*).

TAKE-HOME POINTS

Recognizing Some Common Causes of Neck and Back Pain

Conventional radiographs, CT, and MRI are all used to evaluate the spine, but MRI is the study of choice for most diseases of the spine because of its superior ability to display soft tissues.

Normal features of the vertebral bodies, intervertebral disks, the spinal cord, spinal nerves, and spinal ligaments are described.

Some of the more common causes of back pain are muscle and ligament strain, herniation of an intervertebral disk, degeneration of an intervertebral disk, arthritis involving the synovial joints of the spine, compression fractures from osteoporosis, trauma to the spine, and malignancy involving the spine.

Most *herniated disks* occur posterolaterally in the lower cervical or lower lumbar spine and are best evaluated using MRI.

Postlaminectomy syndrome is persistent pain in the back or legs following spine surgery. Gadolinium-enhanced MRI can be very helpful in detecting the cause.

With increasing age, the nucleus pulposus becomes dehydrated and degenerates, leading to changes of *degenerative disk disease* such as progressive loss of the height of the disk space, marginal osteophyte production, sclerosis of the endplates of the vertebral bodies, and occasionally the appearance of a vacuum disk.

The facet joints are true joints and are subject to changes of osteoarthritis; *facet osteoarthritis* is frequently associated with degenerative disk disease and can lead to radicular pain.

Diffuse idiopathic skeletal hyperostosis is manifest by thick, bridging or flowing calcification/ossification of the anterior longitudinal ligament usually occurring in men over the age of 50. The disk spaces and the facet joints are usually preserved.

Compression fractures of the spine are most often secondary to osteoporosis and are seen more commonly in women. They can be seen on conventional radiographs and, because they usually disproportionately involve the anterior portion of the body, produce an exaggerated kyphosis in the thoracic spine.

Spondylolisthesis is defined as slippage (typically forward) of one vertebral body (and the spine above it) on another; in general it is caused by either bilateral breaks in the pars interarticularis (spondylolysis) or osteoarthritis of the facet joints (degenerative spondylolisthesis).

Spondylolysis is believed secondary to a congenitally dysplastic pars interarticularis which eventually develops a stress fracture; when this occurs, the vertebral body is able to slip forward on the body below it.

Degenerative spondylolisthesis, which is most common at L4-L5, may occur through a complex interaction between the ligaments, disks, and facet joints; there is no break in the pars interarticularis, and the degree of slip is usually less than that seen with spondylolysis.

Spinal stenosis is a narrowing of the spinal canal or the neural foramina secondary to soft tissue or bony abnormalities, either on an acquired or, less commonly, congenital basis; it occurs most frequently in the cervical and lumbar regions.

Metastatic lesions to the spine are common, especially to the blood-rich posterior aspect of the vertebral body including the pedicles; lung (mixed), breast (mixed), and prostate (osteoblastic) metastases are the most common.

Multiple myeloma also frequently involves the spine either with severe osteoporosis, which can produce compression fractures, or lytic destruction of the vertebral body.

Infection of the spine usually starts in the vertebral body endplates in adults and then involves the adjacent disk. Think of **diskitis** when a process involves two adjacent vertebral bodies and the intervening disk.

Three parallel arcuate lines should smoothly connect important landmarks on the lateral cervical spine view and allow for a quick assessment for fracture or subluxation before the patient is moved for further studies.

The findings in a Jefferson fracture, hangman fracture, burst fracture, and locked facets are discussed; the first two are self-decompressing injuries that are usually not associated with neurologic deficit while the latter two are frequently associated with neurologic impairment.

Chapter 25

Recognizing Some Common Causes of Intracranial Pathology

- Advances in neuroimaging have had a remarkable impact on the diagnosis and treatment of neurologic diseases ranging from earlier detection and treatment of stroke to a more timely diagnosis of dementia, from the rapid detection and treatment of cerebral aneurysms to the ability to diagnose multiple sclerosis after a single attack.
- Both CT and MRI are utilized for studying the brain and spinal cord, but MRI is the study of first choice for most clinical scenarios (Table 25-1). Conventional radiography has no significant role in imaging intracranial abnormalities.

NORMAL ANATOMY

- The normal anatomy of the brain is somewhat easier to understand with CT than MRI (Fig. 25-1).
- In the posterior fossa, the **4th** ventricle appears as an inverted U-shaped structure. Like all cerebrospinal fluid (CSF) containing structures, it normally appears black. Superior to the 4th ventricle are the **cerebellar hemispheres**, inferiorly lie the **pons** and **medulla oblongata**. The **tentorium cerebelli** separates the **infratentorial** components of the posterior fossa (medulla, pons, cerebellum, and 4th ventricle) from the **supratentorial** compartment.
- The **interpeduncular cistern** lies in the midbrain and separates the paired **cerebral peduncles** (which emerge from the superior surface of the pons). The **suprasellar cistern** is anterior to the interpeduncular cistern and usually has a five-point or six-point starlike appearance.
- The **sylvian fissures** are bilaterally symmetrical and contain CSF. They separate the temporal from the frontal and parietal lobes.
- The **lentiform nucleus** is composed of the **putamen** (laterally) and **globus pallidus** (medially). The **3rd** ventricle is slitlike and midline. At the posterior aspect of the 3rd ventricle is the **pineal gland**. Farther posterior is the **quadrigeminal plate cistern**.
- The **corpus callosum** connects the right and left cerebral hemispheres and forms the roof of the lateral ventricle. The anterior end is called the **genu** and the posterior end is called the **splenium**.
- The **basal ganglia** are represented by the **subthalamic nucleus**, **substantia nigra**, **globus pallidus**, **putamen**, and **caudate nucleus**. The putamen and caudate nucleus are called the **striatum**.
- The **frontal horns** of the **lateral ventricles** hug the head of the **caudate nucleus**. The two frontal horns are separated by the midline **septum pellucidum**. The **temporal horns**, which are normally very small, are more inferior

and contained in the **temporal lobes**. The posterior horns of the lateral ventricle (**occipital horns**) lie in the occipital lobes. The most superior portion of the ventricular system is formed by the **bodies** of the lateral ventricles.

- The **falx cerebri** lies in the **interhemispheric fissure**, which separates the two **cerebral hemispheres**, and is frequently calcified in adults.
- The surface or **cortex** of the brain is made up of **gray matter** convolutions, which in turn are composed of **sulci** (grooves) and **gyri** (elevations). The medullary **white matter** lies below the cortex.

> On an unenhanced CT scan of the brain, anything that appears "white" will generally either be **bone (calcium)** density or **blood** in the absence of a metallic foreign body (Table 25-2).

- **Calcifications that may be seen on CT of the brain which are nonpathologic:**
  - Pineal gland (Fig. 25-2A)
  - Basal ganglia (see Fig. 25-2A)
  - Choroid plexus (see Fig. 25-1F)
  - Falx and tentorium (Fig. 25-2B)
- **Normal structures that can enhance** after administration of iodinated intravenous contrast:
  - **Venous sinuses**
  - **Choroid plexus**
  - **Pituitary gland and stalk**
- **Metallic densities** in the head can cause artifacts on CT scans. Dental fillings, aneurysm clips, and bullets can all cause *streak artifacts*.

MRI AND THE BRAIN

> In general, **MRI is the study of choice** for detecting and staging intracranial and spinal cord abnormalities. It is usually more sensitive than CT because of its **superior contrast** and **soft tissue resolution**. It is, however, **less sensitive** than CT in detecting **calcification** in lesions and **cortical bone**, which appear as signal voids with MR. It cannot be used in patients with pacemakers.

- MRI is more difficult to interpret because the same structure or abnormality will appear differently depending on the pulse sequence, the scan parameters, and the fact that MRI is more variable in its depiction of differences which occur over the time course of some abnormalities (e.g., hemorrhage) than is CT.

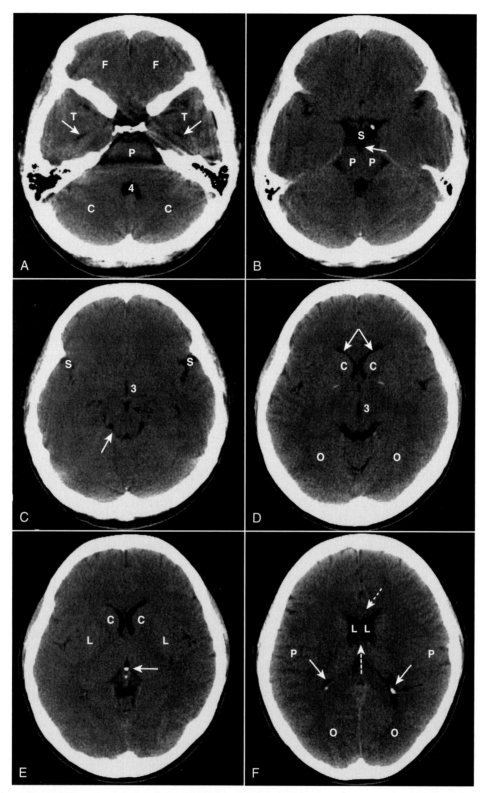

Figure 25-1 **Normal unenhanced CT scans of the head. A,** Frontal lobes (*F*); temporal lobes (*T*); temporal horns (*solid white arrows*); fourth ventricle (*4*); cerebellum (*C*); pons (*P*). **B,** Suprasellar cistern (*S*); cerebral peduncles (*P*); interpeduncular cistern (*solid white arrow*). **C,** Sylvian fissures (*S*); 3rd ventricle (*3*); interpeduncular cistern (*solid black arrow*); quadrigeminal plate cistern (*solid white arrow*). **D,** Anterior horns of the lateral ventricles (*solid white arrows*); caudate nuclei (*C*); 3rd ventricle (*3*); occipital lobes (*O*). **E,** Caudate nuclei (*C*); lentiform nuclei (*L*); calcified pineal gland (*solid white arrow*). **F,** Genu of corpus callosum (*dotted white arrow*); lateral ventricles (*L*); septum pellucidum (*dashed white arrow*); parietal lobes (*P*); occipital horn (*solid black arrow*); calcified choroid plexus (*solid white arrows*); occipital lobes (*O*).

TABLE 25-1 IMAGING STUDIES OF THE BRAIN FOR SELECTED ABNORMALITIES

Abnormality	Study of First Choice	Other Studies
Acute stroke	Diffusion-weighted MR imaging for acute or small strokes, if available	Noncontrast CT can differentiate hemorrhagic from ischemic infarct
Headache, acute and severe	Noncontrast CT to detect subarachnoid hemorrhage	MR-angiography (MRA) or CT-angiography (CTA) if subarachnoid hemorrhage is found
Headaches, chronic	MRI without and with contrast	CT without and with contrast can be substituted
Seizures	MRI without and with contrast	CT without and with contrast can be substituted if MRI not available
Blood	Noncontrast CT	Ultrasound for infants
Head trauma	Nonenhanced CT is readily available and the study of first choice in head trauma	MRI is better at detecting diffuse axonal injury but requires more time and is not always available
Extracranial carotid disease	Doppler ultrasonography	MRA excellent study
Hydrocephalus	MRI as initial study	CT for follow-up
Vertigo and dizziness	Contrast-enhanced MRI	MRA if needed
Masses	Contrast-enhanced MRI	Contrast-enhanced CT if MRI not available
Change in mental status	MRI without or with contrast	CT without contrast is equivalent

- **Initial evaluation of an MRI of the brain** might start with the T1-weighted sagittal view of the brain. On this view the brain looks more like the anatomic specimens or diagrams you are accustomed to looking at (Fig. 25-3). We are fortunate that many structures in the brain are paired, so don't forget to compare one side to the other on axial scans of the brain (Fig. 25-4).
- Table 25-3 summarizes the signal characteristics of various tissues seen on MRI.

HEAD TRAUMA

- **Traumatic brain injuries** extract a huge cost to the patient and society, not only as a result of the acute injury but also for the long-term disability they produce. In the United States, motor vehicle accidents account for nearly half of traumatic brain injuries.
- **Unenhanced CT is the study of choice in acute head trauma.** The primary goal in obtaining the scan is to determine if there is a life-threatening, but treatable, lesion.

  Initial CT evaluation of the brain in the emergency setting focuses on whether there is **mass effect** or **blood**.

- To determine if there is **mass effect**, look for a **displacement or compression** of key structures from their normal positions by analyzing the location and appearance of the **ventricles, basal cisterns** and the **sulci**.
- **Blood** will usually be hyperintense (bright) and might collect in the **basal cisterns, sylvian and interhemispheric fissures, ventricles, the subdural or epidural spaces,** or in the **brain parenchyma (intracerebral)**.

Skull Fractures

- Skull fractures are usually produced by **direct impact** to the skull and they most often occur at the point of impact. They are important primarily because their presence implies a **force substantial enough to cause intracranial injury**.

- In order to visualize skull fractures, you must view the CT scan using the "bone window" settings that optimize visualization of the osseous structures (Fig. 25-5).
- Skull fractures can be described as **linear, depressed, or basilar**.
  - **Linear skull fractures** are the most common and have little importance other than for the intracranial abnormalities that may have occurred at the time of the fracture, such as an epidural hematoma. Fractures of the cranial vault are most likely to occur in the **temporal** and **parietal bones** (see Fig. 25-5B).
  - **Depressed skull fractures** are more likely to be associated with **underlying brain injury**. They result from a high-energy blow to a small area of the skull (e.g., from a baseball bat), most often in the **frontoparietal region** and are **usually comminuted**. They may require **surgical elevation** of the depressed fragment when the fragment lies deeper than the inner table adjacent to the fracture (Fig. 25-6A).

  Basilar skull fractures are the **most serious** and consist of a linear fracture at the base of the skull. They can be associated with **tears in the dura mater** with subsequent **CSF leak**, which can lead to CSF rhinorrhea and otorrhea. They can be suspected if there is air seen in the brain (*traumatic pneumocephalus*), **fluid in the mastoid air cells**, or an **air-fluid level** in the sphenoid sinus (Fig. 25-6B).

Facial Fractures

- **CT is the imaging study of choice** for evaluating **facial fractures**. Multislice scanners allow for reconstruction in the coronal plane so the patient does not have to be repositioned in the scanner.

  Care must be taken in diagnosing facial fractures based upon viewing what appears to be a fracture on only one image since CT scans, by their nature, produce sections so thin, they may not demonstrate the entire contour of the bone in question. Look for a fracture to appear on several contiguous images.

TABLE 25-2 CT DENSITIES

Hypodense (Dark) (AKA Hypointense)	Isodense	Hyperdense (Bright) (AKA Hyperintense)
Fat (not usually present in the head)	Normal brain	Metal (e.g., aneurysm clips or bullets)
Air (e.g., sinuses)	Some forms of protein (e.g., subacute	Iodine (after contrast administration)
Water (e.g., CSF)	subdural hematomas)	Calcium
		Hemorrhage (high protein)

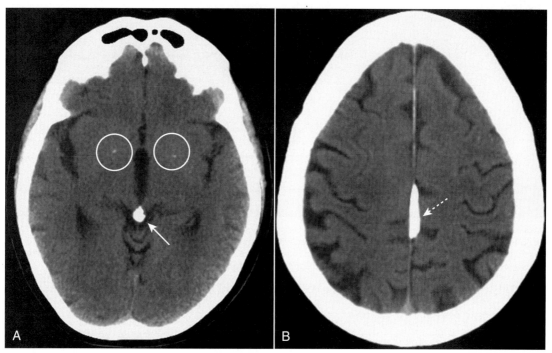

Figure 25-2 Physiologic calcifications. A, There are small, punctate calcifications in the basal ganglia (*white circles*) and calcification of the pineal gland (*solid white arrow*). **B**, Calcification of the falx cerebri is present (*dotted white arrow*). Anything that appears white on a noncontrast enhanced CT of the brain is either calcium or blood. Physiologic calcifications tend to increase in incidence with advancing age.

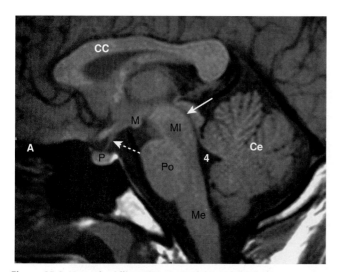

Figure 25-3 Normal midline MRI. Sagittal T1-weighted close-up image demonstrates the midline structures of the brain. For orientation purposes, anterior is to your left (*A*). The corpus callosum (*CC*) is located superiorly. The pituitary gland (*P*) sits in the sella turcica and connects to the hypothalamus via the pituitary stalk or infundibulum (*dotted white arrow*). The mamillary bodies (*M*) are located anterior to the brain stem. The cerebral aqueduct (*solid white arrow*) is superior to the midbrain. The brain stem is composed of the midbrain (*Mi*), the pons (*Po*), and the medulla (*Me*). The 4th ventricle (*4*) communicates with the cerebral aqueduct and lies between the cerebellum (*Ce*) and the brain stem.

- The most common **orbital fracture** is the *blow-out fracture*, which is produced by a **direct impact on the orbit** (e.g., a baseball strikes the eye) that causes a sudden increase in intraorbital pressure leading to a fracture of the inferior orbital floor (into the maxillary sinus) or the medial wall of the orbit (into the ethmoid sinus). Sometimes, the **inferior rectus muscle** can be trapped in the fracture leading to **restriction of upward gaze** and **diplopia**.
- **Recognizing a blow-out fracture of the orbit** (Fig. 25-7A).
  - **Orbital emphysema.** Air in the orbit from communication with one of the adjacent air-containing sinuses, either the ethmoid or maxillary sinus.
  - **Fracture** through either the medial wall or floor of the orbit.
  - **Entrapment of fat and/or extraocular muscle**, which projects downward as a soft tissue mass into the top of the maxillary sinus.
  - **Fluid (blood)** in the maxillary sinus.
- A *tripod fracture*, usually a result of blunt force to the cheek, is another relatively common facial fracture. This fracture involves **separation of the zygoma** from the remainder of the face by **separation of the frontozygomatic suture, fracture of the floor of the orbit**, and fracture of the **lateral wall of the ipsilateral maxillary sinus** (Fig. 25-7B).

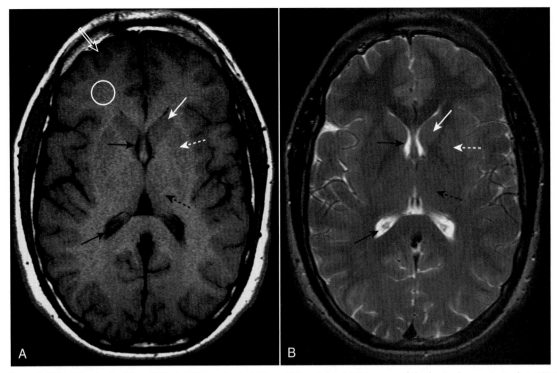

Figure 25-4 **Normal MRI of the brain, T1 and T2.** Axial T1-weighted **(A)** and T2-weighted **(B)** images of the brain demonstrate that CSF in the lateral ventricles is dark on T1 and bright on T2 (*solid black arrows*). Gray matter, which contains the neuronal cell bodies, is actually gray on T1-weighted images (*open white arrow*), and white matter, which contains myelinated axon tracts, is whiter (*white circle*). The caudate nuclei (*solid white arrows*) and lentiform nucleus (*dotted white arrows*) together form the basal ganglia. The thalamus (*dotted black arrows*) is located posterior to the basal ganglia.

TABLE 25-3 SIGNAL CHARACTERISTICS OF VARIOUS TISSUES SEEN ON T1-WEIGHTED AND T2-WEIGHTED MRI SCANS

Bright on T1	Dark on T1	Bright on T2	Dark on T2
Fat	Calcification	Water (edema, CSF)	Fat
Gadolinium	Air		Calcification
High protein	Chronic hemorrhage		Air
Subacute hemorrhage	Acute hemorrhage		Early subacute hemorrhage
	Water (edema, CSF)		Chronic hemorrhage
			Acute hemorrhage
			High protein

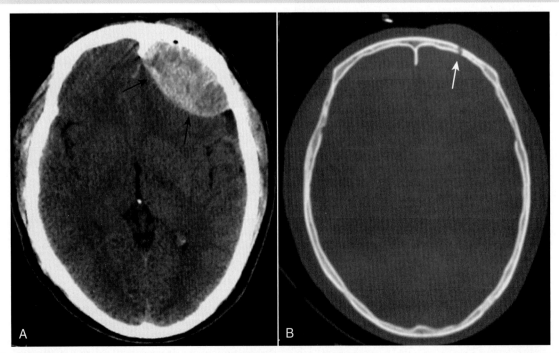

Figure 25-5 **CT, "brain" and "bone" windows.** In order to visualize skull fractures, you must view the CT scan using the "bone" windows. **A,** Using the "brain window," a lenticular-shaped, hyperintense lesion is seen in the left frontal region displaying the typical appearance of an epidural hematoma (*solid black arrows*). **B,** Viewing the same scan at the "bone window" setting shows a fracture (*solid white arrow*) of the left frontal bone at the site of the epidural hematoma.

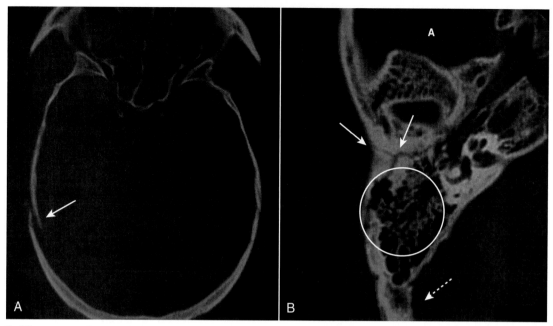

Figure 25-6 Skull fractures. A, There is a depressed fracture of the right parietal bone with the fragment lying deeper than the inner table of the adjacent bone (*solid white arrow*). Depressed skull fractures occur more often in the frontoparietal region. **B,** On this close-up axial CT of the mastoids, there is a comminuted fracture of the right temporal bone (*solid white arrows*), fluid in the mastoid air cells (*white circle*), and air in the brain (pneumocephalus) (*dotted white arrow*). Basilar skull fractures can be associated with tears in the dura mater with subsequent CSF leak. (*A* = Anterior.)

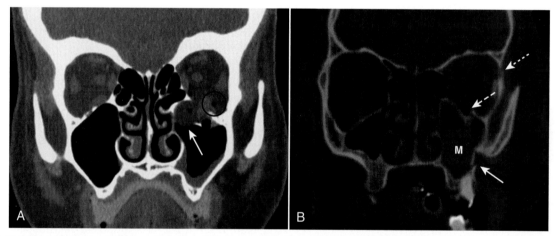

Figure 25-7 Facial bone fractures. A, Blow-out fracture. Air is demonstrated in the left orbit representing orbital emphysema (*black circle*). A fracture of the floor of the orbit is seen, and soft tissue (in this case, fat) extends inferiorly into the top of the maxillary sinus (*solid white arrow*). **B, Tripod fracture.** There is diastasis of the frontozygomatic suture on the left (*dotted white arrow*), a fracture of the floor of the orbit with orbital emphysema (*dashed white arrow*), and a fracture (*solid white arrow*) through the lateral wall of the maxillary sinus (*M*), which is filled with blood.

INTRACRANIAL HEMORRHAGE

- Skull fractures may be associated with **intracranial hemorrhage** and/or **diffuse axonal injury**.
- There are **four types of intracranial hemorrhages** that may be **associated with head trauma**:
  - Epidural hematoma
  - Subdural hematoma
  - Intracerebral hemorrhage
  - Subarachnoid hemorrhage (discussed with aneurysms)

Epidural Hematoma (Extradural Hematoma)

- Epidural hematomas represent **hemorrhage** into the potential space between the **dura mater and the inner table of the skull** (Table 25-4).

- Most cases are due to **injury to the middle meningeal artery** or vein from blunt head trauma, typically from a motor vehicle accident.

> Almost all epidural hematomas (95%) have an associated skull fracture, frequently in the temporal bone. Epidural hematomas may also be caused by disruption of the dural venous sinuses adjacent to a skull fracture.

- Recognizing an epidural hematoma
  - They appear as a **high density, extraaxial, biconvex lens-shaped mass** most often found in the **temporoparietal region** of the brain (Fig. 25-8).
  - Since the dura is normally fused to the calvarium at the margins of the sutures, it is **impossible for an epidural**

TABLE 25-4 THE MENINGES

Layer	Comments
Dura mater	Composed of two layers, an **outer periosteal layer** which cannot be separated from the skull and an inner meningeal layer; the **inner meningeal layer** enfolds to form the tentorium and falx.
Arachnoid	The avascular middle layer, it is separated from the dura by a potential space known as the **subdural space.**
Pia mater	Closely applied to the brain and spinal cord, the pia mater carries blood vessels that supply both; separating the arachnoid from the pia is the **subarachnoid space**; together the **pia and arachnoid** are called the **leptomeninges.**

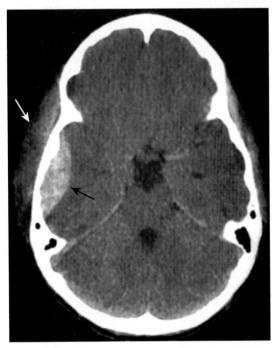

Figure 25-8 Epidural hematoma. Acute epidural hematomas usually occur as a result of a trauma-induced skull fracture. Findings include a high-density, extraaxial, biconvex, lens-shaped mass lesion often found in the temporal-parietal region of the brain (*solid black arrow*). There is a scalp hematoma (*solid white arrow*) also present. The patient had a temporal bone skull fracture seen on bone windows.

hematoma to cross suture lines (subdural hematomas can cross sutures).
- Epidural hematomas can cross the tentorium, but subdural hematomas do not.

Subdural Hematoma (SDH)

- **Subdural hematomas are more common** than epidural hematomas and are usually not associated with a skull fracture. They are most commonly **a result of deceleration injuries in motor vehicle or motorcycle accidents** (younger patients) or **secondary to falls** (older patients).
- Subdural hematomas are usually produced by **damage to the bridging veins** that cross from the cerebral cortex to the venous sinuses of the brain. They represent hemorrhage into the potential space **between the dura mater and the arachnoid.**

➡ Acute subdural hematomas frequently herald the presence of more severe parenchymal brain injury and increased intracranial pressure and are **associated with a higher mortality rate.**

- **Recognizing an acute subdural hematoma**
  - **On CT, acute subdural hematomas are crescent-shaped, extracerebral bands of high attenuation that may cross suture lines** and enter the interhemispheric fissure. They **do not cross the midline.**
  - Typically, a SDH is **concave** inward towards the brain (epidural hematomas are **convex** inward) (Fig. 25-9A).
  - As time passes and they become subacute, or if the subdural blood is mixed with lower attenuating CSF, they may appear **isointense (isodense)** to the remainder of brain, in which case you should look for **compressed or absent sulci** or **sulci displaced away from the inner table as signs of SDH** (Fig. 25-9B).
  - Subdural collections may demonstrate a **fluid-fluid level after 1 week**, as the cells settle under serum.
- **Chronic subdural hematoma**
  - Chronic subdural hematomas are those present more than 3 weeks after injury.
  - Chronic subdural hematomas are usually **low density** compared to the remainder of the brain (Fig. 25-9C).

Intracerebral Hematoma (Intracerebral Hemorrhage)

- Trauma is only one of the mechanisms that can lead to intracerebral hemorrhage. Intracerebral hematomas can also occur from ruptures of **aneurysms, atheromatous disease in small vessels**, or vasculitis.
- Injuries occurring at the **point of impact** (called *coup injuries*) and injuries occurring **opposite the point of impact** (called *contrecoup injuries*) are most common following trauma. **Coup** injuries are most often due to **shearing** of small intracerebral vessels. **Contrecoup** injuries are **acceleration/deceleration injuries** that occur when the brain is propelled in the opposite direction and strikes the inner surface of the skull.

➡ Either of these mechanisms can produce a **cerebral contusion. Contusions are hemorrhages with associated edema** usually found in the **inferior frontal lobes and temporal lobes on or near the surface of the brain** (Fig. 25-10).

- **CT findings of intracerebral hemorrhage change over time and may not be immediately evident on the initial scan.** MRI typically demonstrates the lesions from the time of injury, but may not be available on an emergency basis.
- **Recognizing traumatic intracerebral hemorrhage on CT**
  - Cerebral contusions may appear as multiple, small, well-demarcated areas of **high attenuation** within the brain parenchyma (see Fig. 25-10A).
  - They may be surrounded by a **hypodense rim** from edema (see Fig. 25-10B).
  - **Intraventricular blood** may be present (Fig. 25-11).

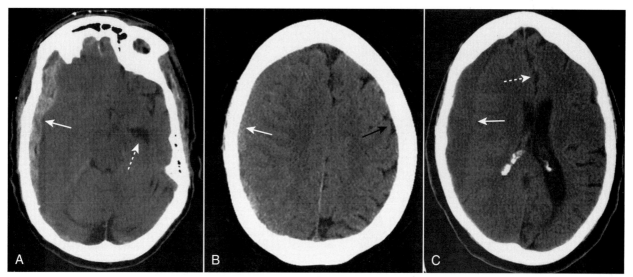

Figure 25-9 Acute, isodense, and chronic subdural hematomas. A, There is a crescent-shaped band of high-density blood concave inward towards the brain (*solid white arrow*). Mass effect is present with herniation of the brain as indicated by the dilated contralateral temporal horn (*dotted white arrow*). **B**, As they become subacute, subdural hematomas become less dense and may be the same density (isodense) as the normal brain tissue (*solid white arrow*). You can recognize an isodense subdural by the unilateral absence or displacement of the sulci away from the inner table of the skull compared to the normal opposite side (*solid black arrow*). **C**, Chronic subdural hematomas (more than 3 weeks old) are usually of low density (*solid white arrow*) compared to the remainder if the brain. There is still mass effect demonstrated by displacement of the interhemispheric fissure (*dotted white arrow*) and compression of the lateral ventricle.

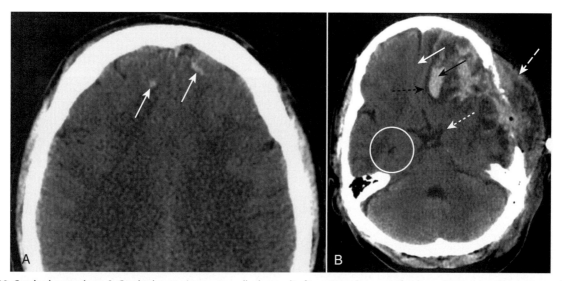

Figure 25-10 Cerebral contusions. A, Cerebral contusions are usually the result of trauma and can manifest by multiple areas of high attenuation hemorrhage (*solid white arrows*) within the brain parenchyma on CT. **B**, Contusions (*solid black arrow*) are frequently surrounded by a rim of hypoattenuation from edema (*dotted black arrow*), and mass effect is common, as is demonstrated here by amputation of the ipsilateral basilar cisterns (*dotted white arrow*), midline displacement (*solid white arrow*) representing subfalcine herniation, and dilatation of the contralateral temporal horn (*white circle*). A portion of the left side of the skull has been surgically removed, and there is a large scalp hematoma present (*dashed white arrow*).

- **Mass effect is common. The mass effect may produce compression** of the **ventricles and shift of the 3rd ventricle and septum pellucidum** to the opposite side. Such displacement can produce severe brain or vascular damage.
- These displacements are called *herniations*. Patients with sufficient mass effect are at risk for *transtentorial* and *subfalcine brain herniation* and death (see Fig. 25-10B).
- **The types of brain herniation** are described in Table 25-5 (Fig. 25-12).

DIFFUSE AXONAL INJURY

- Diffuse axonal injury is **responsible for the prolonged coma following head trauma** and is the head injury with the poorest prognosis.
- Acceleration/deceleration forces **diffusely injure axons deep to the cortex** producing unconsciousness from the moment of injury. This occurs most often as a result of a motor vehicle accident.

 The **corpus callosum is most commonly affected**, and the initial CT scan may be normal or underestimate

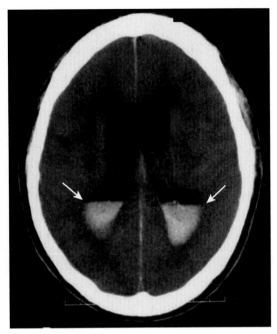

Figure 25-11 Intraventricular hemorrhage. Intraventricular hemorrhage (*solid white arrows*) is common in premature infants but less common in adults. It usually results from break-through bleeding from a brain contusion or subarachnoid hemorrhage and requires a considerable amount of force to produce. Therefore, it is typically associated with severe brain damage and has a poor prognosis.

TABLE 25-5 TYPES OF BRAIN HERNIATION

Type	Remarks
Subfalcine herniation	The supratentorial brain, along with the lateral ventricle and septum pellucidum, herniates beneath the falx and shifts across the midline toward the opposite side (see Fig. 25-12A).
Transtentorial herniation	Usually, the cerebral hemispheres are displaced downward through the incisura beneath the tentorium compressing the ipsilateral temporal horn and causing **dilatation of the contralateral temporal horn** (see Fig. 25-12B).
Foramen magnum/ tonsillar herniation	Infratentorial brain is displaced downward through the foramen magnum.
Sphenoid herniation	Supratentorial brain slides over the sphenoid bone either anteriorly (in the case of the temporal lobe) or posteriorly (for the frontal lobe).
Extracranial herniation	Displacement of brain through a defect in the cranium.

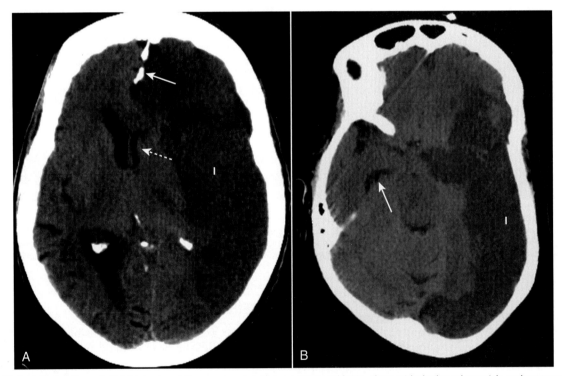

Figure 25-12 Brain herniations. A, Subfalcine herniation occurs when the supratentorial brain, along with the lateral ventricle and septum pellucidum, herniate beneath the falx (*solid white arrow*) and shift across the midline toward the opposite side (*dotted white arrow*). **B,** Transtentorial herniation usually occurs when the cerebral hemispheres are displaced downward through the incisura beneath the tentorium compressing the ipsilateral temporal horn and causing dilatation of the contralateral temporal horn (*solid white arrow*). Both patients had large cerebral infarcts (*I*) with cytotoxic edema.

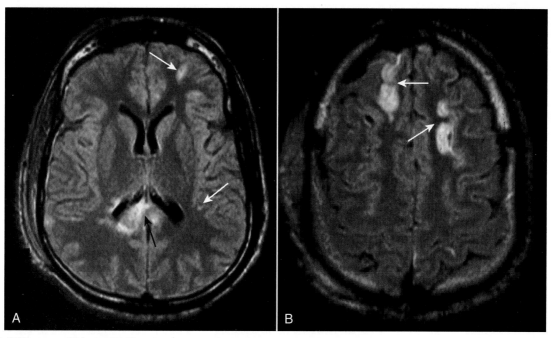

Figure 25-13 Diffuse axonal injury, MRI. These images were obtained using a pulse sequence similar to T2 but with suppression of the bright signal from CSF, which enhances areas of edema (that appear bright). **(A)** and **(B)** are axial images demonstrating multiple foci of abnormal increased signal at the gray-white matter junction (*solid white arrows*) and within the splenium of the corpus callosum (*solid black arrow*) in a patient with diffuse axonal injury.

the degree of injury. CT findings may be similar to those described for intracerebral hemorrhage following head trauma.

- **MR is the study of choice in identifying diffuse axonal injury.**
  - **The small petechial lesions** may be **bright** on **T1-weighted images**.
  - The most common findings are multiple **bright areas on T2-weighted images** at the **temporal or parietal corticomedullary junction** or in the corpus callosum (Fig. 25-13)

INCREASED INTRACRANIAL PRESSURE

- Some of the clinical signs of **increased intracranial pressure are papilledema, headache, and diplopia**.

  In general, increased intracranial pressure is due to either **cerebral edema**, which leads to increased **volume of the brain**, or **hydrocephalus**, which is **increased size of the ventricles**.

- **Cerebral edema**
  - In adults, **trauma, hypertension** (associated as it is with **intracerebral bleeds** and **stroke**) and **masses** are the most common causes of brain edema.
  - Cerebral edema is divided into **two major types: vasogenic** and **cytotoxic**.
    - **Vasogenic edema** represents extracellular accumulation of fluid and is the type that is associated with **malignancy** and **infection**. It is due to **abnormal permeability of the blood brain barrier**. It predominantly affects the **white matter** (Fig. 25-14A).

- **Cytotoxic edema** represents cellular edema and is associated with **cerebral ischemia**. It is due to **cell death**. It affects both the gray and white matter (Fig. 25-14B).
- Recognizing cerebral edema
  - **There is a loss of the normal differentiation between gray and white matter.**
  - **There may be effacement** (compression or obliteration) of the normal **sulci**.
  - **The ventricles may be compressed** (Fig. 25-15).
  - **Herniation** of the brain may manifest, in part, by **effacement of the basilar cisterns** (see Fig. 25-10B).
- Increased intracranial pressure secondary to increase in the size of the ventricles is discussed under Hydrocephalus.

STROKE

General Considerations

- Stroke is a nonspecific term that usually denotes an **acute loss of neurologic function** that occurs when the blood supply to an area of the brain is lost or compromised.

  The diagnosis of stroke is usually a clinical diagnosis. Patients with suspected stroke are imaged to determine if there is **another cause of the neurologic impairment** besides a stroke (e.g., a brain tumor), to **identify the presence of blood** so as to distinguish **ischemic** from **hemorrhagic** stroke, which may determine whether or not thrombolytic therapy will be instituted, and to **identify the infarct** and **characterize it**.

- **Most strokes are embolic in origin**, the emboli arising from the internal **carotid artery** or the common carotid bifurcation. Emboli can also arise in the **heart**.

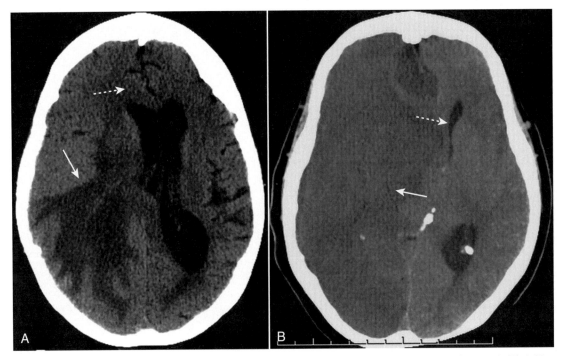

Figure 25-14 Vasogenic and cytotoxic edema. There are two major categories of cerebral edema: vasogenic **(A)** and cytotoxic **(B)**. **A**, Vasogenic edema (*solid white arrow*) represents extracellular accumulation of fluid and is the type that occurs with infection and malignancy, as in this unenhanced scan of a patient with a glioma. It predominantly affects the white matter. **B**, Cytotoxic edema (*solid white arrow*) represents cellular edema and affects both the gray and white matter. Cytotoxic edema is associated with cerebral ischemia, as in this patient with a very large ischemic infarct on the right. In both of these patients, there is increased intracranial pressure as manifest by the herniation of brain to the contralateral side (*dotted white arrows* in both).

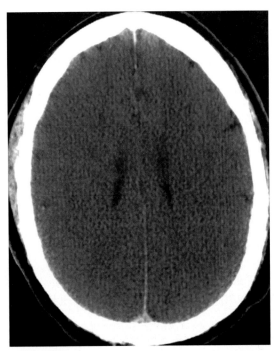

Figure 25-15 Diffuse cerebral edema, CT. Cerebral edema produces loss of normal differentiation between gray and white matter, effacement (narrowing or obliteration) of the normal sulci, and ventricular compression, all of which are visible in this patient with anoxic encephalopathy.

- The other common cause of stroke is **thrombosis**, representing in-situ **occlusion** of the carotid, vertebrobasilar, or intracerebral circulations from **atheromatous lesions**. Thrombosis of the **middle cerebral artery** is particularly common.

- Strokes are divided into two large groups: **ischemic or hemorrhagic**. Ischemic strokes are much more common. The classification is important because rapid treatment of ischemic stroke with **tissue plasminogen activator (t-PA)** or another form of intraarterial recanalization technique can substantially improve the prognosis.

- Most **acute strokes are initially imaged by obtaining a noncontrast enhanced CT scan of the brain** (within 24 hours of the onset of symptoms), mostly because of its availability. CT findings may be present within hours after the onset of symptoms for ischemic stroke and immediately after a hemorrhagic stroke.

- MR imaging has become more widely used for early diagnosis. **Diffusion-weighted MR** imaging is more sensitive and relatively specific for detecting early infarction with the capacity to detect changes within a few minutes of the onset of the event. On MRI, the temporal staging of hemorrhage can be identified based on chemical changes that occur in the hemoglobin molecule as the hemorrhage evolves (Fig. 25-16).

Ischemic Stroke

- **Thromboembolic disease** consequent to **atherosclerosis** is the **most common cause of an ischemic stroke**. The **source of the emboli** can be from atheromatous debris, arterial stenosis and occlusion, or from emboli arising from the left side of the heart (e.g., atrial fibrillation).

- *Vascular watershed* areas are the distal arterial territories that represent the **junctions between areas served by the major intracerebral vessels** such as the region between the anterior cerebral artery distribution and the middle cerebral artery distribution. Reduction in blood flow, for

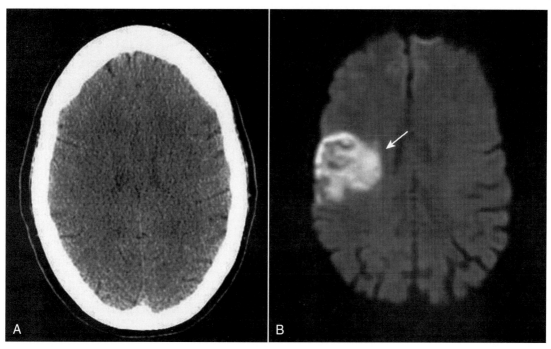

Figure 25-16 CT and diffusion-weighted MRI in acute stroke. A, The CT scan in this patient with symptoms for 2 hours prior to the study is normal. **B**, A diffusion-weighted MRI scan on the same patient a few minutes later shows an area of abnormally bright signal intensity in the right parietal lobe (*solid white arrow*). Diffusion-weighted imaging (DWI) is an MRI sequence that can be rapidly acquired and which is extremely sensitive to detecting abnormalities in normal water movement in the brain so that it can identify a stroke within minutes after the event.

whatever reason, affects these sensitive and susceptible watershed areas the most.

➡ **The most common finding of an acute, nonhemorrhagic stroke is a normal CT scan (less than 24 hours old).** If multiple vascular distributions are involved, emboli or **vasculitis** should be thought of as the cause. If the stroke **crosses or falls between vascular territories**, then hypoperfusion due to hypotension (*watershed infarcts*) should be considered.

■ Table 25-6 briefly summarizes the four major vascular distribution patterns of strokes and some of the symptoms associated with each.
■ **Recognizing ischemic stroke**
  • On CT, the findings will depend on the amount of time that has elapsed since the original event.
  • **12-24 hours:** Indistinct area of low attenuation in a vascular distribution.
  • **>24 hours:** Better circumscribed lesion with mass effect that peaks at 3 to 5 days and usually disappears by 2 to 4 weeks (Fig. 25-17A).
  • **72 hours:** Though contrast is rarely used in the setting of acute stroke, contrast enhancement typically occurs when the mass effect is waning or has disappeared.
  • **>4 weeks:** Mass effect disappears; there is now a well-circumscribed, low attenuation lesion with no contrast enhancement (Fig. 25-17B).

Hemorrhagic Stroke

■ Hemorrhage **occurs in about 15%** of strokes. Hemorrhage is **associated with a higher morbidity and mortality than**

ischemic stroke. Hemorrhage from stroke can occur into the brain parenchyma or the subarachnoid space.
■ In the majority of cases, there is **associated hypertension. About 60% of hypertensive hemorrhages occur in the basal ganglia.** Other areas commonly involved are the thalamus, pons, and cerebellum (Fig. 25-18).

➡ The decision to utilize **thrombolytic** or another **intra-arterial recanalization therapy** is based on algorithms formulated by the initial nonenhanced CT scan findings. The **more rapidly treatment is initiated** (usually less than 4 to 5 hours after the onset of symptoms), the **greater its potential benefit.**

■ **Recognizing intracerebral hemorrhage (in general)**
  • Freshly extravasated whole blood with a normal hematocrit will be visible as **increased density** on nonenhanced CT scans of the brain immediately after the event (see Fig. 25-18). This is due to the protein in the blood (mostly hemoglobin).
  • **Dissection** of blood into the **ventricular system** can occur in hypertensive intracerebral bleeds (see Fig. 25-11).
  • As the clot begins to form, the **blood becomes denser for about 3 days** because of dehydration of the clot.
  • **After the third day**, the **clot decreases in density** and becomes invisible over the next several weeks. The clot loses density from the **outside in** so that it **appears to shrink.**
  • **After about 2 months, only a small hypodensity may remain** (Fig. 25-19; Box 25-1).
■ On MRI, the changes in the appearance of hemorrhage over time are more dramatic. MRI is sensitive to changing effects

TABLE 25-6 VASCULAR DISTRIBUTION TERRITORIES OF STROKE

Circulation	Anatomy Affected	Signs and Symptoms
Anterior cerebral artery (uncommon)	Supplies all of the frontal and parietal lobes (medial surfaces), the anterior four fifths of the corpus callosum, the frontobasal cerebral cortex, and the anterior diencephalon.	Can result in disinhibition and perseveration of speech; produces primitive reflexes (e.g., grasping or sucking), altered mental status, impaired judgment, contralateral weakness (greater in legs than arms).
Middle cerebral artery (common)	Supplies almost the entire convex surface of the brain including the frontal, parietal, and temporal lobes (laterally), insula, claustrum, and extreme capsule. Lenticulostriate branches supply the basal ganglia, including the head of the caudate nucleus, the putamen including the lateral parts of the internal and external capsules.	Produces contralateral hemiparesis or hypesthesia, ipsilateral hemianopsia, and gaze preference toward the side of the lesion; agnosia is common; receptive or expressive aphasia may result if the lesion occurs in the dominant hemisphere; weakness of the arm and face is usually worse than that of the lower limb.
Posterior cerebral artery	Supplies portions of the midbrain, subthalamic nucleus, basal nucleus, thalamus, mesial inferior temporal lobe, and occipital and occipitoparietal cortices.	Occlusions affect vision and thought producing contralateral homonymous hemianopsia, cortical blindness, visual agnosia, altered mental status, and impaired memory.
Vertebrobasilar system	Perfuses the medulla, cerebellum, pons, midbrain, thalamus, and occipital cortex.	Occlusion of large vessels in this system usually leads to major disability or death; small lesions usually have a benign prognosis; may cause a wide variety of cranial nerve, cerebellar, and brain stem deficits; a hallmark of posterior circulation stroke is crossed findings: ipsilateral cranial nerve deficits and contralateral motor deficits (in contrast to anterior stroke).

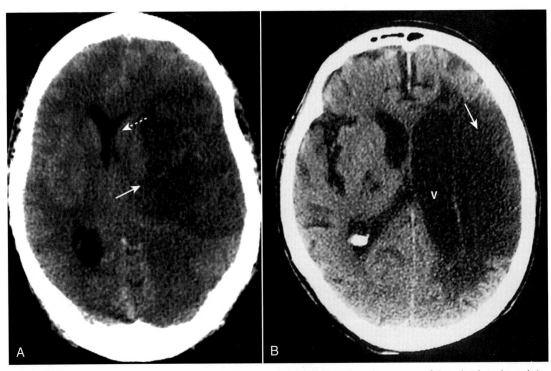

Figure 25-17 Ischemic stroke, newer and older. The findings in ischemic stroke will depend on the amount of time that has elapsed since the original event. **A**, At about 24 hours, the lesion becomes relatively well circumscribed (*solid white arrow*) with mass effect evidenced by a shift of the ventricles (*dotted white arrow*) that peaks at 3 to 5 days and disappears by about 2 to 4 weeks. **B**, As the stroke matures, it loses its mass effect, tends to become an even more sharply marginated low attenuation lesion (*solid white arrow*), and may be associated with enlargement of the adjacent ventricle (*V*) due to loss of brain substance in the infarcted area.

in both the **iron and protein** portions of the hemoglobin molecule in the days and weeks following an acute bleed. Table 25-7 summarizes those changes.

RUPTURED ANEURYSMS

- The most frequent central nervous system aneurysm is the *berry aneurysm*, which develops from a **congenital** weakening in the arterial wall, usually at the sites of vessel branching in the **circle of Willis** at the base of the brain. They can be familial (about 10% of cases) or associated with connective tissue diseases.
- **Hypertension** and **aging** play a role in the growth of aneurysms. **Larger aneurysms bleed more frequently** than do smaller ones.
- The aim is to discover and treat the aneurysm **before** it has undergone a major bleed. In some studies, **10 mm was found to be the critical size for rupture.**

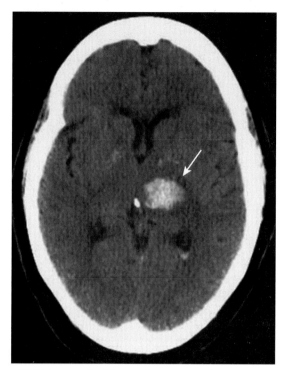

Figure 25-18 Intracerebral hemorrhage, acute. Freshly extravasated whole blood, as this bleed into the thalamus (*solid white arrow*), will be visible as increased density on nonenhanced CT scans of the brain due primarily to the protein in the blood (mostly hemoglobin). As the clot begins to form, the blood becomes denser for about 3 days because of dehydration of the clot. After the third day, the clot gradually decreases in density from the outside in and becomes invisible over the next several weeks.

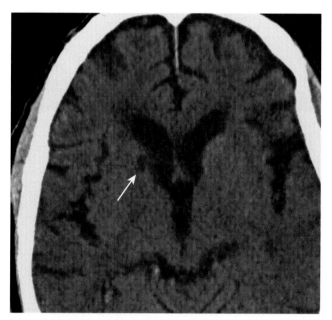

Figure 25-19 Lacunar infarct. A lacunar infarct, or lacune, is a small cerebral infarct produced by occlusion of an end artery. Lacunar infarcts have a predilection for the basal ganglia, internal capsule, and pons, primarily related to hypertension and atherosclerosis. The term lacunar infarct is reserved for low density, cystic lesions, 5 mm to 15 mm in size (*solid white arrow*).

> **Box 25-1 Lacunar Infarcts**
>
> Small cerebral infarcts produced by occlusion of small end arteries accounting for up to 20% of all cerebral infarctions.
>
> They have a predilection for the basal ganglia, internal capsule and pons; they occur in association with hypertension, atherosclerosis, and diabetes.
>
> The term lacunar infarct is reserved for low-density, cystic lesions, about 5-15 mm in size.

TABLE 25-7 CHANGES IN THE APPEARANCE OF BLOOD OVER TIME ON MRI

Phase	Time	T1	T2
Hyperacute	<24 hours	Isointense	Bright
Acute	1-3 days	Isointense	Dark
Early subacute	3-7 days	Bright	Dark
Late subacute	7-14 days	Bright	Bright
Chronic	>14 days	Dark	Dark

- The classical history a patient describes who has had a ruptured aneurysm is "the worst headache of my life."

When aneurysms rupture, the **blood usually enters the subarachnoid space**. Rupture of an aneurysm is the **most common nontraumatic cause of a subarachnoid hemorrhage** (80%) but not the only cause. Trauma, arteriovenous malformations, or breakthrough of an intraparenchymal bleed can also produce subarachnoid hemorrhage.

- Today, most aneurysms are detected by **either CT angiography or MR angiography**. **CT angiography** is performed using a power injector to deliver a rapid bolus intravenous injection of iodinated contrast, a CT scanner capable of rapid acquisition of data and special computer algorithms, and postprocessing techniques that can highlight the vessels and, if desired, display them three-dimensionally (Fig. 25-20).
- **MR angiography** can be done without any contrast, but is usually performed with the intravenous injection of MR contrast (gadolinium) and specialized computer algorithms that allow for highlighting the blood vessels being studied.
- **Recognizing a subarachnoid hemorrhage (from a ruptured aneurysm)**
  - **On CT, blood is hyperdense and may be visualized within the sulci and basal cisterns** (Fig. 25-21 A and B).
  - The region of the **falx may become hyperdense**, widened, and irregularly margined (Fig. 25-21C).
  - Generally, the **greatest concentration of blood indicates the most likely site of the ruptured aneurysm**.
- Other causes of intracerebral hemorrhage besides aneurysms include arteriovenous malformations, tumors, mycotic aneurysms, and amyloid angiopathy (Box 25-2).

HYDROCEPHALUS

- **Hydrocephalus is defined as an expansion of the ventricular system** on the basis of an increase in the volume of cerebrospinal fluid contained within it (Box 25-3).

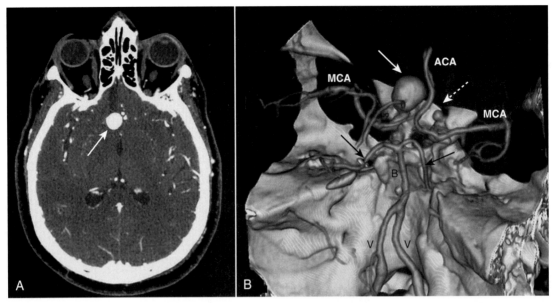

Figure 25-20 Berry aneurysm, axial CT and 3-D reconstruction. A, There is a 2 cm focal outpouching of contrast in the region of the right internal carotid artery (ICA) on this contrast-enhanced CT of the brain (*solid white arrow*). This is consistent with an aneurysm. **B**, A 3-D reconstruction of the circle of Willis from a CT-angiogram demonstrates the aneurysm arising from the supraclinoid segment of the right ICA (*solid white arrow*) and another smaller aneurysm arising from the supraclinoid segment of the left ICA (*dotted white arrow*). V = vertebral artery; B = basilar artery; MCA = middle cerebral arteries; ACA = anterior cerebral arteries; *solid black arrows* point to posterior cerebral arteries.

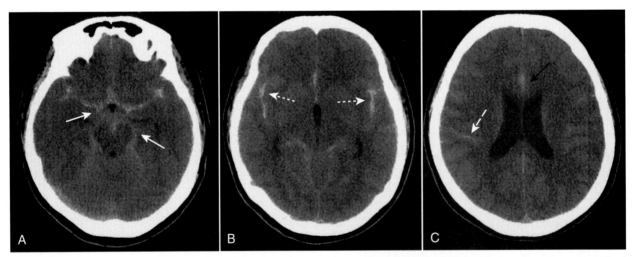

Figure 25-21 Subarachnoid hemorrhage, unenhanced CT scans. Subarachnoid hemorrhage is frequently the result of a ruptured aneurysm. Blood may be most easily visualized within the basal cisterns (*solid white arrows* in **A**), in the fissures (*dotted white arrows* in **B**), and interdigitated in the subarachnoid spaces of the sulci (*dashed white arrow* in **C**). The region of the falx may become hyperdense, widened, and irregularly marginated (*solid black arrow* in **C**).

Box 25-2 Amyloid Angiopathy

Amyloid is a proteinaceous material that can be deposited with increasing age in the media and adventitia of small-sized and medium-sized intracranial vessels, mostly involving the frontal and parietal lobes.

This deposit produces a loss of elasticity of the vessels and increases their fragility.

Hemorrhages from amyloid angiopathy are usually large, involving an entire lobe; they may occur in several areas simultaneously.

There is no association with hypertension and it is not associated with amyloid elsewhere.

Box 25-3 Normal Flow of Cerebrospinal Fluid

Most cerebrospinal fluid is produced by the choroid plexuses in the ventricles, primarily the lateral and 4th ventricles.

The direction of flow is from the lateral ventricles through the foramen of Monro to the 3rd ventricle, then through the aqueduct of Sylvius to the 4th ventricle, and then into the basilar subarachnoid cisterns through the two lateral foramina of Luschka and the medial foramen of Magendie.

CSF can then take one of two paths. It can pass upward over the convexities to be reabsorbed into the bloodstream at the arachnoid villi.

Or CSF can pass inferiorly down the spinal subarachnoid space where it is either reabsorbed directly or ascends back to the brain to the arachnoid villi.

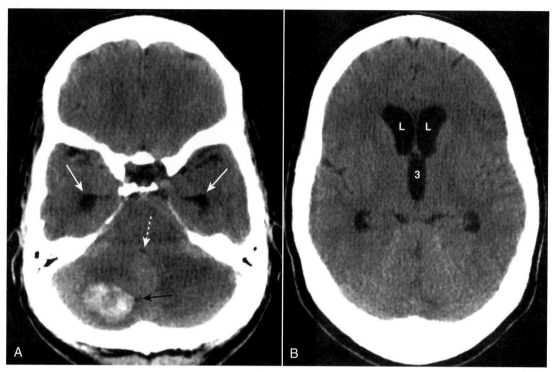

Figure 25-22 Noncommunicating hydrocephalus. A, There is dilatation of the temporal horns (*solid white arrows*) and the 4ᵗʰ ventricle is compressed and nearly invisible (*dotted white arrow*). A hemorrhagic metastatic lesion (*solid black arrow*) is present that is obstructing the 4ᵗʰ ventricle. **B,** The frontal horns of the lateral ventricles (*L*) and 3ʳᵈ ventricle (*3*) are dilated, but note that the sulci are not dilated. This form of hydrocephalus is the result of obstruction to the outflow of cerebrospinal fluid from the ventricles.

 Hydrocephalus may be due to several factors:

- **Underabsorption of cerebrospinal fluid** (*communicating hydrocephalus*)
- **Restriction of the outflow of cerebrospinal fluid from the ventricles** (*noncommunicating hydrocephalus*)
- **Overproduction of cerebrospinal fluid** (rare)
- In hydrocephalus, the **ventricles** are usually **disproportionately dilated** compared to the sulci, whereas **both the ventricles and sulci** are **proportionately enlarged** in **cerebral atrophy**.
- The **temporal horns are particularly sensitive** to increases in CSF pressure. In the absence of hydrocephalus, the **temporal horns are barely visible. With hydrocephalus** the temporal horns may be greater than 2 mm in size (Fig. 25-22).

Obstructive Hydrocephalus

- Obstructive hydrocephalus is divided into two major categories: **communicating (*extraventricular obstruction*)** and **noncommunicating (*intraventricular obstruction*)**.
- **Communicating hydrocephalus** is due to abnormalities that **inhibit the resorption of cerebrospinal fluid**, most often at the level of the arachnoid villi (Fig. 25-23).
  - **CSF flow** through the **ventricles** and **over the convexities** normally occurs **unimpeded**. Reabsorption through the arachnoid villi can become restricted by such things as **subarachnoid hemorrhage** or **meningitis**.

 Classically, the 4ᵗʰ ventricle is **dilated in communicating hydrocephalus** and **normal** in size in **noncommunicating** hydrocephalus.

- Communicating hydrocephalus is **usually treated with a ventricular shunt**.
- **Noncommunicating hydrocephalus** occurs as a result of tumors, cysts, or other physically obstructing lesions that do not allow cerebrospinal fluid to exit from the ventricles.
  - Congenital hydrocephalus is often produced by a blockage between the 3ʳᵈ and 4ᵗʰ ventricles at the level of the **aqueduct of Sylvius (*aqueductal obstruction*)**.
  - When the obstruction is caused by a tumor or a cyst, noncommunicating hydrocephalus is **usually treated by surgically** removing the obstructing lesion (Fig. 25-24).
- **Nonobstructive hydrocephalus** from overproduction of CSF is rare and can occur with a *choroid plexus papilloma*.

Normal-Pressure Hydrocephalus (NPH)

- NPH is a form of **communicating hydrocephalus** characterized by a classical triad of clinical symptoms: **abnormalities of gait, dementia**, and **urinary incontinence**. The age of onset is typically between 50 and 70 years old.

 Its recognition is important because it is usually amenable to treatment using a one-way *ventriculoperitoneal shunt* which allows the CSF to exit the ventricles and drain into the peritoneal cavity where the CSF is reabsorbed.

- Imaging findings are similar to other forms of communicating hydrocephalus and include **enlarged ventricles**, particularly the temporal horns, with **normal or flattened sulci** (Fig. 25-25).

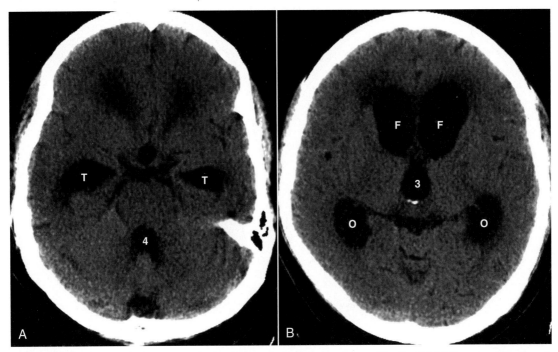

Figure 25-23 Communicating hydrocephalus. Communicating hydrocephalus is due to abnormalities that inhibit the resorption of cerebrospinal fluid, most often at the level of the arachnoid villi. **A,** Classically, the 4th ventricle is dilated in communicating hydrocephalus (*4*) but normal in size in noncommunicating hydrocephalus. The temporal horns (*T*) are particularly sensitive to increases in intraventricular volume or pressure and are dilated in this patient. **B,** The frontal horns (*F*), occipital horns (*O*), and 3rd ventricle (*3*) are markedly dilated. There is a disproportionate dilatation of the ventricles compared to the sulci (which are normal to small in this case). Communicating hydrocephalus is usually treated with a ventricular shunt.

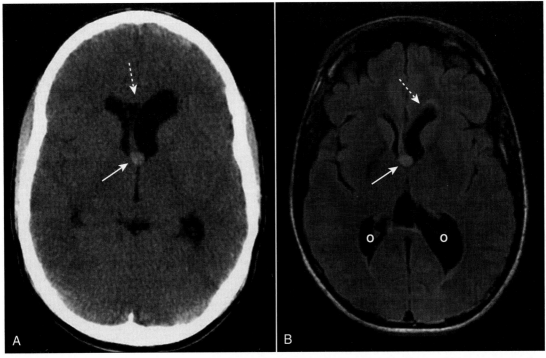

Figure 25-24 Colloid cyst of the 3rd ventricle, CT and MRI. A colloid cyst is a rare, benign lesion of the 3rd ventricle that can cause obstructive hydrocephalus. **A,** There is a hyperdense mass in the anterior aspect of the 3rd ventricle (*solid white arrow*) causing asymmetric obstruction of the left foramen of Monro compared to the right (*dotted white arrow*). **B,** On this T2-like sequence, the lesion has increased signal (*solid white arrow*) and is causing dilatation of the frontal (*dotted white arrow*) and occipital (*O*) horns of the lateral ventricle.

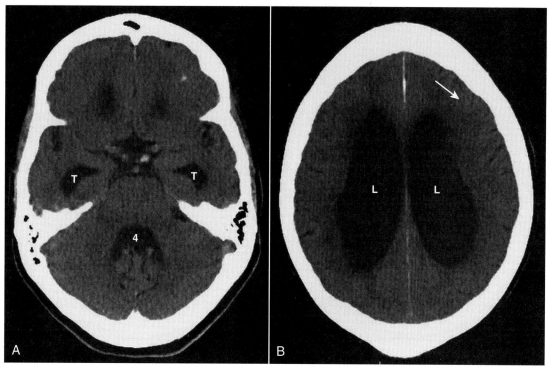

Figure 25-25 Normal pressure hydrocephalus (NPH). NPH is a form of communicating hydrocephalus characterized by a classical triad of clinical symptoms: abnormalities of gait, dementia, and urinary incontinence. **A,** The ventricles are enlarged, particularly the temporal horns (*T*) as well as the 4th ventricle (*4*). **B,** The bodies of the lateral ventricles (*L*) are also markedly enlarged but the sulci are normal or flattened (*solid white arrow*).

CEREBRAL ATROPHY

- Disorders associated with **gross cerebral atrophy** are also associated with **dementia, Alzheimer disease being one of the most common**. Atrophy implies a loss of both gray and white matter.
  - The major finding in patients with Alzheimer disease (though not specific) is **diffuse cortical atrophy**, especially in the **temporal lobes**.

 As in hydrocephalus, the **ventricles dilate** in cerebral atrophy but do so because a loss of normal cerebral tissue produces a vacant space that is filled passively with CSF. Unlike hydrocephalus, the **dynamics of CSF** production and absorption are **normal in atrophy**.

- In general, cerebral atrophy leads to **proportionate enlargement of both the ventricles and the sulci** (Fig. 25-26).

BRAIN TUMORS

Gliomas of the Brain

- **Gliomas are the most common primary, supratentorial, intraaxial mass in an adult. They account for 35% to 45% of all intracranial tumors.** *Glioblastoma multiforme* accounts for more than half of all gliomas, astrocytomas about 20%, with the remainder split between *ependymoma*, *medulloblastoma*, and *oligodendroglioma*.
- Glioblastoma multiforme occurs **more commonly in males** between 65 and 75 years of age, especially in the **frontal and temporal lobes**. It has the **worst prognosis** of all gliomas.

- It **infiltrates** adjacent areas of the brain along **white matter tracts** making it difficult to resect, but, like most brain tumors, it **does not produce extracerebral metastases**.

 Recognizing glioblastoma multiforme

- As the most aggressive of tumors, glioblastoma multiforme frequently demonstrates **necrosis** within the tumor.
- The tumor **infiltrates** the surrounding brain tissue, frequently **crossing** the white matter tracts of the **corpus callosum** to the opposite cerebral hemisphere producing a pattern called a *butterfly glioma*.
- It tends to produce considerable **vasogenic edema** and **mass effect** and **enhances with contrast**, at least in part (Fig. 25-27).

Metastases

- Solitary intraaxial masses are about evenly split between **solitary metastases** and **primary brain tumors**. About **40% of all intracranial neoplasms** are metastases. **Lung, breast**, and **melanoma** are the most common primary malignancies to produce brain metastases.

Recognizing metastases to the brain

- Metastases to the brain are frequently **well-defined, round masses near the gray-white junction**.
- They are **usually multiple, but can be solitary**.
- They are **typically hypodense or isodense on nonenhanced CT**.

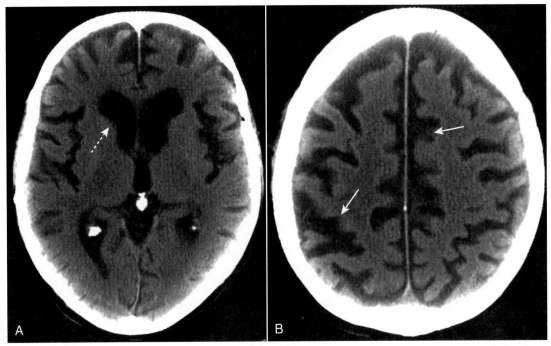

Figure 25-26 Diffuse cortical atrophy. In general, cerebral atrophy produces enlargement of the sulci and the ventricles secondarily. CSF dynamics are normal in atrophy, compared to hydrocephalus. Disorders that cause gross cerebral atrophy are also associated with dementia, Alzheimer disease being one of the most common. **A,** The lateral ventricles (*dotted white arrow*) are enlarged. **B,** Unlike hydrocephalus, the sulci are also enlarged (*solid white arrows*).

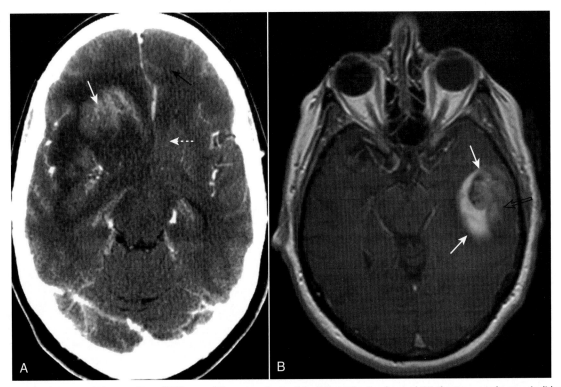

Figure 25-27 Glioblastoma multiforme, CT and MRI, two different patients. A, In this contrast-enhanced CT, the tumor enhances (*solid white arrow*), produces considerable vasogenic edema (*dotted white arrow*), and infiltrates the surrounding brain tissue. There is either edema or tumor that has crossed over to the left frontal lobe (*solid black arrow*). **B,** Axial T1-weighted postgadolinium image in another patient demonstrates an enhancing mass in the left temporal lobe (*solid white arrows*). The internal enhancement of the mass is somewhat heterogeneous (*open black arrow*), which implies intratumoral necrosis or cystic change.

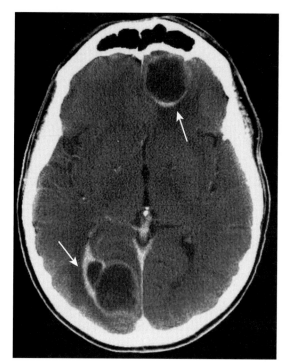

Figure 25-28 Metastases, contrast-enhanced CT. About 40% of all intracranial neoplasms are metastases. They typically produce well-defined, round masses near the gray-white junction and are usually multiple. With intravenous contrast, they can enhance, sometimes demonstrating ring enhancement (*solid white arrows*). Lung, breast, and melanoma are the most common primary malignancies to produce brain metastases. This patient had lung cancer.

- With intravenous contrast, they can **enhance**, sometimes with a pattern of **ring-enhancement**.
- Most evoke some **vasogenic edema**, frequently out of proportion to the size of the mass (Fig. 25-28).

Meningioma

- Meningiomas are the **most common extraaxial mass**, usually occurring in middle-aged women. Their most common locations are **parasaggital**, **over the convexities**, the sphenoid wing, and the cerebellopontine angle cistern, in decreasing frequency.
- They tend to be **slow-growing** with an **excellent prognosis** if surgically excised.
- When **multiple**, they may have an association with *neurofibromatosis type 2*.

> **Recognizing a meningioma on CT scan of the brain**

- On **unenhanced CT**, over **half are hyperdense** to normal brain and about **20% contain calcification** (Fig. 25-29).
- On contrast-enhanced studies, **meningiomas enhance markedly**.
- They **may have edema** surrounding them.

Vestibular Schwannoma (Acoustic Neuroma)

- **Vestibular schwannomas** are the most common schwannomas of all of the cranial nerves. Their most common

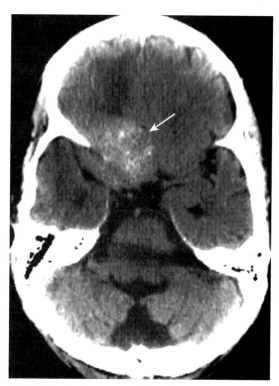

Figure 25-29 Meningioma, nonenhanced CT. Meningiomas usually occur in middle-aged women and are the most common extraaxial mass. This meningioma is arising from the right sphenoid wing, a relatively common site of origin. On unenhanced CT, over half are hyperdense to normal brain and about 20% contain calcification, as does this lesion that appears as a dense mass (*solid white arrow*). On contrast-enhanced studies, meningiomas markedly enhance.

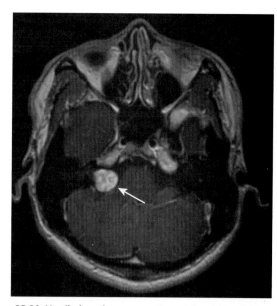

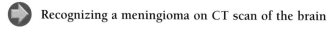

Figure 25-30 Vestibular schwannoma, T1-weighted MRI with contrast. There is a homogeneously enhancing soft tissue mass at the right cerebellopontine angle (*solid white arrow*), classical for a vestibular schwannoma. These tumors occur most commonly along the course of the 8th nerve. Hearing loss is the most common presenting symptom.

symptom is **hearing loss**, but they also produce tinnitus and disturbances in equilibrium.
- They occur most commonly along the **course of the 8th nerve** within the **internal auditory canal** at the **cerebellopontine angle** (Fig. 25-30).

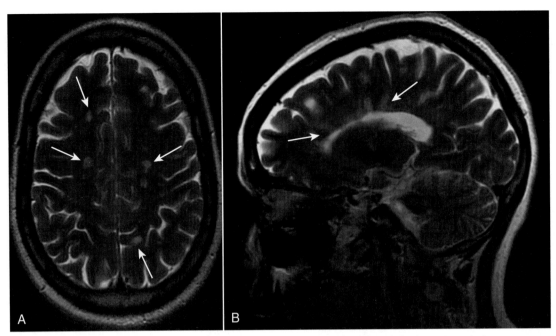

Figure 25-31 Multiple sclerosis, axial and sagittal MRI. Lesions of multiple sclerosis have a predilection for the periventricular area, corpus callosum, and optic nerves (*solid white arrows*). **A,** The lesions produce discrete, globular foci of high-signal intensity (white) on T2-weighted images. **B,** Ovoid lesions with their long axis perpendicular to the ventricular surface seen in multiple sclerosis are called *Dawson fingers* (*solid white arrows*). MRI is the study of choice in imaging multiple sclerosis because of its greater sensitivity than CT in demonstrating plaques both in the brain and spinal cord.

TABLE 25-8 TERMINOLOGY

Term	Remarks
Intraaxial/extraaxial	Intraaxial lesions originate in the brain parenchyma; extraaxial lesions originate outside of the brain substance (i.e., meninges, intraventricular)
Infratentorial	Beneath the tentorium cerebelli that includes the cerebellum, brain stem, 4th ventricle, and cerebellopontine angles
Supratentorial	Above the tentorium cerebelli which includes the cerebral hemispheres (frontal, parietal, occipital, and temporal lobes) and the sella
Transient ischemic attack (TIA)	Sudden neurologic loss that persists for a short time and resolves within 24 hours
Completed stroke	Neurologic deficit lasts for >21 days
Open versus closed head injuries	*Open:* communication of intracranial material outside of the skull *Closed:* no external communication
Increased attenuation/hyperattenuation/ hyperdense/hyperintense	Terms that might be used to describe any tissue brighter than its surrounding tissues
Decreased attenuation/hypoattenuation/ hypodense/hypointense	Terms that might be used to describe any tissue darker than its surrounding tissues
Diffusion-weighted imaging (DWI)	An MRI sequence that can be rapidly acquired and which is extremely sensitive to detecting abnormalities in normal water movement in the brain so that it can identify a stroke within minutes after the event. DWI also helps differentiate acute infarction from more chronic infarction

- Like meningiomas, they can be multiple (i.e., bilateral) and associated with **neurofibromatosis type 2**.

⮕ **Contrast-enhanced MRI** is the **most sensitive** imaging study for detecting vestibular schwannomas which virtually **always enhance**, usually **homogeneously**. On nonenhanced MR, they may be of the same density as the adjacent pontine tissue and difficult to detect.

MULTIPLE SCLEROSIS

- Multiple sclerosis is considered to be **autoimmune** in origin and is the **most common demyelinating disease**. Any neurologic function can be affected by the disease, with some patients having mostly cognitive changes, while others present with ataxia, paresis, or visual symptoms.
- MS is characterized by a **relapsing and remitting course**. There are specific clinical criteria that must be met for establishing this diagnosis, but imaging by MRI along with ancillary tests now permit the diagnosis to be made after a single episode.
- It characteristically affects **myelinated (white matter) tracks** with lesions known as **plaques**. Lesions of multiple sclerosis have a **predilection for the periventricular area, corpus callosum, and optic nerves**.

⮕ **MRI is the study of choice** in imaging multiple sclerosis because of its greater sensitivity than CT in demonstrating plaques both in the brain and spinal cord.

- The lesions produce **discrete, globular foci of high signal intensity (white) on T2-weighted images**.
- On T1-weighted, nonenhanced images, they are isointense to hypointense, but **in acute MS, the lesions enhance with gadolinium on T1-weighted images**.
- The lesions tend to be oriented with their long axes perpendicular to the ventricular walls (Fig. 25-31).

TERMINOLOGY

- See Table 25-8.

WEBLINK

Registered users may obtain more information on Recognizing Some Common Causes of Intracranial Pathology on StudentConsult.com.

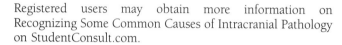

TAKE-HOME POINTS

Recognizing Some Common Causes of Intracranial Pathology

The normal anatomy of the brain is more easily recognized on CT scans, although MRI is generally the study of choice for detecting and staging intracranial and spinal cord abnormalities because of its superior contrast and soft tissue resolution.

Unenhanced CT is usually the study of first choice in acute head trauma. The search for findings should initially focus on finding mass effect or blood.

Linear skull fractures are important mainly for the intracranial abnormalities that may have occurred at the time of the fracture; *depressed skull fractures* can be associated with underlying brain injury and may require elevation of the fragment; *basilar skull fractures* are more serious and can be associated with CSF leaks.

Blow-out fractures of the orbit result from a direct blow and may present with orbital emphysema, fracture through either the floor or medial wall of the orbit, and entrapment of fat and extraocular muscles in the fracture.

There are four types of intracranial hemorrhages that may be associated with trauma: epidural hematoma, subdural hematoma, intracerebral hemorrhage, and subarachnoid hemorrhage.

Epidural hematomas represent hemorrhage into the potential space between the dura mater and the inner table of the skull and are usually due to injuries to the middle meningeal artery or vein from blunt head trauma; almost all (95%) have an associated skull fracture. When acute, epidural hematomas appear as hyperintense collections of blood that typically have a lenticular shape; as they age, they become hypodense to normal brain.

Subdural hematomas most commonly result from deceleration injuries or falls; they represent hemorrhage into the potential space between the dura mater and the arachnoid; acute subdural hematomas portend the presence of more severe brain injury. Subdural hematomas are crescent-shaped bands of blood that may cross suture lines and enter the interhemispheric fissure although they do not cross the midline; they are typically concave inward to the brain and may appear isointense (isodense) to the remainder of the brain as they become subacute and hypodense when chronic.

Traumatic *intracerebral hematomas* are frequently from shearing injuries and present as petechial or larger hemorrhages in the frontal or temporal lobes; they may be associated with increased intracranial pressure and brain herniation.

Brain herniations include subfalcine, transtentorial, foramen magnum/tonsillar, sphenoid, and extracranial herniations.

Diffuse axonal injury is a serious consequence of trauma in which the corpus callosum is most commonly affected; CT findings are similar to those for intracerebral hemorrhage following head trauma; MRI is the study of choice in identifying diffuse axonal injury.

In general, *increased intracranial pressure* is due to either increased volume of the brain (cerebral edema) or increased size of the ventricles (hydrocephalus).

There are two major categories of *cerebral edema*: vasogenic and cytotoxic.

Vasogenic edema represents extracellular accumulation of fluid and is the type that occurs with malignancy and infection and affects the white matter more.

Cytotoxic edema represents cellular edema, is due to cell death, and affects both the gray and white matter; cytotoxic edema is associated with cerebral ischemia.

Stroke denotes an acute loss of neurologic function that occurs when the blood supply to an area of the brain is lost or compromised. MRI is more sensitive to the early diagnosis of stroke than CT. There are certain patterns of ischemia that develop depending on which vascular territory is involved.

Strokes are usually due to *embolic* (more common) or *thrombotic* events and are typically divided into *ischemic* (more common) and *hemorrhagic* varieties (poorer prognosis); hypertension is frequently associated.

Intracerebral hemorrhage will display increased density on nonenhanced CT scans of the brain; as the clot begins to form, the blood becomes denser for about 3 days because of dehydration of the clot and then decreases in density, becoming invisible over the next several weeks; after about 2 months, only a small hypodensity may remain.

Berry aneurysms are usually formed from congenital weakening in the arterial wall; when they rupture, the blood typically enters the subarachnoid space presenting in the basilar cisterns and in the sulci. The aneurysm itself can be detected on either CTA or MRA.

Hydrocephalus represents an increased volume of CSF in the ventricular system and may be due to overproduction of cerebrospinal fluid (rare), underabsorption of cerebrospinal fluid at the level of the arachnoid villi (*communicating*), or obstruction of the outflow of cerebrospinal fluid from the ventricles (*noncommunicating*).

Normal-pressure hydrocephalus is a form of communicating hydrocephalus characterized by a classical triad of abnormalities of gait, dementia, and urinary incontinence that may be improved by insertion of a ventricular shunt.

Cerebral atrophy is a loss of both gray and white matter that may resemble hydrocephalus except that the CSF fluid dynamics are normal in atrophy and, in general, cerebral atrophy produces proportionate enlargement of both the ventricles and the sulci; there is diffuse cerebral atrophy associated with Alzheimer disease.

Glioblastoma multiforme is a highly malignant glioma that occurs most commonly in the frontal and temporal lobes producing a very aggressive, infiltrating, partially enhancing, sometimes necrotic mass that may cross the corpus callosum to the opposite cerebral hemisphere.

Metastases to the brain are frequently well-defined, round masses near the gray-white junction, usually multiple, typically hypodense or isodense on nonenhanced CT that enhance with contrast; they can provoke vasogenic edema out of proportion to the size of the mass; lung, breast, and melanoma are the most frequent sources of brain metastases.

Meningiomas usually occur in middle-aged women in a parasaggital location; they tend to be slow-growing with an excellent prognosis if surgically excised; on CT, they characteristically can be dense without contrast because of calcification within the tumor and may enhance dramatically.

Vestibular schwannomas occur most commonly along the course of the 8th cranial nerve within the internal auditory canal at the cerebellopontine angle and are best identified on MRI, where they homogeneously enhance.

Multiple sclerosis is the most common demyelinating disease, characterized by a relapsing and remitting course and a predilection for the periventricular area, corpus callosum, and optic nerves; it is best visualized on MRI and produces discrete, globular foci of high-signal intensity (white) on T2-weighted images.

Appendix

Recognizing What to Order

The following guidelines for which imaging study to order under certain clinical circumstances are used with permission from the American College of Radiology's Appropriateness Criteria®. These guidelines were developed by a series of expert panels consisting of diagnostic radiologists, interventional radiologists, radiation oncologists, and leaders from other specialties. They are evidence-based guidelines designed to assist health-care providers in making the most appropriate imaging or treatment decision for a specific clinical condition.

THORACIC IMAGING

Indication	Procedure	Comment (If Any)
Cough, sputum, chest pain, shortness of breath, ± fever	Chest radiograph	
Asthma, suspected pneumonia or pneumothorax	Chest radiograph	
COPD worsening with elevated white blood cell count, pain, associated coronary artery disease (CAD) or CHF	Chest radiograph	
Complicated pneumonia	Chest radiograph	Then CT of chest if pneumonia doesn't resolve
HIV+; acute respiratory illness	Chest radiograph	If chest radiograph is negative, then CT chest without contrast
HIV+; + chest x-ray	CT chest without contrast	
Chronic shortness of breath	Chest radiograph	Infiltrative lung disease may be present with a negative chest x-ray; get CT chest without contrast
Hemoptysis	Chest radiograph	Then chest CT with contrast
Hemoptysis-massive	Chest radiograph followed by CT of chest with contrast	
Rib fractures	Chest radiograph	Frontal chest is sufficient to rule out pneumothorax, contusion

Indication	Procedure	Comment (If Any)
After insertion of ETT, CVC, PICC, Swan-Ganz catheter, DHT, chest tube	Chest radiograph, portable	
Screening for lung metastases from renal cell, testicular, melanoma, head and neck malignancies	Chest radiograph and CT chest as baseline	
Screening for lung metastases from soft tissue or bone sarcomas	CT chest without contrast	
Solitary pulmonary nodule, >1 cm, low suspicion for cancer	CT chest without contrast	To detect occult calcifications, fat, bronchus sign, etc. If indeterminate, consider PET scan
Solitary pulmonary nodule, ≥1 cm, moderate to high clinical suspicion for cancer	CT chest without contrast	To detect occult calcifications, fat, bronchus sign, etc. If indeterminate, consider PET scan
Solitary pulmonary nodule, ≤1 cm, low clinical suspicion for cancer	CT chest without contrast	
Solitary pulmonary nodule, ≤1 cm, moderate to high clinical suspicion for cancer	CT chest without contrast	
Staging for non–small-cell lung cancer	CT chest with contrast; chest radiograph for baseline	Consider also whole body PET scan
Staging for small-cell lung cancer	Chest radiograph; chest CT with contrast; MRI head with contrast	

CARDIAC IMAGING

Indication	Procedure	Comment (If Any)
Acute chest pain, low probability of CAD	Chest radiograph	Single photon emission computer tomography (SPECT) scan if cardiac etiology suspected

Indication	Procedure	Comment (If Any)
Chest pain, suggestive of acute coronary syndrome	Coronary arteriography or SPECT MPI (myocardial perfusion imaging) rest and stress	
Acute chest pain, suspicion of aortic dissection	Chest radiograph only if time permits; CT angiogram (CTA)	CTA recommended as definitive test for dissection; MR angiography (MRA) if patient allergic to contrast
Acute chest pain, suspect pulmonary embolism	Chest radiograph to exclude other causes of acute chest pain; CT pulmonary angiogram (CT-PA)	V/Q scan if chest x-ray negative with high index of suspicion and CT-PA not available
Chronic chest pain, high probability of CAD	Chest radiograph to exclude other causes	SPECT scan
Chronic chest pain—lower probability of CAD	Chest radiograph to exclude other causes	Echocardiography; CTA of the coronary arteries
CHF, new or worse or currently stable	Chest radiograph	
Shortness of breath, cardiac origin	Chest radiograph	Echocardiography; SPECT scan
Suspected congenital heart disease in an adult	Chest radiograph and US transthoracic echocardiography with Doppler	Done in combination

Indication	Procedure	Comment (If Any)
Blunt trauma with hematuria	CT chest, abdomen, and pelvis with contrast	
Dysphagia	Barium swallow (with dynamic imaging if dysphagia is unexplained)	
Jaundice, abdominal pain	US abdomen	
Jaundice, painless	CT abdomen without and with contrast	
Jaundice, obstruction unlikely or confusing picture	US abdomen	
RUQ pain ± fever	US abdomen	
LLQ pain, acute or chronic	CT abdomen and pelvis with contrast	Oral contrast helpful
LLQ pain, woman of childbearing age	US abdomen to exclude gynecologic abnormality	
RLQ pain, acute or chronic	CT abdomen and pelvis with contrast	Oral contrast helpful
RLQ pain, pregnant woman or child	RLQ abdominal US	
Palpable abdominal mass	CT abdomen with or without contrast	
Suspected liver metastases	CT abdomen most commonly done without and with contrast	If negative and suspicion is high, then MRI abdomen with contrast
Small bowel obstruction	CT abdomen and pelvis with IV contrast	No oral contrast; conventional radiographs still being done first

GASTROINTESTINAL IMAGING

Indication	Procedure	Comment (If Any)
Acute abdominal pain and fever; possible abscess	CT abdomen and pelvis with contrast	
Postoperative patient with persistent fever	CT abdomen and pelvis with contrast	
Acute abdominal pain and fever, pregnant patient	US abdomen	
Acute pancreatitis, first episode or no fever	US abdomen	
Acute pancreatitis, worsening, with fever	CT abdomen with or without contrast	
Trauma, blunt, unstable	Chest radiograph; focused assessment with sonography for trauma (FAST); abdomen/pelvis x-ray	Patient's condition permitting
Trauma, blunt, stable	CT chest, abdomen, and pelvis with contrast	

MUSCULOSKELETAL IMAGING

Indication	Procedure	Comment (If Any)
Acute hand or wrist trauma	Conventional radiographs (CR)	If negative and still suspicious: choice of casting with repeat radiograph in 10-14 days or doing MRI or CT
Acute shoulder pain, any etiology	Conventional radiographs	MRI if CR is noncontributory or pain is persistent
Shoulder pain, after arthroplasty or rotator cuff repair	MRI or US	Considered equivalent
Acute knee trauma with clinical findings	Conventional radiographs	MRI if CR is noncontributory or pain is persistent
Chronic ankle, elbow, foot, hip, or wrist pain	Conventional radiographs	MRI next study under most clinical circumstances (if radiography is unremarkable or equivocal and clinical concern warrants)

Indication	Procedure	Comment (If Any)
Knee pain, nontraumatic	Conventional radiographs	If knee radiograph is nondiagnostic, then MRI
Cervical spine trauma, acute; meets clinical criteria for imaging	CT cervical spine without contrast	CR cervical spine, lateral only, if CT not available; if ligamentous injury suspected, then MRI
Chronic neck pain	Conventional radiographs	MRI next study under most clinical circumstances
Suspected metastatic bone disease	Tc 99m whole body bone scan; if negative and results will change treatment, then FDG-PET whole body scan	Radiographs obtained after bone scan if needed for further lesion characterization
Suspected metastatic bone disease to spine	Conventional radiographs	Then MRI if radiographs are negative
Multiple myeloma suspected in spine	Conventional radiographs	Then MRI if radiographs are negative
Soft tissue mass, clinically suspected	Conventional radiographs (will probably still require additional imaging)	MRI area of interest; US may be used to differentiate solid from cystic masses
Osteomyelitis of foot, suspected in diabetic	Conventional radiographs followed by MRI with contrast, if indicated	Radiographs and MRI are complementary. Both are indicated
Low back pain (see Neuro)		

GENITOURINARY IMAGING

Indication	Procedure	Comment (If Any)
Acute flank pain, suspicion of stone	CT abdomen and pelvis without contrast	Stone search study
Recurrent stone symptoms	Either CT abdomen and pelvis without contrast or US kidneys and bladder	
Acute scrotal pain without trauma	US scrotum with Doppler	
Acute pyelonephritis with complications (diabetes, immunocompromised, prior stones)	Either CT abdomen and pelvis without and with contrast or US kidneys and bladder	
Hematuria	CT abdomen and pelvis without and with contrast	Study is known as CT urogram
Hematuria with known renal parenchymal disease	US kidneys and bladder	

Indication	Procedure	Comment (If Any)
Renal trauma, blunt with hematuria	CT abdomen and pelvis with contrast	
Renal trauma, penetrating, with or without hematuria	CT abdomen and pelvis with contrast	
Pelvic trauma, blunt	Abdominal radiographs	Then retrograde cystography or CT pelvis with bladder contrast (CT cystography)
Pelvic trauma, penetrating	Either retrograde cystogram or CT pelvis with bladder contrast (CT cystography)	Equivalent studies; if already doing CT, then do CT cystogram
Renovascular hypertension	MRA abdomen with contrast or CTA abdomen	If diminished renal function, also can use US kidney with Doppler
Obstructive voiding symptoms from enlarged prostate	US pelvis (bladder and prostate) transabdominal	If BUN is elevated, then US of kidneys to evaluate for hydronephrosis
Renal mass of indeterminate benignancy	Either CT abdomen without and with contrast or MRI abdomen without and with contrast	Either CT or MRI is appropriate

NEUROLOGIC IMAGING

Indication	Procedure	Comment (If Any)
Head trauma, minimal clinical findings	CT head without contrast	Known to be low yield
Head trauma, with clinical findings; may include skull fracture	CT head without contrast	MRI for problem solving
Head trauma, penetrating	CT head without contrast	
Head trauma, distant, with neurologic findings	MRI of head without contrast	
Headache, chronic	CT or MRI head without and with contrast	Yield is relatively low
Headache, acute, severe ("worst headache of life")	CT head without contrast	Then either CTA head or MRA head with or without contrast. Use of CT or MRI subject to local preference and availability
Headache, new, + HIV	MRI head without contrast	
Headache, new, pregnant	MRI head without contrast	

Indication	Procedure	Comment (If Any)
Headache, new, suspect meningitis	MRI head without and with contrast or CT without contrast	Use of CT or MRI subject to local preference and availability
CVA, new deficit, <3 hours	CT head without contrast	Noncontrast head CT to exclude acute intracranial hemorrhage is needed prior to thrombolytic therapy
CVA, new deficit, >3 hours	MRI head with or without contrast, or MRA head and neck with or without contrast, or CT head with or without contrast, or CTA head and neck	Use of CT or MRI subject to local preference and availability
Subarachnoid hemorrhage, proven by imaging or lumbar puncture	Cerebral arteriography or CTA of head	
CVA, suspected cerebral hemorrhage	CT head without contrast	
Seizure, alcohol or drug related	MRI head without and with contrast	CT can be substituted if MRI not available in emergency
Seizure, new onset, 18-40 years	MRI head without and with contrast	CT can be substituted if MRI not available in emergency
Seizure, new onset, over age 40	MRI head without and with contrast	CT can be substituted if MRI not available in emergency
Seizure, new onset, focal neurological deficit	MRI head without and/or with contrast	CT can be substituted if MRI not available in emergency
Low back pain, low velocity trauma, osteoporosis	MRI lumbar spine without contrast	Lumbar spine radiographs will still likely be done first
Low back pain, malignancy, or infection	MRI lumbar spine without and with contrast	
Low back pain, surgical candidate	MRI lumbar spine without contrast	
Low back pain, prior lumbar surgery	MRI lumbar spine without and with contrast	
Dementia, suspected Alzheimer, NPH	MRI head without contrast	
Focal neurologic deficits, single or multiple	MRI head without or MRI head without and with contrast	
Focal neurologic deficit, sudden onset	MRI head without, MRI head without and with contrast, or CT head without contrast	
Change in mental status	MRI head without or with contrast or CT head without contrast	

Indication	Procedure	Comment (If Any)
Vision loss, sudden, painless or painful	MRI head and/or orbit without and with contrast	
Vision loss with head trauma	CT head and/or orbit with or without contrast	In subacute trauma, contrast may be useful

PEDIATRIC IMAGING

Indication	Procedure	Comment (If Any)
Fever, with or without respiratory symptoms	Chest radiograph	
Headache with positive neurologic signs	CT head without contrast or MRI head without contrast	CT or MRI should be performed in every patient
Headache, acute, severe	CT or MRI of the head without contrast	CT or MRI should be performed in every patient
Hematuria, isolated	US kidneys and bladder	
Hematuria, painful	CT abdomen and pelvis without contrast	
Hematuria, traumatic, microscopic or macroscopic	CT abdomen and pelvis with contrast	
Limp, 0-5 years, no focal signs	Radiographs of pelvis and lower extremity	
Septic arthritis, suspected	Radiograph and possibly US area of interest	
Seizures, neonate	US head	
Seizures, post-traumatic	CT head without contrast	
Seizures, first generalized or refractory	MRI head without contrast	
Sinusitis, chronic or recurrent	CT paranasal sinuses without contrast	
Urinary tract infection	US kidneys and bladder	
Vomiting, bilious, up to 1 week old	Abdominal radiographs	
Vomiting, bilious, 1 week to 3 months	Upper GI series	
Vomiting, nonbilious since birth	Upper GI series	
Vomiting, projectile, new onset	US abdomen (UGI tract)	
Child abuse	Skeletal survey radiographs	If head injury suspected, CT head without contrast; if seizures or neurologic signs, MRI head
Child abuse, thoracic or abdominal injuries discrepant with history	CT abdomen and pelvis with contrast	

REPRODUCTIVE IMAGING

Indication	Procedure	Comment (If Any)
Vaginal bleeding, postmenopausal	US pelvis	
Vaginal bleeding, abnormal, premenopausal	US pelvis	
Pelvic pain, acute	US pelvis	Both transvaginal and transabdominal US should be performed if possible
Adnexal mass, clinically suspected	US pelvis	
Adnexal mass, complex or solid, enlarging	MRI pelvis with or without contrast	If conservative (nonsurgical) management is elected and malignancy cannot be excluded

Indication	Procedure	Comment (If Any)
First trimester bleeding	US pelvis	
Second and third trimester bleeding	US pregnant uterus	
Ovarian cancer screen, high risk	US pelvis	

A set of guidelines cannot possibly cover the myriad of clinical combinations with which patients present. Whenever possible, be sure to consult with the radiologist when you have a question about how best to tailor an imaging examination to fit the needs of the patient.

These guidelines are reprinted with permission of the American College of Radiology. No other representation of this material is authorized without expressed, written permission from the American College of Radiology. Refer to the ACR website at www.acr.org/ac for the most current and complete version of the ACR Appropriateness Criteria®.

Bibliography

TEXTS

Arnold W, DeLegge M, Schwaitzberg S: *Enteral Access: The Foundation of Feeding*, 2002, Kendall Hunt.

Blickman H: *Pediatric Radiology: The Requisites*, ed 2, St. Louis, 1998, Mosby.

Fraser RS, Pare P, Fraser RG, Pare PD: *Synopsis of Diseases of the Chest*, ed 2, Philadelphia, 1994, W.B. Saunders.

Goodman LR: *Principles of Chest Roentgenology*, ed 3, Philadelphia, 2007, Saunders.

Greenspan A: *Orthopedic Radiology: A Practical Approach*, ed 3, Philadelphia, 2000, Lippincott Williams and Wilkins.

Grossman RL, Yousem DM: *Neuroradiology: The Requisites*, St. Louis, 1994, Mosby.

Guyton AC, Hall J: *Textbook of Medical Physiology*, ed 11, Philadelphia, 2005, W.B. Saunders.

Harris JH, Harris WH: *The Radiology of Emergency Medicine*, ed 4, Philadelphia, 2000, Lippincott Williams and Wilkins.

Juhl JH, Crummy AB: *Essentials of Radiologic Imaging*, ed 6, Philadelphia, 1993, Lippincott.

Love M: *An Introduction to Diagnostic Ultrasound*, Springfield, Il, 1980, Charles C. Thomas.

Manaster BJ, Disler DG, May DA: *Musculoskeletal Imaging: The Requisites*, ed 2, St. Louis, 2002, Mosby.

McLoud TC: *Thoracic Radiology: The Requisites*, St. Louis, 1998, Mosby.

Meyers MA: *Dynamic Radiology of the Abdomen: Normal and Pathological Anatomy*, ed 2, New York, 1982, Springer-Verlag.

Resnick D, Niwayama G: *Diagnosis of Bone and Joint Disorders*, ed 2, Philadelphia, 1981, W.B. Saunders.

Resnick D: *Diagnosis of Bone and Joint Disorders*, ed 4, Philadelphia, 2002, W.B. Saunders.

Rumack C, Wilson S, Charboneau JW: *Diagnostic Ultrasound*, ed 2, St. Louis, 1998, Mosby.

Schultz RJ: *The Language of Fractures*, Huntington, NY, 1972, Robert E. Krieger.

Webb WR, Brant WE, Helms CA: *Fundamentals of Body CT*, Philadelphia, 1991, W.B. Saunders.

Weissleder R, Wittenberg J, Harisinghani MG: *Primer of Diagnostic Imaging*, ed 3, St. Louis, 2003, Mosby.

JOURNAL ARTICLES

Aberle DR, Wiener-Kronish JP, Webb WR, Matthay MA: Hydrostatic versus increased permeability pulmonary edema: diagnosis based on radiographic data in critically ill patients, *Radiology* 168:73-79, 1988.

Amjadi K, Alvarez GG, Vanderhelst E, Velkeniers B, Lam M, Noppen M: The prevalence of blebs or bullae among young healthy adults: a thoracoscopic investigation, *Chest* 132(4):1140-1145, 2007.

Bates D, Ruggieri P: Imaging modalities for evaluation of the spine, *Radiol Clin North Am* 29(4):675-690, 1991.

Boudiaf M, Soyer P, Terem C, Pelage J, Maissiat E, Rymer R: CT evaluation of small bowel obstruction, *RadioGraphics* 21:613-624, 2001.

Burney K, Burchard F, Papouchado M, Wilde P: Cardiac pacing systems and implantable cardiac defibrillators (ICDs): a radiological perspective of equipment, anatomy and complications, *Clin Radiol* 59(8):699-708, 2004.

Cohen SM, Kurtz AB: Biliary sonography, *Radiol Clin North Am* 29(6):1171-1198, 1991.

Dalinka MK, Reginato AJ, Golden DA: Calcium deposition disease, *Semin Roentgenol* 17(1):39-47, 1982.

Dyer DS, Moore EE, Mestek MF, Bernstein SM, Iklé DN, Durham JD, Heinig MJ, Russ PD, Symonds DL, Kumpe DA, Roe EJ, Honigman B,

McIntyre RC, EJ: Can chest CT be used to exclude aortic injury? *Radiology* 213:195-202, 1999.

Edeiken J: Radiologic approach to arthritis, *Semin Roentgenol* 17(1):8-15, 1982.

Ellis K, Austin J, Jaretzki A: Radiologic detection of thymoma in patients with myasthenia gravis, *AJR* 151:873-881, 1988.

Garcia MJ: Could cardiac CT revolutionize the practice of cardiology? *Cleve Clin J Med* 72(2):88-89, 2005.

Gaskill MF, Lukin R, Wiot JG: Lumbar disc disease and stenosis, *Radiol Clin North Am* 29(4):753-764, 1991.

Haus BM, Stark P, Shofer SL, Kuschner WG: Massive pulmonary pseudotumor, *Chest* 124(2):758-760, 2003.

Hendrix RW, Rogers LF: Diagnostic imaging of fracture complications, *Radiol Clin North Am* 27(5):1023-1033, 1989.

Henry M, Arnold T, Harvey J: British Thoracic Society guidelines for the management of spontaneous pneumothorax, *Thorax* 58(suppl 2):39-52, 2003.

Henschke CI, Yankelevitz DF, Wand A, Davis SD, Shiau M: Accuracy and efficacy of chest radiography in the intensive care unit, *Radiol Clin North Am* 34(1):21-31, 1996.

Horrow MM: Ultrasound of the extrahepatic bile duct: issues of size, *Ultrasound Quarterly* 26(2):67-74, 2010.

Indrajit IK, Shreeram MN, D'Souza JD: Multislice CT: a quantum leap in whole body imaging, *Indian J Radiol Imaging* 14(2):209-216, 2004.

Ingram MD, Watson SG, Skippage PL, Patel U: Urethral injuries after pelvic trauma: evaluation with urethrography, *RadioGraphics* 28:1631-1643, 2008.

Johnson JL: Pleural effusions in cardiovascular disease, *Postgrad Med* 107(4):95-101, 2000.

Kundel HL, Wright DJ: The influence of prior knowledge on visual search strategies during the viewing of chest radiographs, *Radiology* 93:315-320, 1969.

Lingawi SS: The naked facet sign, *Radiology* 219:366-367, 2001.

MacMahon H, Austin JHM, Gamsu G, Herold CJ, Jett JR, Naidich DP, Patz EF, Swensen SJ: Guidelines for management of small pulmonary nodules detected on CT scans: a statement from the Fleischner Society, *Radiology* 237:395-400, 2005.

Old JL, Calvert M: Vertebral compression fractures in the elderly, *Am Fam Physician* 69(1):111-116, 2004.

Pathria MN, Petersilge CA: Spinal trauma, *Radiol Clin North Am* 29(4):847-865, 1991.

Riddervold HO: Easily missed fractures, *Radiol Clin North Am* 30(2):475-494, 1992.

Shifrin RY, Choplin RH: Aspiration in patients in critical care units, *Radiol Clin North Am* 34(1):83-96, 1996.

Steenburg SD, Ravenel JG: Acute traumatic thoracic aortic injuries: experience with 64-MDCT, *AJR* 191:1564-1569, 2008.

Thomas EL, Lansdown EL: Visual search patterns of radiologists in training, *Radiology* 81:288–292, 1963.

Tie MLH: Basic head CT for intensivists, *Crit Care Resusc* 3(1):35-44, 2001.

Tocino I, Westcott JL: Barotrauma, *Radiol Clin North Am* 34(1):59-81, 1996.

Yu S, Haughton VM, Rosenbaum AE: Magnetic resonance imaging and anatomy of the spine, *Radiol Clin North Am* 29(4):691-710, 1991.

Yuh WT, Quets JP, Lee HJ, Simonson TM, Michalson LS, Nguyen PT, Sato Y, Mayr NA, Berbaum KS: Anatomic distribution of metastases in the vertebral body and modes of hematogenous spread, *Spine* 21(19):2243-2250, 1996.

Index

The Last Printed Page

So, we meet again. Now, tell the truth: Did you finish the whole book or did you skip right to this page? The former might indicate someone of great self-discipline who seeks the essential core of knowledge, the latter an inquisitive yet impulsive individual with an unquenchable curiosity. Whatever your path to enlightenment, behold the answers.

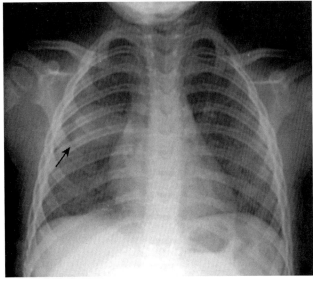

Figure A Round pneumonia, conventional radiography. This was discussed in Chapter 7, *Recognizing Pneumonia*. Occurring mostly in children, round pneumonias are usually caused by *Haemophilus influenzae, Streptococcus,* and *Pneumococcus*. They typically occur in the lower lobes, posteriorly (*solid black arrow*). This pneumonia is in the superior segment of the right lower lobe.

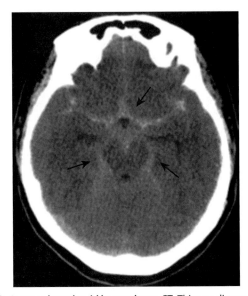

Figure B Acute subarachnoid hemorrhage, CT. This was discussed under "Ruptured Aneurysms" in Chapter 25, *Recognizing Some Common Causes of Intracranial Pathology*. On CT scans, acute hemorrhage is dense and can best be seen in the basilar cisterns (*solid black arrows*), fissures, and sulci. When not caused by trauma, subarachnoid hemorrhage is usually due to a ruptured berry aneurysm at the base of the brain, which was the case in this patient.

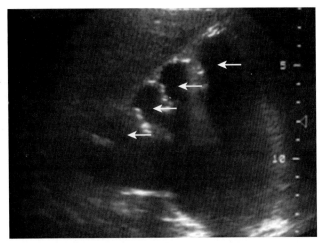

Figure C Hydronephrosis, ultrasound. This was discussed in Chapter 19, *Ultrasound: Understanding the Principles and Recognizing the Normal and Abnormal Findings*. In this sagittal sonogram of the right kidney, the calyces are markedly dilated (*solid white arrows*). The patient had an obstructing right ureteral calculus.

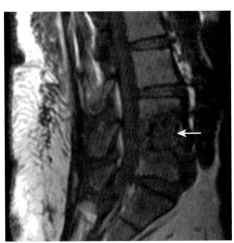

Figure D Discitis and osteomyelitis, MRI of the lumbar spine. This was discussed in Chapter 24, *Recognizing Some Common Causes of Neck and Back Pain*. A sagittal, T1-weighted image of the lumbar spine demonstrates extensive abnormal signal (*solid white arrow*) indicating destruction of the endplates of the L4 and L5 vertebral bodies and the intervening disk. The patient was an intravenous drug abuser in whom hematogenous seeding led to diskitis and osteomyelitis.